FOCUS ON MENTAL RETARDATION RESEARCH

FOCUS ON MENTAL RETARDATION RESEARCH

MARINA I. CARSON
EDITOR

Nova Science Publishers, Inc.
New York

LIBRARY OF CONGRESS CATALOGING-IN-PUBLICATION DATA

Focus on mental retardation research / Marina I. Carson (editor)
p. ; cm.
Includes bibliographical references and index.
ISBN-13: 978-1-60021-647-3 (hardcover)
ISBN-10: 1-60021-647-1 (hardcover)
1. Mental Retardation. I. Carson, Marina I.
[DNLM: 1. Mental Retardation – etiology. 2. Mental Retaration – complications. WM300 F6525 2007]
RC570.F63 2007
616.85'880072-dc22

Published by Nova Science Publishers, Inc. ✢ New York

CONTENTS

PREFACE

Mental retardation is a term for a pattern of persistently slow learning of basic motor and language skills ("milestones") during childhood, and a significantly below-normal global intellectual capacity as an adult. One common criterion for diagnosis of mental retardation is a tested intelligence quotient (IQ) of 70 or below.This new book examines new and critical research and issues in the field.

Chapter 1 - The targets or objectives of the pharmacotherapy of mental retardation are varied and often vague; moreover, they are influenced by the developmental stage and severity of mental retardation. Additionally, diverse etiologies and pathogenetic mechanisms, as well as medical and neurological co-morbidities, influence medication selection. Thus, for toddlers and preschool children, frequent therapeutic objectives include promotion of socialization and self-care skills (e.g., toileting), fostering of language, and improvement of attention, memory and cognitive performance. Targets that may appear in children, adolescents and adults include, but are not limited to, stereotypic movements, mannerisms, agitation, self-injurious behaviors, combativeness and psychosis (especially auditory hallucinations and responding to internal stimuli). A common, but not invariant, neurological co-morbidity is seizure disorder; the pharmacological treatment of seizures occasionally addresses behavioral target symptoms, but not uncommonly is itself associated with cognitive side effects and sleepiness. Cognitive dulling and sleepiness are also concerns with the utilization of antipsychotic medications for behavioral management, especially the conventional ones with a profile of scopolamine-like antimuscarinic cholinergic receptor properties. Clearly, pharmacotherapy is only one (small) component of the multimodal approach to the treatment of mental retardation that often must include speech and language therapy, special education, operant behavioral interventions and social skills training.

Because there are many etiologies resulting in mental retardation, there are few generalities that can be made with respect to its pharmacotherapy. Essentially, all of the major classes of psychiatric medications are used and they are often chosen empirically, usually at the prompting of the physician by the school or parents because of behavioral "dyscontrol." Although generalities are difficult, exciting developments with respect to the author's knowledge about the plasticity and allosteric modulation of major inhibitory and excitatory neurotransmitter systems in brain, mediated by gamma aminobutyric acid (GABA) and L-glutamate, respectively, support development and testing of novel medication strategies for mental retardation and other neuropsychiatric disorders. Also, the role that a selective subtype of nicotinic acetylcholine receptor plays in the normal physiology of attention and cognition and, possibly, the pathophysiology of schizophrenia, Alzheimer's disease and Down's syndrome encourages investigation of novel nicotinic acetylcholine receptor "agonist" medication strategies. Unfortunately, examples of mental retardation associated with defined inborn errors of metabolism may involve damage to the developing brain prior to birth; thus, therapeutic gains to be expected from pharmacotherapeutic interventions in these disorders must be modest. However, this is not always true as neurodevelopmental sequelae in many children with phenylketonuria are addressed with a specialized dietary intervention. Clearly, elucidation of metabolic disturbances resulting from discrete biochemical lesions in inborn errors of metabolism associated with mental retardation may suggest very specific types of intervention. However, because the etiology and pathophysiology of most presentations of mental retardation are unknown, nonspecific approaches to "modulating" global functioning of the brain must be considered even though they are likely to be less-than fully effective. GABAergic, glutamatergic and nicotinic acetylcholine receptor-mediated neurotransmission influence diffuse and highly integrated areas of the brain. Ideally, interventions based on modulation of neurotransmission mediated by GABA, L-glutamate and acetylcholine will show positive therapeutic impact for a large group of mentally retarded persons, whose retardation is varied with respect to etiology, severity and target symptoms of concern. Importantly, disturbances of neurotransmission mediated by these three neurotransmitters are implicated in a variety of neuropsychiatric disorders, including Alzheimer's disease and Down's syndrome that serve as examples of a neurodegenerative disorder and mental retardation, respectively.

This chapter will focus on the general pharmacology of the $GABA_A$ receptor complex, an example of a ligand-gated ion channel receptor, N-methyl-D-aspartic acid (NMDA) receptor, a class of glutamate-gated ion channel receptor, and α_7 nicotinic acetylcholine receptor, an ion channel receptor that is gated by acetylcholine. Where appropriate, the chapter will allude to neuropsychiatric disorders whose pathophysiology involves presumptive disturbance of neurotransmission mediated by these neurotransmitters; symptoms of these disorders include disturbances of attention, memory and cognition. A "functional" circuit that integrates all of these neurotransmitter receptors, at least in the hippocampus, and serves as an important heuristic model for medication development will also be described. Hopefully, medications that are under active development for influencing these three neurotransmitter receptor systems will have roles in the treatment and management of at least some examples of mental retardation. Conducting clinical trials with mentally retarded persons, a special vulnerable population, presents ethical and "human subject protection" challenges, especially with respect to recruitment and obtaining meaningful informed consent or, in the case of minors, assent with parental consent. These extremely important and sensitive issues must be addressed before institutional review boards (IRBs) approve clinical trials. The human subject protection issues will not be covered because they are beyond the scope of this chapter.

Chapter 2 - Mental retardation (MR) often occurs with other developmental disabilities (e.g. autism, cerebral palsy, epilepsy), yet historically, epidemiologic study of MR and of these other conditions has given little attention to examining co-occurrence as a strategy for revealing causal pathways and mechanisms. Co-occurrence of MR and other conditions may suggest alternative causes compared to the occurrence of MR in isolation. Failure to consider such co-occurrence may mask important within group differences and in turn, slow epidemiologic progress. Findings characterizing the prevalence of MR occurring in isolation and with these other conditions are presented as is our data and that of other investigators revealing differing patterns of epidemiologic risk when co-occurrence with other disabilities is considered. Data revealing potential causal pathways and mechanisms when other co-occurrence groupings such as co-occurrence with birth defects are discussed as are advances pointing to gene-environment interactions wherein better understanding and consideration of co-occurrence and phenotype have advanced identification of genetic causes of MR – including fragile X syndrome. Strategies for increasing commitment to the consideration of co-occurrence in epidemiologic studies of MR are outlined.

Chapter 3 - Genomic imprinting is a prime example of epigenetic change leading to variable gene expression. Angelman syndrome (AS) and Prader-Willi syndrome (PWS) are disorders associated with failure of genomic imprinting at the same locus but exhibiting different clinical presentations. The loss of maternal imprint at the chr15q11-q13 locus leads to AS, while lack of paternal patterning results in PWS. Individuals with AS exhibit severe to profound mental retardation (MR) in combination with epilepsy, abnormal EEG patterns, movement disorders, inappropriate smiling or laughter, a happy demeanor, minimal speech, and an easily excitable personality. People with PWS typically present with mild MR, behavior problems, hypotonia, hyperphagia and obesity, and delayed or incomplete sexual development.

Comprehensive clinical and laboratory studies have been undertaken into the medical profiles and life experiences of patient cohorts with AS (n = 34) and PWS (n = 46) in Western Australia. The members of the study cohorts ranged in age from 0.9 years to 48.3 years, with a mean age of 21.2 years. A majority of the group were mentally retarded with only four of the 80 individuals exhibiting IQ levels greater than 84 points which is regarded as the borderline for MR. The results clearly indicated age-specific comorbidities, and specialist care needs were associated with both AS and PWS.

Although the oldest member of the cohorts was under 50 years, it seems probable that people with these disorders will live to significantly older ages in the future. In turn, this will require greater attention to the health, residential and social requirements both of individuals with AS and PWS, and their family carers. Further investigations into the specific etiologies, underlying genetic mechanisms and age- and condition-dependent morbidities that are associated with each syndrome should enable the provision of better care regimes.

Chapter 4 - Mental Retardation (MR) is a cognitive impairment affecting 3% of global population, characterized by subnormal intellectual functioning and impaired behavior. A large percent of individuals with mental deficiency have a significant chromosomal abnormality. Of these, Down syndrome (DS) is the major genetic cause of MR and contributes to about 30% of all moderate-to-severe cases of MR. This invalidating aspect of DS has hard impacts in public health and poses significant challenges for clinicians and scientists.

MR caused by trisomy 21 is mainly a consequence of brain developmental alterations in neurogenesis determined directly from the overexpression of the human chromosome 21 (HC21) gene products or indirectly from the interaction of these HC21 gene products with the whole genome, transcriptome and proteome. The Human genome project has delivered the complete DNA sequence allowing the HC21 gene identification. Molecular studies have been conducted to elucidate how trisomy 21 affects expression of these genes, by mRNA or protein quantifications. Gene dosage effect was found for some genes, but not for others for which there may be additional regulatory factors that over-ride a mere gene dosage effect.

Actually, some genes are considered candidate genes for MR: *SIM2*, *DOPEY2* and *DYRK1A,* localized in the Down syndrome Critical Region 1 (DCR-1), and *SOD1*, *S100b* and *DSCR1,* localized outside the DCR-1. These candidate genes are overexpressed in the trisomic human and transgenic mouse brains, indicating their contribution in the pathogenesis of neurological alterations and MR in DS.

Two opposing hypotheses have been advanced to explain the molecular mechanism of the MR phenotype: "gene dosage effect" and "amplified developmental instability". According to the first hypothesis, the DS critical region DCR-1 was defined as the minimal interval of HC21 carrying a subset of triplicated dosage-sensitive genes directly responsible for this phenotype. The second hypothesis claims that dosage imbalance of hundreds of HC21 genes determine a non-specific genomic transcriptional regulation. This global disruption of the gene expression balance in pathways regulating brain development alters the normal developmental homeostasis and determines MR.

The MR may results from neurodevelopmental and biochemical primary alterations in the brain determined by the presence of 3 copies of HC21 genes. The authors hypothesize a global molecular mechanism in which dosage-dependent genes, expressed 1.5 fold the normal level as a direct consequence of the 1.5 gene dosage, could directly determine primary phenotypes in trisomic brain. Contrarily, some of these dosage-dependent genes could modulate the expression of target genes on the chromosome 21 or the others. The modulation of the target gene expression could be different of 1.5 fold up-regulation or could be down-regulated, determining a secondary gene dosage effect. In parallel, all or some HC21 genes showing expression changes, could participate to the amplified developmental instability of the genome in DS, determining a general gene expression disequilibrium that could also be responsible of primary phenotypes in the brain and participate to pathogenesis of MR.

Actually, the first molecular pathway for MR in DS is elucidated and involves two HC21 dosage-sensitive genes: DYRK1A and DSCR1. Both participate to the control of NFAT phosphorylation, determining converging effects on NFAT-depending gene activation pathways.

Drug treatment identifications for MR in DS need understanding of the molecular mechanisms underlying this cognitive phenotype. In this golden period for DS research, with the development of animal and molecular models, and new techniques for transcriptional regulation, we could hope to rescue the basic molecular defects giving rise to MR.

Chapter 5 - Down's syndrome (DS) is the most frequent genetic disorder associated with mental retardation. The syndrome is the phenotypic result of a triplicated chromosome 21, or from a triplication of its restricted regions. Despite entire DNA sequence of human chromosome 21 is now complete, little is known about the mechanisms by which the increased gene copy number leads to the characteristic DS phenotype. The phenotype can be variable in severity, on the basis of allelic composition of chromosome 21 genes and of the interaction with environment and with expression of genes that are not located on chromosome 21. Dysregulation of the immune system is one characteristic pathological feature of the syndrome and likely contributes to increased susceptibility to viral and bacterial infections, autoimmune diseases, and haematologic malignancies. Chromosome 21 contains the interferon cytokine receptors cluster of genes that are structurally and functionally related. Interferon has pleiotropic effects that manifest mainly on immune system but even in the brain, as shown in DS and in its animal model, the trisomy 16 mouse. Interferon-γ plays a pivotal role in the polarization of immunity towards Th1-mediated responses, which are mainly involved in protection from virus infection and in autoimmunity. It could also cause neurodegeneration and β-amyloid production in DS, thus accounting for cognitive impairment. Notwithstanding these recent discoveries, most of the studies on immunological aspects in DS are old. Investigation with upgraded technologies is needed to improve knowledge in this field. In particular, studies on the expression of proteins, whose genes are encoded on chromosome 21 and that are directly or indirectly involved in immunity, may provide a better understanding of genotype-phenotype correlation in DS and, possibly, a rationale for therapeutic strategies aimed at contrasting the immune derangement and neurodegeneration that are typical of this syndrome.

Chapter 6 - Mental retardation (MR) has long been known to be a common and etiologically heterogeneous disorder, affecting 2-3% of the general population. Over 10% of MR cases with a Mendelian pattern of inheritance have been assigned to the X chromosome, even though it carries less than 4% of all human genes, leading to a recognized excess of hemizygous males with intellectual disability than females. Clinically, X-Linked Mental Retardation (XLMR) appears as syndromic (MRXS) and non-syndromic (MRX) forms, according to the presence or absence of somatic, neurological, behavioral, or metabolic findings in addition to the MR. Therefore, at molecular level this usual classification is questionable as mutations in some genes have been found in both syndromic and nonsyndromic XLMR. Genetic and epigenetic mutations that give rise to XLMR are not evenly distributed along the X-chromosome and seem to cluster in regions Xp11, Xp22 and Xq26-q28. Recent breakthroughs have shown that genes located at these specific regions encode for proteins involved in signaling pathways, responsible for regulate cytoskeleton organization and synaptic efficacy, besides acting in other essential functions, like chromatin remodeling and microRNAs-mediated modulation. In this chapter, the authors provide an up-to-date review of the remarkable progress in the XLMR field, its promise for understanding neural function, memory and learning, and the implications of this research area for developing new diagnostic tools and pharmacological approaches for therapeutic intervention.

Chapter 7 - Mental retardation is characterized by significantly sub-average intellectual functioning, existing concurrently with related limitations in two or more of the applicable adaptive skill areas (communication, self care, home living, social skills, community use, self-direction, health and safety, functional academics, leisure and work). Causes of mental retardation can be broken into several categories (chromosomal abnormalities, genetic and inherited metabolic disorders, trauma, infections, toxic, nutritional, environmental and unexplained causes). The autonomic control of cardiac and respiratory activity in children with mental retardation is defective but pathogenesis of this alteration depend on different causes of mental retardation. Physiological control mechanisms of cardiac autonomic activity (sympathetic and parasympathetic divisions) involve complex interactions between the central autonomic neuronal network, the cerebellum and the cerebral cortex. This network may be altered at various levels in relations to different causes of mental retardation with various clinical expression. Rett syndrome is a classical example of cardiac dysautonomia in mental retardation but many other diseases with mental retardation show clinical signs of alterations in sympatho-vagal balance.

In: Focus on Mental Retardation Research
Editor: Marina I. Carson, pp. 1-27
ISBN: 978-1-60021-647-3

Chapter 1

Pharmacological Modulation of GABA, Glutamate and Acetylcholine Receptor-Mediated Neurotransmission Holds Promise for the Development of Novel Medication Strategies for Mental Retardation: Overview and Hypotheses

Stephen I. Deutsch,[1,2*] Richard B. Rosse,[1,2] Barbara L. Schwartz,[1,2] John Mastropaolo,[1] Katrice D. Long[1] and Brooke L. Gaskins[1]
[1]Mental Health Service Line, Department of Veterans Affairs Medical Center, 50 Irving Street, NW, Washington, DC 20422, USA
[2]Department of Psychiatry, Georgetown University School of Medicine, 3800 Reservoir Road, NW, Washington, DC 2007, USA

Abstract

The targets or objectives of the pharmacotherapy of mental retardation are varied and often vague; moreover, they are influenced by the developmental stage and severity of mental retardation. Additionally, diverse etiologies and pathogenetic mechanisms, as well as medical and neurological co-morbidities, influence medication selection. Thus, for toddlers and preschool children, frequent therapeutic objectives include promotion of socialization and self-care skills (e.g., toileting), fostering of language, and improvement of attention, memory and cognitive performance. Targets that may appear in children, adolescents and adults include, but are not limited to, stereotypic movements, mannerisms, agitation, self-injurious behaviors, combativeness and psychosis (especially

* Corresponding Author: Stephen I. Deutsch, M.D., Ph.D. Associate Chief of Staff for Mental Health, Department of Veterans Affairs Medical Center, 50 Irving Street, NW, Washington, DC 20422; 202 745 8156 (office); 202 745 8169 (facsimile); Stephen.Deutsch@med.va.gov

auditory hallucinations and responding to internal stimuli). A common, but not invariant, neurological co-morbidity is seizure disorder; the pharmacological treatment of seizures occasionally addresses behavioral target symptoms, but not uncommonly is itself associated with cognitive side effects and sleepiness. Cognitive dulling and sleepiness are also concerns with the utilization of antipsychotic medications for behavioral management, especially the conventional ones with a profile of scopolamine-like antimuscarinic cholinergic receptor properties. Clearly, pharmacotherapy is only one (small) component of the multimodal approach to the treatment of mental retardation that often must include speech and language therapy, special education, operant behavioral interventions and social skills training.

Because there are many etiologies resulting in mental retardation, there are few generalities that can be made with respect to its pharmacotherapy. Essentially, all of the major classes of psychiatric medications are used and they are often chosen empirically, usually at the prompting of the physician by the school or parents because of behavioral "dyscontrol." Although generalities are difficult, exciting developments with respect to our knowledge about the plasticity and allosteric modulation of major inhibitory and excitatory neurotransmitter systems in brain, mediated by gamma aminobutyric acid (GABA) and L-glutamate, respectively, support development and testing of novel medication strategies for mental retardation and other neuropsychiatric disorders. Also, the role that a selective subtype of nicotinic acetylcholine receptor plays in the normal physiology of attention and cognition and, possibly, the pathophysiology of schizophrenia, Alzheimer's disease and Down's syndrome encourages investigation of novel nicotinic acetylcholine receptor "agonist" medication strategies. Unfortunately, examples of mental retardation associated with defined inborn errors of metabolism may involve damage to the developing brain prior to birth; thus, therapeutic gains to be expected from pharmacotherapeutic interventions in these disorders must be modest. However, this is not always true as neurodevelopmental sequelae in many children with phenylketonuria are addressed with a specialized dietary intervention. Clearly, elucidation of metabolic disturbances resulting from discrete biochemical lesions in inborn errors of metabolism associated with mental retardation may suggest very specific types of intervention. However, because the etiology and pathophysiology of most presentations of mental retardation are unknown, nonspecific approaches to "modulating" global functioning of the brain must be considered even though they are likely to be less-than fully effective. GABAergic, glutamatergic and nicotinic acetylcholine receptor-mediated neurotransmission influence diffuse and highly integrated areas of the brain. Ideally, interventions based on modulation of neurotransmission mediated by GABA, L-glutamate and acetylcholine will show positive therapeutic impact for a large group of mentally retarded persons, whose retardation is varied with respect to etiology, severity and target symptoms of concern. Importantly, disturbances of neurotransmission mediated by these three neurotransmitters are implicated in a variety of neuropsychiatric disorders, including Alzheimer's disease and Down's syndrome that serve as examples of a neurodegenerative disorder and mental retardation, respectively.

This chapter will focus on the general pharmacology of the $GABA_A$ receptor complex, an example of a ligand-gated ion channel receptor, N-methyl-D-aspartic acid (NMDA) receptor, a class of glutamate-gated ion channel receptor, and α_7 nicotinic acetylcholine receptor, an ion channel receptor that is gated by acetylcholine. Where appropriate, the chapter will allude to neuropsychiatric disorders whose pathophysiology involves presumptive disturbance of neurotransmission mediated by these neurotransmitters; symptoms of these disorders include disturbances of attention, memory and cognition. A "functional" circuit that integrates all of these neurotransmitter receptors, at least in the hippocampus, and serves as an important heuristic model for medication development will also be described. Hopefully, medications that are under active development for influencing these three neurotransmitter receptor systems will have roles in the treatment and management of at least some examples of mental retardation. Conducting clinical trials with mentally retarded persons, a special vulnerable population, presents ethical and "human subject protection" challenges, especially with respect to recruitment and obtaining meaningful informed consent or, in the case of minors, assent with parental consent. These extremely important and sensitive issues must be addressed before institutional review boards (IRBs) approve clinical trials. The human subject protection issues will not be covered because they are beyond the scope of this chapter.

Introduction

The psychiatrist or psychopharmacologist engaged in the evaluation and care of a person with mental retardation must clarify the reason(s) for the referral and the goals of the evaluation and treatment recommendations. Importantly, no sole practitioner will be in a position to address all or most of the concerns raised by the parents, residential setting or school seeking the psychopharmacology consultation. The treatment recommendations will be influenced by the age of the person (the treatment goals of a toddler or preschool-age child with mental retardation differ from those of an adult), setting (i.e., home, residential treatment facility, school), etiology of the retardation (e.g., in some rare instances of a known genetic syndrome, treatment may include dietary, vitamin or hormonal interventions), severity of the retardation, and behavioral and motor symptoms (e.g., mood lability, mannerisms, stereotypies, agitation, aggression and hyperactivity), among other factors. For the young child, the goals always include promotion of social, cognitive and language development; unfortunately, medications selected to address some target symptoms (e.g., agitation, aggression and stereotypies) may interfere with cognition and school performance. Also, some medications may be selected because in addition to targeting behavioral symptoms, they may be indicated for co-morbid medical or neurological conditions, especially seizures; the latter are often associated with adverse cognitive side effects. The medications will often be selected empirically because the results of controlled clinical trials or the consensus opinion of experts do not exist; in these circumstances, the psychopharmacologist is dependent on the observational skills and objective reporting of the parents, caregivers, nursing assistants and teachers to guide medication selection and dose titration. Oftentimes, the psychopharmacologist will educate the "raters," who are able to observe the patient for long periods of time in naturalistic settings (e.g., home, residential treatment facility, school), as opposed to the limited observations that are possible in the "artificial" office setting during a 30 minute to one hour evaluation, about the specific symptoms and behaviors that are targeted for treatment, and adverse medication side effects that may emerge during the course of treatment. Whenever possible, these collaborative discussions can be facilitated by the use of objective rating instruments. The raters should also maintain a log or diary of specific problem behaviors, noting their frequency, intensity and circumstances of occurrence; this type of log can be invaluable in determining the effectiveness of specific medications and possible operant contingencies contributing to their maintenance (e.g., head banging). The authors cannot over-emphasize the importance of fostering and maintaining collaborative therapeutic relationships with parents, caregivers, nursing assistants and teachers in order to achieve optimal and effective pharmacotherapeutic goals. The psychopharmacologist should be optimistic, empathic (acknowledging the difficulties caregivers have with the daily management of many of these patients), and exquisitely honest about limitations of the field and current understanding of pathophysiology and treatment. Additionally, the psychopharmacologist must recognize that an effective (i.e., optimal) treatment plan is an interdisciplinary effort; no single individual can deliver all of the indicated modalities of treatment. Not uncommonly, thoughtfully developed treatment plans are undermined by an inability of the interdisciplinary team to work collaboratively and respectfully with each other.

Unfortunately, in the majority of cases, the etiology and pathophysiological mechanisms responsible for the presentation of "retardation," which should be regarded as a syndrome with cognitive, behavioral and motor components, are not known. Moreover, medications from a variety of pharmacological classes (e.g., antipsychotic medications, antidepressants, anxiolytic agents, psychostimulants and mood stabilizers and antiepilepsy drugs) will be selected empirically and less-than-fully effective. The written and explicit consent of the parent or legal guardian and (the assent of the) patient should be obtained if the medications are prescribed for "off-label" indications or in spite of specific "black box" warnings. The psychopharmacologist must also be very vigilant about laboratory monitoring for therapeutic blood levels (if known and appropriate) and abnormalities that may relate to electrolyte disturbances, impairment of glucose homeostasis, cardiac (including measurement of QT and $QT_{corrected}$ intervals), thyroid, liver and renal abnormalities. At the time of each scheduled appointment (or more frequently via phone if necessary), the psychopharmacologist should attempt to elicit both spontaneously and formally the emergence of possible medication association side effects (there are formal instruments for rating the emergence of treatment emergent side effects). In any event, the psychopharmacological treatment and management of persons with mental retardation have become an important area of concern for psychiatrists, child and adolescent psychiatrists, pediatricians and pediatric subspecialists, and neurologists and pediatric neurologists. Although manipulation of major neurotransmitter systems lacks "specificity" and, in most instances, does not target etiology or presumptive pathophysiological mechanisms, they are a promising and fertile area of current and future investigation. Clearly, influencing the global inhibitory and excitatory "tone" in the brain should have measurable effects on attention, cognition, memory, disruptive behaviors and motor symptoms. Also, a specific subtype of nicotinic acetylcholine receptor, designated α_7, is enriched in selective areas of the brain and is involved in normal mechanisms of attention and cognition. The selective stimulation of this receptor, which is enriched presynatpically and on the surface of GABAergic inhibitory interneurons, may be a strategy for enhancing the signal to noise ratio along complex synaptic circuits. Ideally, the careful titration of highly selective pharmacological interventions will be shown to be associated with desired therapeutic outcomes.

Table 1. Mental Retardation: Assessment and Treatment Planning

Multimodal, Interdisciplinary With Clearly Defined Short- and Long-Term Treatment and Rehabilitation Goals
Geneticist and Genetic Counselor
Developmental Pediatrician/Behavioral Pediatrician/Pediatric Neurologist
Pediatric Neuropsychologist (including Psychoeducational and Vocational Assessment and Planning)
Special Education
Speech and Language Specialist
Child Psychiatrist/Psychiatrist
Psychologist (Implementation of Operant/Behavioral Strategies and Procedures)
Social Work/Service Evaluation and On-Going Support
Parents and/or Caregivers (Involved as Co-Therapists, Co-Educators, Trainers)

Table 2. Mental Retardation: Pharmacotherapeutic Targets*

Cognition	
	Attention
	Distractibility
	Memory
	Abstraction
Hypoactivity/Hyperactivity	
Impulsivity	
Speech and Language	
Socialization	
Self-Care	
	Personal Hygiene
	Dressing
	Feeding, Meal Planning and Preparation
	Toileting
Motor Stereotypies	
Mannerisms, Posturing	
Agitation	
Aggression	
Sleep Disturbance	
Mood Lability	
Psychosis, especially Auditory Hallucinations	

* Primary pharmacotherapeutic targets are influenced by age, developmental stage, etiology and severity of mental retardation.

LIGAND-GATED ION CHANNEL RECEPTORS: GENERAL PRINCIPLES

The maintenance of unequal ion concentration gradients across the lipid bilayer of cell membranes is critical to life. These ion gradients represent an enormous amount of potential energy and a variety of ATP energy-dependent "pumps" exist to maintain and rapidly restore any disruption of these gradients. Ion channels are essentially potential holes or pores extending through the lipid bilayer that have filtering characteristics enabling solutes of particular sizes (hydration radius) and charge flux along their electrochemical gradients. The consequences of the permeation of ions of a particular hydration radius and charge density include changing the membrane resting potential, making the cell either more quiescent (hyperpolarization) or excitable (depolarization). Also, in the case of an influx of calcium ions, a cascade of biochemical events subsequent to their binding to various calcium ion binding proteins may occur; in addition, calcium ions are necessary for enzyme-catalyzed reactions within the cell independently of their complexing with calcium ion binding proteins.

There are several gating mechanisms that regulate the frequency and duration of channel opening; ion channels can open as a result of changing the cell's resting membrane potential (voltage-gated), the binding of neurotransmitter or other ligand (ligand-gated) or application of mechanical forces such as stretching. Changes in the resting membrane potential and intraneuronal concentrations of ions as a result of the binding of neurotransmitter can occur within a timeframe of 100 milliseconds or less and is referred to as "fast" synaptic transmission. Importantly, ligand-gating of ion channel opening is highly regulated by a number of mechanisms and at different levels of regulation: genetic (including the regionally selective transcription of specific receptor polypeptide subunits in response to stress and other experiences and according to the developmental stage of the brain), post-transcriptionally (RNA splice variants), post-translationally (especially phosphorylation of intracellular loops of receptor polypeptide subunits via specific kinases), and allosteric modulators and other types of modulation (e.g., neurosteroids, polyamines, nitrosylation, zinc ion binding, etc).

The ligand-gated ion channel receptors differ from each other with respect to the specific neurotransmitters, whose binding results in channel opening, and channel characteristics (e.g., some channels are selective filters for positively charged ions like sodium and calcium, whereas others are selective for the negatively charged chloride ion). Nonetheless, from a functional, if not also structural, perspective they are quite similar to each other. The receptor itself is a potential channel, resulting from the alignment of specific hydrophobic domains of each of the constituent polypeptides. The binding of the appropriate ligand to an extracellular domain on the heteromeric protein increases the likelihood that the ion channel will transiently assume an open configuration. The efficiency of this coupling between ligand binding and channel opening is influenced and modified by a variety of the factors mentioned above. The allosteric modulatory sites are obvious fertile targets for medication development efforts to adjust the gain or fine tune ligand-gated receptor-mediated neurotransmission. Of relevance to mental retardation and other neuropsychiatric disorders (e.g., schizophrenia), there is interest in promoting GABAergic, Glutamatergic (i.e., NMDA receptor-mediated) and nicotinic cholinergic (i.e., α_7 nicotinic acetylcholine receptor-mediated) neurotransmission very selectively for therapeutic purposes. This chapter will review the rationale underlying these strategies, which offer much promise for the pharmacotherapy of mental retardation.

$GABA_A$ RECEPTOR: A TARGET FOR THE PHARMACOTHERAPY OF MENTAL RETARDATION

γ-amino-butyric acid (GABA), the major inhibitory neurotransmitter in the brain, is derived from L-glutamate via the action of L-glutamic acid decarboxylase (GAD) in a one-step decarboxylase reaction; there are two genetically distinct GAD enzymes. L-Glutamate itself is also a neurotransmitter within the brain, serving as its major excitatory neurotransmitter. Astrocytic stores of glutamine serve as the major source for the neurotransmitter pools of GABA and L-glutamate. The importance of GABA and L-glutamate for the maintenance of general inhibitory and excitatory tone, respectively, within the brain is highlighted by the fact that neurons within the brain use or respond to these two amino acid neurotransmitters or are no more than one neuron removed from a cell that does (Olsen, 2002). Further, the pathophysiology of many neuropsychiatric disorders is thought to involve, at least in part, a disruption of the delicate balance between inhibitory and excitatory tone maintained by GABA and L-glutamate, respectively.

GABA, like L-glutamate and acetylcholine, interacts with two broad categories of neurotransmitter receptor complex: a ligand-gated ion channel receptor and a receptor coupled to a GTP-binding protein. The former is designated the $GABA_A$ receptor complex and is responsible for mediating "fast synaptic transmission," which is reflected in the generation of inhibitory post-synaptic potentials in a timeframe of 100 milliseconds or less subsequent to the calcium ion- and depolarization-dependent release of GABA from the presynaptic nerve terminal. The rapid generation of inhibitory post-synaptic potentials results from the transient opening of a potential pore or channel that traverses the lipid bilayer of the post-synaptic membrane, allowing for the rapid and selective permeation of chloride ions that usually results in hyperpolarization of the cell membrane; the latter reflecting the resting membrane potential for chloride ions, whose extracellular concentration is usually higher than its intracellular concentration. GABAergic inhibitory interneurons are components of cortical circuits innervating the soma and dendrites of "principal" neurons or other inhibitory interneurons and, thereby, regulate the integrated activity of these circuits (Ben-Ari and Holmes, 2005).

Interestingly, during the development of the brain and in pathological conditions such as epilepsy, the "polarity" of action mediated by $GABA_A$ receptors is excitatory, as opposed to, inhibitory (Ben-Ari and Holmes, 2005). This shift in "polarity" may explain the diminished or relative ineffectiveness of many antiepileptic medications in temporal lobe epilepsy. The altered polarity during development and in many examples of epilepsy reflects elevation of the intracellular concentration of chloride ions; thus, gated opening of the ion channel results in depolarization when intracellular chloride ion concentrations are elevated. In developing neurons, elevated intracellular chloride ion concentrations reflect differences in the developmentally programmed expressions of two "cotransporters," involved in extruding (i.e., K^+/Cl^- cotransporter [KCC2]) and accumulating (i.e., $Na^+,K^+/2Cl^-$ [NKCC1]) intracellular chloride ions; the former appears later in the development of the brain, while the latter is functional during an earlier stage of brain development. The switching on and off of these transporters is genetically programmed and results in elevated intracellular chloride ion concentrations and a change in the polarity of GABA's more familiar synaptic action from inhibition to excitation during fetal development. This altered polarity during development may be critical for forming appropriate synaptic connectivity. Epileptogenesis may also involve an altered polarity of GABA's familiar actions from inhibition to excitation that could be associated with a downregulation of KCC2 and diminished ability to extrude intracellular chloride ions (Ben-Ari and Holmes, 2005). Altered polarity of GABA's action during the development of the brain and epileptogenesis has implications for the administration of GABA "agonists," such as benzodiazepines or valproic acid, to pregnant woman, which may promote excitotoxic damage to the developing fetal brain, and some patients with atypical or refractory presentations of epilepsy (Ben-Ari and Holmes, 2005).

$GABA_A$ Receptor: Combinatorial Diversity Contributes to Sensitivity to Allosteric Modulation

The $GABA_A$ receptor is a heteropentameric receptor comprised of combinations of constituent polypeptide subunits. These subunits are grouped into families based on the degree of shared sequence homology (e.g., α, β, γ, δ, and ε); receptor subunits within a family reflect distinct genes, as opposed to normally-occurring polymorphisms of a single gene. Thus, there may be as many as six α receptor subunits, and three β and γ receptor subunits. Also, subunits from different families share sequence homology, although significantly less homology than members of the same family, reflecting the fact that they are all derived from a common ancestral protein. In fact, the $GABA_A$ receptor subunits share significant homology with nicotinic acetylcholine receptor subunits, supporting the existence of a superfamily of receptor subunits and degeneracy with respect to the architecture and function of ligand-gated ion channel receptors. Subunits are integral membrane proteins that have an N-terminal glycosylated extracellular domain, four membrane-spanning hydrophobic domains (M1-4) of about 25 amino acids in length, a "large" intracellular loop between the third and fourth membrane spanning domain, and a small C-terminal extracellular loop. The potential pore, whose opening is gated by GABA, is formed by the alignment of the second membrane spanning domain of each of the five constituent polypeptides. The benzodiazepine ligands bind at the interface between α and γ subunits, and GABA appears to bind at the interface between α and β subunits (Wisden and Stephens, 1999).

The most prevalent $GABA_A$ receptors are composed of α, β, and γ subunits in a ratio of 2:2:1 (Jones –Davis et al., 2005); however, subpopulations of receptors exist with the γ subunits replaced with δ and θ subunits that have unique pharmacological properties and anatomic distributions. For example, the δ subunit does not (usually) contribute to benzodiazepine binding or modulation (Jones-Davis et al., 2005). When benzodiazepine ligands act as allosteric modulators, their binding to an interface between α and γ subunits results in a conformational change that leads to a coupling between binding of GABA and increased frequency of channel opening (in most cases, this allosteric modulatory effect on frequency of channel opening is dependent on the binding of GABA to an interface between α and β subunits). Using molecular biological strategies, chimeric subunits have been created from alternatively spliced portions of specific γ subunits (e.g., γ_2L), which bind benzodiazepines and couple this binding to increased frequency of channel opening, and the δ subunit in order to identify the distinct domains of the receptor subunit contributing to the binding of benzodiazepines and their coupling to increased frequency of channel opening; these domains are dissociable from each other (Jones-Davis et al., 2005). At least with respect to the γ_2L subunit, two domains were identified that are critical for the "coupling" of benzodiazepine binding to increasing the frequency of channel opening: an extracellular M1 domain (an area nearer to the N-terminus leading into the first transmembranous "loop") and an M2 domain leading into the M2-M3 extracellular loop. Importantly, analogous or homologous domains that transduce binding of allosteric modulators to changes in channel properties may be shared "structural machinery" or properties of all members of the superfamily of ligand-gated ion channel receptors (Jones-Davis et al., 2005).

In addition to the combinatorial diversity resulting in receptors with differing pharmacological properties based on differences in the combinations of their constituent polypeptide subunits, splice variants modulate pharmacological properties (e.g., conferring heightened sensitivity or resistance to the acute effects of alcohol and affecting allosteric modulatory properties of benzodiazepines, among other effects). For example, the two splice variants of the γ2 subunit differ with respect to the presence of a consensus sequence of eight amino acids in the intracellular loop that serves as a substrate for protein kinase C- dependent phosphorylation. However, with respect to combinatorial diversity, there are some constraints such that most of the pentameric receptors contain two of the same α subunit, two of the same β subunit, and a γ subunit (Olsen, 2002). $GABA_A$ receptors containing α_4 or α_6 subunits do not bind benzodiazepine agonists (i.e., compounds related to diazepam), and the presence of γ subunits is usually essential for the binding of benzodiazepines. Combinatorial diversity and genetically-regulated expression of specific receptor subunits, alternative splicing, intracellular phosphorylation and extracellular glycosylation are genetic and post-translational modifications that influence pharmacological properties of the receptor. Additionally, the receptor contains allosteric modulatory binding sites that bind allosteric modulators in a reversible and rapid manner, allowing for rapid fine tuning and adjustment of GABA-gated chloride ion conductance. These allosteric modulators influence the likelihood and extent to which GABA is effective in promoting chloride ion conductance; they include benzodiazepines, barbiturates and neurosteroids. For example, benzodiazepine agonists bind at the surface of the cell to increase the efficiency of coupling between the binding of GABA and channel opening, affecting the frequency of channel opening, whereas barbiturates, such as pentobarbital, bind to a hydrophobic site within the channel domain and affect the duration of channel opening. Further, in contrast to benzodiazepines that depend on the presence of GABA for their pharmacological actions, barbiturates are capable of opening the channel at higher concentrations in the absence of GABA; this may account for the higher risk for lethality of barbiturates, as compared to benzodiazepine agonists. The ability of benzodiazepine agonists to improve the efficiency of coupling between the binding of GABA and channel opening, resulting in an increased frequency of channel opening, is thought to account for their diverse pharmacological properties, including anxiolysis, sedation, muscle relaxation and antiseizure effects. Interestingly, a series of ligands have been identified that bind with high-affinity and stereoselectivity to the benzodiazepine binding site on the $GABA_A$ receptor complex but have properties opposite to those of the classical benzodiazepine receptor agonists; that is, these compounds elicit anxiety and lower the seizure threshold (Olsen, 2002). They are referred to as inverse receptor agonists and are to be distinguished from pure benzodiazepine receptor antagonists (e.g., flumazenil); the latter are devoid of any pharmacological actions or effects on their own, but can block (i.e., competitively antagonize) the effects of agonists (e.g., drugs like diazepam) or inverse agonists (e.g., some β-carboline derivatives). Benzodiazepine agonists acting on $GABA_A$

receptors located within the hippocampus can cause an anterograde amnesia, which is a nuisance side-effect associated with this class of medications; conceivably, selective inverse benzodiazepine receptor agonist, whose actions are localized to the hippocampus, can be identified that would facilitate memory performance, attention and other aspects of cognition. Neurosteroids are synthesized in the periphery as well as in situ within the brain by glial cells; they are derived from the translocation of cholesterol from the cytoplasm into mitochondria, the rate-limiting step in their synthesis. These neurosteroids are both positive and negative allosteric modulators of GABA-gated chloride ion conductance, whose actions are mediated rapidly by the $GABA_A$ receptor on the surface of the cell, as opposed to binding to cytosolic steroid receptors, whose actions depend on translocation into the nucleus and regulation of transcriptional events. Alphaxolone is a synthetic neurosteroid analogue that potentiates GABA-gated chloride ion conductance that has been developed as an anesthetic medication.

Of the six or so alpha $GABA_A$ receptor subunits at least four are sensitive to the positive allosteric modulatory effects of benzodiazepine agonists (i.e., α_1, α_2, α_3, and α_5), whereas α_4 and α_6 are insensitive to these allosteric modulatory properties of benzodiazepines (Rudolph et al., 1999). Interestingly, a single histidine amino acid residue located at the 101 position of the mouse α_1 subunit is responsible for benzodiazepine-sensitivity; the α_4 and α_6 subunits, which are insensitive to benzodiazepines, have an arginine residue in this corresponding position (Rudolph et al., 1999). Introducing a targeted histidine to arginine point mutation in position 101 of the α_1 subunit into the germline of mice led to the creation of homozygous mutant, heterozygous and wild-type mice showing varying degrees of sensitivity to the allosteric modulatory properties of benzodiazepines. The α_1 subunit is the most abundant in the brain and is particularly enriched in cortical areas and thalamus (Rudolph et al., 1999); thus, creation of these mutant mice allowed for the examination of the consequences of selective insensitivity to benzodiazepines. The results of in vitro and behavioral investigations showed that the benzodiazepine modulatory site on $GABA_A$ receptors containing α_1 subunits is responsible for mediating sedative, amnestic and some of the antiseizure properties of benzodiazepines; the benzodiazepine modulatory site associated with this subunit does not seem to be involved in the anxiolytic, muscle relaxant, motor incoordinating or ethanol-potentiating effects of the benzodiazepine agonists. Although the targeted histidine to arginine point mutation in position 101 of the α_1 subunit results in insensitivity to benzodiazepines, the receptor retains its sensitivity to the modulatory effects of 3α-hydroxy-5β-pregnan-20-one, a neurosteroid, and sodium pentobarbital (Rudolph et al., 1999). The creation of mice with targeted point mutations in $GABA_A$ receptor subunits should lead to the development of highly-selective benzodiazepine agonists and inverse receptor agonists that may be able to avoid such adverse medical side effects as anterograde amnesia and improve aspects of memory and vigilance, respectively. For example, a series of 8-substituted imidazobenzodiazepines have been synthesized that show highly selective binding to the α_5 subunit that is enriched in a subpopulation of neurons in dorsal hippocampus, relative to other brain regions (Skolnick et al., 1997; Cook et al., 2005). Further, a relatively selective α_5 inverse benzodiazepine receptor agonist antagonizes reinforcing and motor-impairing effects of alcohol (Cook et al., 2005). The latter data implicate hippocampal "outputs" in at least some of the acute pharmacological actions of alcohol. More importantly, the data are "proof of concept" that highly selective benzodiazepine agonists, inverse receptor agonists and antagonists may be developed that could very selectively fine-tune or adjust the gain of GABAergic neurotransmission at the level of the receptor in discrete regions of brain (where specific $GABA_A$ receptor subtype are enriched) (Skolnick et al., 1997; Costa et al., 2002; Cook et al., 2005).

Genetic Evidence Consistent with the Involvement of the $GABA_A$ Receptor in the Pathogenesis of Syndromes of Mental Retardation

There is now converging and growing evidence that altered expression of $GABA_A$ receptor subunits, particularly those whose genes are located in the q11 to q13 or q14 region of chromosome 15, may contribute to a heterogeneous group of neurodevelopmental disorders (Ungaro et al., 2001). This group includes, but is not limited to, Angelman and Prader-Willi syndromes, hereditary spastic paraplegia and, perhaps, a subgroup of patients with autism, among other disorders. Importantly, mutant $GABA_A$ receptor subunit genes may not be responsible for at least some of these disorders; rather, linkage between a disorder and the region on chromosome 15 that includes genes for these subunits is consistent with altered regulation of expression and rate of expression of normal polymorphisms for these receptor subunits. The plasticity and pharmacological properties of the $GABA_A$ receptor complex result from the combinatorial diversity related to genetically regulated expression of different subunits; distinct combinations of subunits comprising this heteropentameric receptor influence channel properties and GABA-gated chloride ion conductance and modulation of this gated chloride ion conductance by benzodiazepine ligands, barbiturates, neurosteroids and ethanol, among other modulators. The genes for the α_5, β_3, and γ_3 $GABA_A$ receptor subunits are located on chromosome 15 in the q11-q13 region; they are referred to as GABRA5, GABRB3, and GABRG3, respectively. Interestingly, the gene for the α_7 subunit of the nicotinic acetylcholine receptor is also located on chromosome 15 in the q13-q14 region and altered regulation of its expression is linked to, or associated with, schizophrenia and sensory impairment observed in this disorder (Freedman et al., 1997, 2001; Leonard et al., 2002). The pathophysiology of schizophrenia may be due to "neurotransmitter imbalance" with disturbances of the delicate balance between neurotransmission mediated by multiple neurotransmitters, including GABA and the acetylcholine signal transduced by the α_7 nicotinic acetylcholine receptor. Perhaps, disturbances in nontranscribed or untranslated regions of chromosome 15q affect the rate of expression of normal gene products in this region, including specific receptor subunits for $GABA_A$ and nicotinic acetylcholine receptors.

Maternally or paternally-derived de novo cytogenetic deletions of the proximal q11-q13 region of chromosome 15 underlie the etiology of Angelman and Prader-Willi syndromes, respectively (Knoll et al., 1989). Patients with Angelman and Prader-Willi syndrome manifest symptoms that are also found in patients with autism; for example, patients with Prader-Willi syndrome may show resistance to a change in routine and patients with Angelman's syndrome may manifest hand flapping (Sutcliffe and Nurmi, 2003). The emergence of discrete and different syndromes depending on whether the affected "homologue" is of maternal or paternal origin led to recognition of "imprinting" and the identification of at least three "hotspots" for chromosome breakage resulting in deletions (and duplications and triplications). In addition to deletions resulting in these well-defined syndromes, duplications and triplications have also been identified and syndromes may differ depending on whether the maternal or paternal chromosome is affected. Curiously, children with paternally-derived duplications of the q11-q13 region may have normal phenotypes in contrast to those with maternally-derived duplications, which are associated with developmental delays and autistic behaviors (Ungaro et al., 2001; Maggouta et al., 2003). Maternally and paternally-derived triplications are associated with abnormal phenotypes and profound neurodevelopmental delays. Alterations of the expression of a number of genes in the triplicated regions have been shown and differences in expression are also influenced by whether the region of the maternal or paternal chromosome is triplicated, which may be due, in part, to differences in the methylation of CpG-enriched islands of the maternal and paternal chromosomes. In any event, the region contains the cluster of three genes for GABA $_A$ receptor subunits and $GABA_A$ receptors are important for neurodevelopment and maintenance of inhibitory tone in the brain. Thus, GABAergic abnormalities may accompany Angelman and Prader-Willi syndromes, which are associated with deletions of 15q11-q13, and other abnormal phenotypes resulting from duplications, triplications, translocations, inversions and the formation of supernumerary marker chromosomes of this region spanning approximately 4 Mb (Ungaro et al., 2001; Maggouta et al., 2003).

Mouse A9 hybrid cells were created that contained a single human chromosome, either a maternally or paternally derived chromosome 15 (Meguro et al., 1997). These cells were used to study the phenomenon of genetic imprinting, which suggests that there is a functional inequality between maternally and paternally-derived regions of some chromosomes. Although they are not fully-known, the bases of this inequality could include DNA methylation, the structure of chromatin and asynchronous replication. Using this system, it was shown that expression of the three $GABA_A$ receptor subunits (α_5, β_3, and γ_3) was exclusively from the paternal chromosome. Ordinarily, the level of expression of these subunits is low and restricted to specific brain regions, making it difficult to determine the imprinting status of these genes; thus, the Mouse A9 hybrid cell is a useful methodology for determining whether genes are preferentially expressed from the maternal or paternal chromosome. Also, the 5' region of the GABARB3 gene on the paternal chromosome, which is located upstream in the 5'direction to the other two receptor subunit alleles, is hypermethylated; there was no hypermethylation of the GABARB3 gene on the maternally-derived chromosome (Meguro et al., 1997). Methylation of CpG islands is a mechanism of regulating gene expression; with respect to the three $GABA_A$ receptor subunits on the 15q11-q13 region of the paternal chromosome, this may represent a mechanism of positive regulation of paternally expressed imprinted genes. There are also data showing that the paternal q11-q13 region of chromosome 15 containing the GABARB3 gene may replicate earlier than the same region on the maternal chromosome; this reciprocal asynchronous replication may be another mechanism contributing to imprinting, resulting in Prader-Willi syndrome with deletion of the paternal q11-q13 segment of chromosome 15 and Angelman syndrome with deletion of the maternal segment of this chromosome. In any event, the data suggest that deficient expression of the $GABA_A$ receptor subunits encoded on chromosome 15 in the q11-q13 region, especially the β_3 subunit, may contribute to the pathogenesis and pathophysiology of Prader-Willi syndrome (Meguro et al., 1997).

Although hereditary spastic paraplegia (HSP) may be inherited in an autosomal dominant manner, it presents as a heterogeneous group of disorders with a variable age of onset (e.g., between 12 and 35 years), whose primary features include progressive lower extremity weakness and spasticity (Fink et al., 1996). Using microsatellite polymorphisms on chromosome 15q, linkage was found between HSP and the 15q region that contains the genes for the α_5 and β_3 subunits in an extended kindred with autosomal dominant HSP. Linkage to the 15q region was replicated in this extended kindred using two different microsatellite markers located in an approximately 100-kb region between the genes for the α_5 and β_3 subunits and a marker located within an untranslated region of the gene for α_5 itself. The subunit genes themselves were ruled out as the cause of HSP in this kindred because "obligate recombinants" were identified who manifest illness without inheriting the markers for specific polymorphisms of these genes; thus, linkage of HSP to the 15q region was shown while linkage to the genes for these receptor subunits was ruled out (Fink et al., 1996). An explanation that implicates disturbance of GABAergic neurotransmission in HSP is altered (rates of) expression of normal genes for the α_5 and β_3 subunits. Altered regulation of expression is consistent with the variable age of onset observed in this extended HSP kindred.

Chromosomal abnormalities in neuropsychiatric disorders may define chromosomal regions of interest that contain candidate genes conferring risk and/or involved in the pathophysiology of the disorder (Nurmi et al., 2003; Sutcliffe and Nurmi, 2003). The most common chromosomal abnormalities in autism are duplications of the q11-q13 region of the maternally-derived chromosome 15; thus, "imprinted" gene expression of the maternally-derived proximal region of the long arm of chromosome 15, as opposed to duplications of this region derived from the paternal chromosome, and a possible gene "dosage" effect may contribute to risk and/or the pathophysiological mechanism responsible for autism. The duplications of the 15q11-q13 region are of two types: tandem duplication or "supernumary pseudodicentric, inverted, and duplicated regions of chromosome 15," often referred to as idic(15) (Sutcliffe and Nurmi, 2003). Relative to the tandem duplication, the phenotypes of patients with idic(15) are more severe, which is probably related to a larger gene dosage effect because this duplication spans a larger genomic interval and has a greater copy number of the 15q11-q13 region (i.e., gene dosage effect refers to overexpression of genes in this duplicated region). Autistic patients with the idic(15) duplication are more severely cognitively impaired and more often present with seizures, and motor stereotypies. Importantly, the data on duplications of the maternal 15q11-q13 region show that this is not a necessary or sufficient condition for autism; only a minority of persons with maternal duplication of 15q11-q13 meet criteria for pervasive developmental disorder and only about 1% to 3% of patients with autism have evidence of maternal duplication. However, linkage of the autism phenotype to this region that contains genes for three $GABA_A$ receptor subunits (i.e., α_5, β_3, and γ_3) in chromosomally "normal" autism families has been reported and the β_3 subunit in particular is emerging as a candidate gene (Nurmi et al., 2003; Sutcliffe and Nurmi, 2003). Stratifying of autistic patients enrolled in the Collaborative Linkage Study of Autism (CLSA) according to the cluster of "savant skills" derived from a principal components analysis of the Autism Diagnostic Interview (ADI) showed a higher likelihood of linkage of this phenotypic subset with the 15q11-q13 region; moreover, the peak score for linkage was to a microsatellite marker located within the GABARB3 (i.e., β_3 subunit). Thus, genetic linkage of probands with savant skills to the 15q11-q13 region is more likely in general, and to the locus of the GABARB3 gene in particular. Savant skills, which are abilities that are significantly higher than expected given the patient's poor cognitive performance, are not commonly observed in autism, although they occur more frequently in autism than in other developmental disorders (Nurmi et al., 2003). Savant skills are usually very circumscribed and limited to a discrete domain of cognitive or motor function; they include rote memory, arithmetic and calendrical calculations, musical ability and visuo-spatial skills (e.g., puzzle assembly). As discussed, the β_3 $GABA_A$ receptor subunit is a good candidate gene because of the role $GABA_A$ receptors play in the development of the brain and maintenance of inhibitory tone (Nurmi et al., 2003).

Functional consequences of deletion of maternally-derived 15q11-q13 were shown in a positron emission tomography (PET) study of four patients with Angelman syndrome (Holopainen et al., 2001). The study suggested that this chromosomal deletion is associated with reductions in the expression of $GABA_A$ receptors in frontal cortex, parietal cortex, hippocampus, and cerebellum, as reflected in the decreased binding of ^{11}C-flumazenil, a relatively pure competitive benzodiazepine antagonist. Diminished ^{11}C-flumazenil binding was observed in one patient with a more restricted deletion that included the gene locus for only the β_3 subunit, but not the genes for α_5 or γ_3 subunits, supporting a primary role for the β_3 subunit in reduced binding. The authors proposed that a reduction in the density of $GABA_A$ receptors accounted for the reduced binding, as opposed to a change in the affinity of the receptor for ^{11}C-flumazenil, because β subunits do not affect the affinity of the receptor for benzodiazepines and a reduced density of receptors is found in the brains of GABRB3 (β_3) subunit knockout mice (Holopainen et al., 2001). The results are somewhat tentative because of the small number of patients that were studied and the potentially confounding effects of epilepsy, treatment with anti-epileptic medications, and anesthesia prior to the PET procedure; nonetheless, the data suggest that a deletion of the maternal 15q11-q13 chromosomal fragment that contains the gene for the β_3 subunit has functional consequences. Diminished inhibitory tone in the brains of these patients with Angelman syndrome could account for seizures, cognitive impairment and motor abnormalities. These symptoms may also result, at least in part, from a neurodevelopmental disruption of normal synaptic connectivity associated with diminished expression of $GABA_A$ receptors.

Because ethosuximide possessed relatively specific efficacy for seizures manifested by the GABARB3-deficient knockout mouse, it was successfully used to treat refractory atypical absence seizures in two patients with Angelman syndrome; ethosuximide was added to valproate. Serum concentrations of ethosuximide in these two patients that were associated with suppression of irregular high-voltage delta waves with multifocal spikes ranged between 116.9 μg/ml and 133.6 μg/ml. The data suggest that ethosuximide may have a special indication for refractory seizures in patients with Angelman syndrome and may diminish the consequences of reduced inhibitory tone resulting from absent expression of the β_3 subunit and diminished density of $GABA_A$ receptors.

As discussed, alterations in the combinations of $GABA_A$ receptor units result in differences in pharmacological properties that are sometimes very subtle and apparent only after provocation or pharmacological "challenge" with a specific benzodiazepine agonist; thus, in the absence of a benzodiazepine, differences in ion conductance properties between "combinatorially" distinct receptors may not be evident (Ranna et al., 2006). Moreover, although the α_1 subunit is most commonly incorporated into functional $GABA_A$ receptors, absence of its expression is not lethal, supporting the notion that fine tuning of central inhibitory tone in a regionally-selective manner is crucial for optimal (and, perhaps, normal) functioning of the brain (Ranna et al., 2006). Regionally-selective expression of specific receptor subtypes may be an opportunity for targeting subpopulations of receptors for specific therapeutic objectives. For example, locus coeruleus (LC) is a bilateral brainstem nucleus located in the floor of the fourth ventricle that gives rise to a diffuse network of noradrenergic projections; LC plays important roles in regulation of vigilance, anxiety, attention and memory (Ranna et al., 2006). The LC receives a very dense GABAergic innervation; it is estimated that GABAergic nerve terminals account for 50% of the nerve terminals in this area. Importantly, ε and θ, two relatively uncommon $GABA_A$ receptor subunits, are enriched and selectively expressed in LC. In terms of the genetic regulation of their expression, it is of interest that the genes for ε and θ, as well as the α_3 subunit are clustered together on the q28 region of the X chromosome. This clustering suggests that their expression may share some common regulatory features, including regulation of anatomically-selective expression (e.g., in LC). Of interest, there does not appear to be expression of α_1, α_4, α_5, or α_6 in the LC; in situ hybridization data support expression of α_3 and α_2 in LC.

The availability of expression systems, such as Xenopus oocytes and human embryonic kidney 293T cells, has allowed the study of the pharmacological and electrophysiological properties of human recombinant $GABA_A$ receptors constructed from specific receptor subunits. These types of studies have shown that the reduced GABA-sensitivity of the α_3 subunit, relative to the α_1 subunit, can be increased by inclusion of the ε subunit; this modulatory effect of the ε subunit on GABA-sensitivity depends on the specific α subunit because the sensitivity of the α_1 subunit-containing $GABA_A$ receptor, in contrast to the α_3 subunit-containing receptor, was not increased by the ε subunit in a Xenopus oocyte expression system (Ranna et al., 2006). The introduction of the ε subunit was also associated with diminished modulatory effects of several compounds including flurazepam (a benzodiazepine receptor agonist) and pregnanolone (a neurosteroid), whereas it did not influence the modulatory effect of pentobarbital (Ranna et al., 2006). Also, the ion channels of receptors containing the ε subunit were "leakier" with respect to chloride ion currents, suggesting that the open configuration of the channel is energetically more favorable with inclusion of the ε subunit. The expression of the δ subunit may be regionally-enriched in cerebellar granule cells, followed by thalamus and olfactory bulb and its inclusion in $GABA_A$ receptors results in insensitivity to the allosteric modulatory actions of benzodiazepines (Costa et al., 2002).

$GABA_A$ Receptor Combinatorial Diversity: Therapeutic Implications

In any event, the use of in vitro expression systems and the construction of pharmacologically-active, "combinatorially-distinct" receptors permit tabulation of the sensitivity to the modulatory effects of benzodiazepine ligands (including imidazenil and its derivatives) on chloride ion currents and GABA binding for a variety of distinct receptors (Costa et al., 2002). These studies will identify candidate medications that can target specific receptor combinations in regionally-selective areas of brain. The therapeutic goals of selective GABAergic interventions would include improved attention, improved memory performance, improved sleep, diminished impulsivity, diminished distractibility and diminished anxiety, among other therapeutic targets. Clearly, defective or deficient GABAergic neurotransmission is associated with altered neural function and may be causative in genetic syndromes associated with mental retardation, such as Prader-Willi and Angelman's syndromes. Therapeutic compounds would include specific benzodiazepine ligands, neurosteroids, inhibitors of the glial and neuronal reuptake of GABA (e.g., tiagabine), and inhibitors of the intraneuronal metabolism of GABA (e.g., vigabatrin), the latter should increase the quantity of GABA available for synaptic release (Bowery and Smart, 2006). The effectiveness of benzodiazepine agonists (e.g., lorazepam and diazepam) in resolving catatonia, a syndrome characterized by cognitive and motor impairments that occurs in association with schizophrenia, affective disorders, and medical and neurological conditions, demonstrate the profound therapeutic value that can be achieved by pharmacological manipulation of central inhibitory tone (Hung and Huang, 2006).

NMDA RECEPTOR: A TARGET FOR THE PHARMACOTHERAPY OF MENTAL RETARDATION

Biochemical Pharmacology and Allosteric Modulation

The N-methyl-D-aspartic acid (NMDA) receptor complex is an example of a heteromeric (probably pentameric) L-glutamate-gated ion channel receptor that also possesses properties of voltage-gating. The process of coupling the binding of L-glutamate and glycine, its obligatory co-agonist, to channel opening is very highly-regulated with multiple allosteric modulatory ligands influencing the likelihood that channel opening will occur (Bonhaus et al., 1987; Fagg, 1987; Foster and Wong, 1987; Long et al., 2006, in the press; Millan, 2005). The functional properties of the complex can also be (rapidly) influenced by intracellular phosphorylation sites, extracellular glycosylation, nitrosylation sites (which suggests an interaction with nitric oxide dependent mechanisms), "redox" sites, and zinc ion binding sites; the complexity of regulating glutamate-gated (calcium) ion conductance is consistent with the vitally important role this neurotransmitter complex plays in regulation of cognition, mood and motor behavior (Millan, 2005).

Further, the astrocyte is a critical component of the anatomy of this glutamatergic synapse and is an active participant in the orchestration of the depolarization- and calcium ion-dependent release of glutamate from presynaptic nerve terminals and channel opening. Specifically, astrocytes participate in the regulation of the synaptic availability of L-glutamate and glycine themselves, as well as synaptic levels of D-serine, a glycine agonist, and kynurenic acid, a glycine antagonist (Millan, 2005). As discussed already with respect to the $GABA_A$ receptor complex, astrocytes are also involved in maintaining the neurotransmitter pool of L-glutamate, via shuttling of glutamine between these cells and glutamatergic neurons, and local synaptic levels of neurosteroids. Voltage-gating is another important local mechanism for regulating the effectiveness of glutamate-gated calcium ion conductance. Ordinarily, at the resting membrane potential of the neuron, the NMDA receptor-associated ionophore is obstructed by bound hydrated magnesium ions. In order to relieve this magnesium ion blockade, allowing L-glutamate to be effective in promoting the inward conductance of calcium ions, the membrane must begin to depolarize. Thus, membrane depolarization due to the coordinated action of other neurotransmitters (e.g., acetylcholine) and other classes of L-glutamate-gated ion channel receptors (i.e., AMPA/Kainate receptors) and other ion channels (i.e., voltage-gated channels) must take place in the same topographic area on the surface of the neuron to enable NMDA receptor-mediated neurotransmission to occur.

The NMDA receptor complex, like the other examples of ligand-gated ion channel receptors, is constructed from constituent polypeptide subunits, each of which has extracellular, transmembranous hydrophobic and intracellular domains; the latter have consensus sequences of amino acids that serve as substrates for phosphorylation (Millan, 2005). Because various kinases are activated by GTP-coupled, neurotransmitter receptor-mediated reactions, the extent to which the NMDA receptor is phosphorylated reflects "cross-talk" between different neurotransmitter receptor systems. Thus, neurotransmitters, whose chemical signal is transduced by a GTP-coupled receptor that is a large single protein with seven transmembranous hydrophobic domains, may influence the gating properties of L-glutamate and glycine by stimulating (or inhibiting) the phosphorylation of NMDA receptors in a protein kinase A or protein kinase C-dependent manner. The NMDA receptor complex contains various combinations of NR1 and NR2A-B subunits (combinatorial diversity); the NR1 subunit contains the glycine$_B$ binding site and specific NR2 receptor subtypes often determine the pharmacological properties of the ion channel receptors, including affinity of the glycine binding site on the NR1 subunit for glycine, efficacy of glycine and the kinetics of receptor desensitization (Akbarian et al., 1996; Deutsch et al., 2001; Grimwood et al., 1999; Humphries et al., 1996; Huntsman et al., 1998; Long et al., 2006, in the press; Millan, 2005). Glycine can oppose the desensitization of the receptor to L-glutamate and increase the duration and frequency of opening of the receptor-associated ion channel (thus, in addition to being a co-agonist, glycine has allosteric modulatory properties). The various NR2 receptor subunits represent distinct alleles; however, in addition to combinatorial diversity, the plasticity of the NMDA receptor is also affected by alternative splicing and splice variants of the NR2 subunits. Regulators of genetic expression determine the subunit combinations that are expressed; moreover, the combinations are not homogeneously distributed throughout the brain. Specifically, NMDA receptor complexes containing specific subunits are enriched in discrete regions: NR1 and NR2A-containing subunits are concentrated in hippocampus, thalamus and frontal cortex; and NR2C and NR2D are enriched in cerebellum and brain stem, respectively. The developmental stage of the brain also influences expression of receptor polypeptide subunits, such as the NR3 subunit. It is possible that pathological states are associated with abnormal regulation and altered expression of polypeptide subunits.

Astrocyte and Endogenous Modulation of the NMDA Receptor

The astrocyte may be the principal source of synaptic glycine in the local area of the NMDA receptor (Millan, 2005). Within the astrocyte, glycine can be derived from L-serine via serine hydroxymethltransferase, and its release may be dependent on the "reversal" of glycine trnasporters. Glycine transporters, which are sodium ion- and chloride ion-dependent and enriched in the areas of NMDA receptors, accomplish synaptic inactivation of glycine via astrocytic reuptake. Also, the mitochondrial glycine cleavage enzyme system prevents excess accumulation of intracellular levels of glycine Deutsch et al., 1990, 1998). In addition to its likely metabolic role in one-carbon metabolism, sarcosine is a naturally-occurring inhibitor of the specific GlyT-1 glycine transporter and is under active investigation as a glycinergic intervention designed to facilitate NMDA receptor-mediated neurotransmission (Long et al., 2006, in the press). The astrocyte may also be the source of D-serine, derived from L-serine by the action of D-serine racemase. D-Serine is not incorporated into proteins and may serve as an important locally-derived glycine agonist at the strychnine-insensitive glycine$_B$ binding site on the NMDA receptor complex (Long et al., 2006, in the press). In fact, there are certain combinations of NMDA receptor subunits that render the receptor more sensitive to D-serine than glycine itself. D-Serine racemase is enriched in areas with a high density of NMDA receptors, such as the hippocampus and cerebral cortex, consistent with its role as an obligatory co-agonist. Moreover, there are a variety of glial and neuronal transporters involved in the reuptake of D-serine from the synaptic cleft; the glial enzyme D-serine amino acid oxidase (D-AAO) also participates in the regulation of levels of D-serine in the local synaptic region of the NMDA receptor.

The dipeptide N-acetyl-aspartate-glutamate (NAAG) is another local modulator of glutamatergic neurotransmission, whose availability is regulated by the activity of two forms of glutamate carboxypeptidase (CGPII and III) on the surface of astrocytes, with activities at both the presynaptic glutamatergic nerve terminal and postsynaptic NMDA receptor (Millan, 2005). Presynaptically, NAAG stimulates "metabotropic" glutamate receptors (i.e., glutamate receptors that are not ion channels and coupled to a biochemical effector [e.g., cAMP production]) that inhibit the presynaptic release of glutamate, whereas, postsynaptically, NAAG is an NMDA receptor antagonist, antagonizing glycine and D-serine. Moreover, the astrocyte cleavage of NAAG by CGPII/III generates a local source of L-glutamate and, ultimately, L-aspartate, a 4-carbon dicarboxylic excitatory amino acid that is also active at glutamate-gated ion channel receptors. The modulatory activity of NAAG and regulation of its local levels highlight the critical and intimate role of the astrocyte in NMDA receptor-mediated neurotransmission.

An "alternate" pathway of tryptophan metabolism that generates kynurenic acid, a competitive glycine antagonist at the glycine$_B$ strychnine-insensitive site, is present within the astrocyte (Millan, 2005; Rosse et al., 1992). The more familiar pathway is the generation of serotonin after the sequential hydroxylation and decarboxylation of tryptophan. Further, the pathway resulting in kynurenic acid can also lead to the generation of quinolinic acid, an excitotoxic compound that acts at glutamate receptors. Astrocytes are also the in situ source for the production of neurosteroids; they are derived as a result of the translocation of cholesterol across the mitochondrial membrane and rapidly modulate NMDA receptor-mediated neurotransmission after binding to an allosteric modulatory site on the receptor. In summary, the astrocyte influences the local availability of L-glutamate, glycine, and modulators that increase (e.g., D-serine) and decrease (e.g., kynurenic acid) the efficiency of coupling between its binding and channel opening.

Implications of Anatomic Circuitry for the Pharmacotherapy of Mental Retardation

As noted, L-glutamate is one of the most abundant neurotransmitters in the brain. L-Glutamate is an important chemical mediator of intracortical (cortico-cortical) association pathways (presumably, it is involved in the bilateral integration of information from various cortical regions), and cortical efferent projection pathways (Deutsch et al., 1989, 2001). Glutamatergic projections to the striatum and hippocampus have been well-described. Within the hippocampus, the NMDA receptor is necessary for the induction of long-term potentiation, an important electrophysiological basis or underlying mechanism for many types of learning and memory. L-Glutamate is also used in many intra-hippocampal projection pathways and by important hippocampal efferent projections. Glutamatergic projections onto NMDA receptors located on the surface of GABAergic inhibitory interneurons located within the striatum regulate inhibitory tone on important glutamatergic projections originating within the thalamus that, in turn, project to the cortex (striato-thalamic-cortical circuit) (Deutsch et al., 2001). Conceivably, the selective modulation of NMDA receptor functioning within the cerebral cortex could improve striatothalamic filtering of sensory input to the cortex (thereby, improving the signal to noise ratio and heightening appreciation of, and attention to, relevant environmental stimuli). Further, the inhibitory tone of dopaminergic projections originating in the midbrain (i.e., substantia nigra and ventral tegmental area) is determined by L-glutamate-gated NMDA receptors on the surface of striatal GABAergic inhibitory neurons that innervate these dopaminergic cell bodies. There are also direct "reciprocal" connections between glutamatergic and dopaminergic neurons involved in the regulation of dopamine release. Independently of L-glutamate, dopaminergic neurotransmission has important roles in the regulation of higher cognitive functions (e.g., dopamine D1 and D5 receptors in the cerebral cortex), mood (e.g., dopamine D2, D3 and D4 receptors in limbic structures) and motor functions (e.g., dopamine D2 receptors in the basal ganglia). Thus, L-glutamate's modulation of dopaminergic activity in discrete regions of brain may impact cognition, mood and motor functions that are often disturbed in presentations of mental retardation.

The challenge is the development of highly selective strategies for modulating only some combinatorially-distinctive NMDA receptors that are enriched in discrete areas of the brain; also, this modulation must be in the right direction (e.g., in some regions and some instances, facilitation of NMDA receptor-mediated neurotransmission may be desirable, whereas, in other examples, antagonism may be desired). Importantly, the circuitry utilizing NMDA receptors must be better understood in order to appreciate "downstream" consequences of facilitating or antagonizing NMDA receptor-mediated neurotransmission (Deutsch et al., 2001). Thus, for example, an important pathophysiological consequence of NMDA receptor hypofunction in schizophrenia may be disinhibition of glutamatergic projections that are downstream from GABAergic inhibitory interneurons, resulting in excitotoxic stimulation of AMPA/kainate receptors, which are other examples of L-glutamate-gated ion channel receptors. An appreciation of this circuitry has stimulated thinking about a therapeutic role for selective potentiation of the GABAergic inhibitory interneurons that synapse on these "downstream" glutamatergic projections and AMPA/kainate receptor antagonists in the treatment of schizophrenia. Theoretically, modulating neurotransmission along circuits utilizing NMDA receptors holds much promise for improving sustained attention and diminishing distractibility (e.g., targeting NMDA receptors in cortex, some of which receive glutamatergic projections from the thalamus), improving working memory (e.g., NMDA receptors in the cerebral cortex), enhancing the learning of new information (e.g., NMDA receptors in the hippocampus), and diminishing mood and motor abnormalities (e.g., targeting NMDA receptors on the surface of striatal GABAergic inhibitory interneurons that project to midbrain [A9, A10, and substantia nigra] nuclei of dopaminergic cell bodies). There are a number of candidate NMDA receptor interventional strategies that can be explored in the pharmacotherapy of mental retardation (Schwartz et al., 1991, 1992, 1996).

A$_7$ Nicotinic Acetylcholine Receptor: A Target for the Pharmacotherapy of Mental Retardation

Acetylcholine is one of the earliest neurotransmitters to be identified. Because of the free rotation around single carbon bonds in aqueous solutions, acetylcholine can rapidly assume different configurations; presumably, the affinity and stereoselectivity of its binding to various acetylcholine receptors is determined by specific configurations that the molecule can assume. There are two broad classes of neurotransmitter receptors that recognize acetylcholine: muscarinic and nicotinic acetylcholine receptors. The muscarinic acetylcholine receptors are members of the superfamily of receptors with seven transmembranous hydrophobic domains, whose ultimate actions depend on the role GTP-binding proteins play in the coupling of the binding of acetylcholine at the surface of the cell to biochemical consequences within the cell (e.g., turnover of membrane phosphoinosides leading to generation of inositol tris-phosphate [IP3], increased intracellular concentrations of calcium ions, and activation of protein kinase C). Muscarinic acetylcholine receptors are implicated in normal memory and cognition because of the cognitive dulling and impaired memory performance associated with scopolamine and other drugs possessing the property of binding to muscarinic acetylcholine receptors. Importantly, Alzheimer's disease, a progressive neurodegenerative disorder that is the leading cause of dementia, is associated with prominent degeneration of anatomic projection pathways that utilize acetylcholine as their principal neurotransmitter (e.g., projections from the diagonal band of Brocca and nucleus basalis of Meynert to the hippocampus and frontal cortex, respectively). "Scopolamine-induced dementia" serves as a useful pharmacological model for studying at least some aspects of Alzheimer's disease and testing potential therapeutic compounds. There are at least two muscarinic acetylcholine receptors in the human brain that are under consideration as pharmacotherapeutic targets to improve cognition, designated M1 and M4. However, in addition to the role that muscarinic acetylcholine receptors play in memory, cognition and the pathophysiology of Alzheimer's disease, there is emerging interest in a specific subtype of nicotinic acetylcholine receptor, designated α_7, which may also serve as a therapeutic target for improvement of attention and cognition (or at least complex cognitive processes dependent on intact attention) (Deutsch et al., 2005).

As reviewed earlier, nicotinic acetylcholine receptors are ligand-gated ion channel receptors that mediate "fast" synaptic transmission, as opposed to the "slow" synaptic transmission mediated by muscarinic acetylcholine receptors (Albuquerque et al., 1997; Alkondon et al., 1997; Broide and Leslie, 1999; Deutsch et al., 2005; Lena and Changeux, 1998; Lindstrom, 1997; Weiland et al., 2000). They are members of a large superfamily of ligand-gated ion channel receptors that includes the $GABA_A$ receptor complex. The receptors are pentameric proteins that are anchored in the membrane and constructed from constituent polypeptide subunits, each of which shares significant amino acid homology and similar functional domains: extracellular domain, transmembranous hydrophobic domains consisting of about 20-25 neutral or relatively nonpolar amino acids, and an intracellular loop that has consensus sequences of amino acids for specific kinase-mediated phosphorylations between the third and fourth transmembranous hydrophobic domains. From an evolutionary perspective, the α_7 subunit is an ancestral one and using in vitro expression systems was shown to be capable of forming a functional channel by itself (i.e., forming a homopentameric receptor ion channel that can be gated by acetylcholine). Moreover, receptors containing the α_7 subunit have unique channel properties, including high calcium ion permeability and rapid desensitization, resulting in a unique electrophysiological signature in patch-clamp recordings, referred to as type 1A.

α_7 Nicotinic Acetylcholine Receptor: Implicated in Sensory Inhibition and Regionally-Selective Inhibitory Tone

The α_7 nicotinic acetylcholine receptor is located on the presynaptic nerve terminal where it participates in the depolarization-dependent regulation of release of multiple neurotransmitters. Additionally, the receptor is located on the surface of GABAergic inhibitory neurons, where it plays a very important role in modulating the inhibitory tone of the brain (Albuquerque et al., 1997). The α_7 nicotinic acetylcholine receptor is enriched in a number of areas of the brain, including the hippocampus, frontal cortex and thalamus. This receptor is implicated very importantly in a fundamental mechanism of attention that is critical for attending to relevant environmental stimuli, while "ignoring" irrelevant ones; the phenomenon is called sensory inhibition. Sensory inhibition is measured formally in an auditory evoked electrophysiological paradigm. In this paradigm, positive potentials that are evoked about 50 milliseconds after an auditory stimulus are measured in response to a pair of identical auditory stimuli presented exactly 500 milliseconds apart from each other. Ordinarily, the amplitude of the "P50" response evoked in response to the presentation of the second of the two paired stimuli is reduced to less than 50% of the amplitude evoked in response to the first stimulus of the pair. These evoked responses that are measured from the vertex of the head and the gated sensory inhibition (i.e., the normally blunted amplitude of the P50 response to the second of the identically-paired stimuli) are dependent on α_7 nicotinic acetylcholine receptors located in the hippocampus (Deutsch et al., 2005). Patients with schizophrenia and their closely-related biological relatives have impaired sensory inhibition, as measured with the P50 paradigm, and autopsy studies show that the expression of this receptor is diminished in hippocampus (and other regions) in the brains of patients with schizophrenia (Leonard et al., 2002). Moreover, there are genetically inbred strains of mice that differ from each other in the related paradigm with mice (i.e., measuring of the P20-N40 from extracellular electrodes placed in the hippocampus). Using these genetically inbred mouse strains, an inverse relationship was observed between the density of α_7 nicotinic acetylcholine receptors in the hippocampus and the magnitude of the impairment of sensory inhibition (Deutsch et al., 2005). These data strongly implicate the α_7 nicotinic acetylcholine receptor located in the hippocampus in the process of sensory inhibition; moreover, the data suggest that diminished expression or faulty transduction of the acetylcholine signal by the α_7 nicotinic acetylcholine receptors may cause problems with sensory gating of auditory stimuli. Not uncommonly, persons with mental retardation have difficulties with sustained attention and distractibility. Presumably, the α_7 nicotinic acetylcholine receptor is "recruited" into the normal process of improving signal to noise detection; a failure to do so may be experienced by the patient as "sensory flooding," which makes it difficult on a neurological basis to extract relevant information from an environment that is enriched in noises, sounds and smells.

α_7 Nicotinic Acetylcholine Receptor: Implicated in the Pathogenesis of Down's Syndrome

$A\beta_{1-42}$ is a pathogenetic 42 amino acid amyloidogenic split product of the amyloid precursor protein (APP), whose insoluble deposition leads to the formation of neuritic plaques, a histopathological hallmark of Alzheimer's disease and Down's syndrome. APP is a large integral membrane protein (i.e., membrane spanning protein with extracellular and intracellular domains), whose functions are uncertain, that is encoded on chromosome 21; the gene dosage effect related to the extra copy of chromosome 21 in persons with Down's syndrome favors its pathological degradation and accelerated formation of $A\beta_{1-42}$. At least some of the acute and long-term pathological consequences of the $A\beta_{1-42}$ peptide are mediated by the α_7 nicotinic acetylcholine receptor; there are data suggesting that insoluble $A\beta_{1-42}$ can form a stable high-affinity complex with the α_7 nicotinic acetylcholine receptor, serving as a nidus for the insoluble deposition of the pathogenetic split product in the β-pleated sheet configuration (Deutsch et al., 2003, 2005; Liu et al., 2001; Wang et al., 2000). The complexing of the $A\beta_{1-42}$ split product with the receptor could interfere with the transduction of the acetylcholine signal by the α_7 nicotinic acetylcholine receptor, leading to impairment of sensory inhibition and cognitive processes dependent on this fundamental attentional mechanism. Moreover, in vitro data suggest that the $A\beta_{1-42}/\alpha_7$ nicotinic acetylcholine receptor complex is neurotoxic to cells expressing the receptor on their surface. The cytotoxicity of the $A\beta_{1-42}$ peptide for transfected human neuroblastoma cells overexpressing the α_7 nicotinic acetylcholine receptor could be attenuated by nicotinic acetylcholine receptor agonists; $A\beta_{1-42}$ was relatively nontoxic to cultured control cells not expressing this transcript (Deutsch et al., 2003, 2005; Liu et al., 2001; Wang et al., 2000). Thus, with respect to Down's syndrome specifically, α_7 nicotinic acetylcholine receptor agonists may prevent cytotoxicity and the progression of Alzheimer-like pathological processes, in addition to correcting impairment of sensory inhibition and improvement of cognitive processes dependent on this fundamental mechanism of attention.

α_7 Nicotinic Acetylcholine Receptor Agonist Interventional Strategies for Improved Cognition

Strategies for medication development of an α_7 nicotinic acetylcholine receptor agonist must address the need for its chronic administration in mental retardation and the rapid agonist-induced desensitization of the receptor (Mastropaolo et al., 2004). Fortunately, positive allosteric modulatory sites on the α_7 nicotinic acetylcholine receptor exist and could be exploited to improve the efficiency of coupling between the binding of acetylcholine itself or a more selective α_7 agonist such as an anabaseine derivative or choline and channel opening, while preserving the receptor in a responsive, as opposed to a refractory (desensitized), state. Choline, the hydrolytic split product and precursor of acetylcholine, is a locally-derived (in the region of the α_7 nicotinic acetylcholine receptor synapse) highly selective agonist, and galantamine is a positive allosteric modulator of nicotinic acetylcholine receptors (Deutsch et al., 2005; Rosse and Deutsch, 2002). Thus, it may be possible to provide "proof of concept" for the effectiveness of an α_7 nicotinic acetylcholine receptor agonist interventional strategy for mental retardation in general, and Down's syndrome in particular.

Table 3. Novel Pharmacotherapeutic Considerations

GABA

1. $GABA_A$ Receptor Subtype Selective Benzodiazepine Ligands
   Agonists (Positive Allosteric Modulators)
   Inverse Agonists
   Antagonists
2. Neurosteroids
   Positive Allosteric Modulators
   Negative Allosteric Modulators

NMDA

1. Guanosine, Derivatives and Analogues (Promotion of Glial Reuptake of Glutamate)
2. Glycinergic Interventions
   D-Serine (Competitive Glycine Agonist)
   Sarcosine, Derivatives and Analogues (Glycine Reuptake Inhibitors)
3. Polyamines
4. Neurosteroids

α_7 Nicotinic Acetylcholine Receptor Agonist Interventions

1. Anabaseine Derivatives and Analogues
2. Choline (CDP-Choline)
3. Galantamine and Selective Positive Allosteric Modulators of α_7 Nicotinic Acetylcholine Receptors

Selective AMPA/KA Interventions

1. Antagonists
2. Agonists

CONCLUSIONS

The syndromes of mental retardation present enormous challenges to the practitioner providing psychopharmacological assessment and treatment (e.g., family practitioner, pediatrician, psychiatrist or neurologist). Because the etiology of the mental retardation is often unknown (as is the pathophysiology), medication approaches are selected empirically. For this reason, the psychopharmacologist is dependent on the close collaboration of others (e.g., parents, caregivers, nursing assistant, residential treatment facility managers, and teachers) for accurate information about disabling symptoms, especially their frequency of occurrence and setting in which they occur. There are major neurotransmitter systems in the brain that modulate excitatory and inhibitory tone, especially ligand-gated ion channel receptors such as the $GABA_A$, NMDA and α_7 nicotinic acetylcholine receptors. These ligand-gated ion channel receptors have multiple allosteric modulatory sites that may be targeted selectively in discrete regions of the brain to facilitate excitatory and inhibitory tone. Ideally, the manipulation of excitatory and inhibitory tone within discrete regions of the brain would improve symptoms in various domains of psychopathology associated with mental retardation, including cognitive, mood, and motor domains. The development of medications designed to modulate ligand-gated ion channel receptors with unique polypeptide receptor subunits, targeting the "combinatorial diversity" of these receptors offers much therapeutic promise. It is anticipated that clinical trials of novel medications based on these principles will be actively pursued. The goal is to promote social, cognitive and language development, stabilize mood, and eliminate socially-disabling motor symptoms (such as stereotypies). Effective interventions will reduce caregiver burden and improve the quality of life for persons with mental retardation.

ACKNOWLEDGMENTS

The authors would like to acknowledge Elana Orlofsky for providing much of the inspiration behind the ideas developed and expressed in this book chapter. We would also like to acknowledge the consistent support we have received from the Mental Illness Research, Education and Clinical Center (MIRECC) of the integrated network of Veterans Affairs Medical Centers in the mid-Atlantic Region (VISN5) under the direction of Dr. Alan S. Bellack.

REFERENCES

Albuquerque EX, Alkondon M, Pereira EFR, Castro NG, Schrattenholz A, Barbosa CTF, Bonfante-Cabarcas R, Aracava Y, Eisenberg HM, Maelicke A. Properties of neuronal nicotinic acetylcholine receptors: Pharmacological characterization and modulation of synaptic function. *J Pharmacol Exp Ther* 1997; 280: 1117-1136.

Alkondon M, Pereira EFR, Cortes WS, Maelicke A, Albuquerque EX. Choline is a selective agonist of α7 nicotinic acetylcholine receptors in the rat brain neurons. *Eur J Neuroscience* 1997; 9: 2734-2742.

Akbarian S, Sucher NJ, Bradley D, Tafazzoli A, Trinh D, Hetrick WP, Potkin SG, Sandman CA, Bunney WE Jr., Jones EG. Selective alterations in gene expression for NMDA receptor subunits in prefrontal cortex of schizophrenics. *Journal of Neuroscience* 1996; 16: 19-30.

Ascher P, Johnson JW. The NMDA receptor, its channel, and its modulation by glycine. In: Collingridge GL, Watkins JC, eds. *The NMDA Receptor (2nd Edition)*. Oxford-New York-Tokyo: Oxford University Press, 1994, pp 177-205.

Ben-Ari Y, Holmes GL. The multiple facets of γ-aminobutyric acid dysfunction in epilepsy: review. *Current Opinion in Neurology* 2005; 18(2): 141-145.

Bonhaus SW, Burge BC, McNamara JO. Biochemical evidence that glycine allosterically regulates an NMDA receptor-coupled ion channel. *Eur J Pharmacol* 1987; 142: 489-490.

Bowery NG, Smart TG. GABA and glycine as neurotransmitters: a brief history. *British Journal of Pharmacology* 2006; 147: S109-S119.

Broide RS, Leslie FM. The α7 nicotinic acetylcholine receptor in neuronal plasticity. *Molecular Neurobiology* 1999; 20: 1-16.

Costa E, Auta J, Grayson DR, Matsumoto K, Pappas GD, Zhang X, Guidotti A. $GABA_A$ receptors and benzodiazepines: a role for dendritic resident subunit mRNAs. *Neuropharmacology* 2002; 43: 925-937.

Deutsch SI, Mastropaolo J, Schwartz BL, Rosse RB, Morihisa JM. A "glutamatergic hypothesis" of schizophrenia: rationale for pharmacotherapy with glycine. *Clinical Neuropharmacology* 1989; 12: 1-13.

Deutsch SI, Deutsch LH, Weizman R. Nonketotic hyperglycinemia: a paradigm for the application of neuroscience to the understanding and treatment of a developmental disorder. In: Deutsch SI, Weizman A, Weizman R, eds. *Application of basic neuroscience to child psychiatry*. New York: Plenum Publishing Corporation, 1990, pp. 165-180.

Deutsch SI, Rosse RB, Mastropaolo J. Current status of NMDA antagonist interventions in the treatment of nonketotic hyperglycinemia. *Clinical Neuropharmacology* 1998; 21(2): 71-79.

Deutsch SI, Rosse RB, Schwartz BL, Mastropaolo J. A revised excitotoxic hypothesis of schizophrenia: therapeutic implications. *Clinical Neuropharmacology* 2001; 24: 43-49.

Deutsch SI, Rosse RB, Mastropaolo J, Chilton M. Progressive worsening of adaptive functions in Down syndrome may be mediated by the complexing of soluble Aβ peptides with the α_7 nicotinic acetylcholine receptor: therapeutic implications. *Clinical Neuropharmacology* 2003; 26(5): 277-283.

Deutsch SI, Rosse RB, Schwartz BL, Weizman A, Chilton M, Arnold DS, Mastropaolo J. Therapeutic implications of a selective $\alpha_7$nicotinic receptor abnormality in schizophrenia. *Israel Journal of Psychiatry* 2005; 42(1): 33-44.

Fagg GE. Phencyclidine and related drugs bind to the activated N-methyl-D-aspartate receptor-channel complex in rat brain membranes. *Neurosci Lett* 1987; 76: 221-227.

Fink JK, Jones SM, Sharp GB, Lange BM, Otterud B, Leppert M. Hereditary spastic paraplegia linked to chromosome 15q: analysis of candidate genes. *Neurology* 1996; 46: 835-836.

Foster AC, Wong EHF. The novel anticonvulsant MK-801 binds to the activated state of the N-methyl-D-aspartate receptor in rat brain. *Br J Pharmacol* 1987; 91: 403-409.

Freedman R, Coon H, Myles-Worsley M, Orr-Urtreger A, Olincy A, Davis A, Polymeropoulos M, Holik J, Hopkins J, Hoff M, et al. Linkage of a neurophysiological deficit in schizophrenia to a chromosome 15 locus. *Proc Natl Acad Sci USA* 1997; 94: 587-592.

Freedman R, Leonard S, Gault JM, Hopkins J, Cloninger CR, Kaufmann CA, Tsuang MT, Farone SV, Malaspina D, Svrakic DM, et al. Linkage disequilibrium for schizophrenia at the 15q13-14 locus of the α7-nicotinic acetylcholine receptor subunit gene (CHRNA7). *Am J Med Genet (Neuropsychiatr Genet)* 2001; 105: 20-22.

Holopainen IE, Metsahonkala E-L, Kokkonen H, Parkkola RK, Manner TE, Nagren K, Korpi ER. Decreased binding of [^{11}C]flumazenil in Angelman syndrome patients with $GABA_A$ receptor β_3 subunit deletions. *Ann Neurol* 2001; 49: 110-113.

Humphries C, Mortimer A, Hirsch S, de Belleroche J. NMDA receptor mRNA correlation with antemortem cognitive impairment in schizophrenia. *Neuroreport* 1996; 7(12): 2051-2055.

Hung Y-Y, Huang T-L. Lorazepam and diazepam rapidly relieve catatonic features in major depression. *Clinical Neuropharmacology* 2006; 29(3): 144-147.

Huntsman, MM, Tran BV, Potkin SG, Bunney WE Jr, Jones EG. Altered ratios of alternatively spliced long and short $gamma_2$ subunit mRNAs of the gamma-amino butyrate type A receptor in prefrontal cortex of schizophrenics. *Proceedings of the National Academy of Sciences USA* 1998; 95: 15066-71.

Jones-Davis DM, Song L, Gallagher MJ, Macdonald RL. Structural determinants of benzodiazepine allosteric regulation of $GABA_A$ receptor currents. *J Neurosci* 2005; 25(35): 8056-8065.

Knoll JH, Nicholls RD, Magenis RE, Graham JM Jr, Lalande M, Latt SA. Angelman and Prader-Willi syndromes share a common chromosome 15 deletion but differ in parental origin of the deletion. *Am J Med Genet* 1989; 32(2): 285-290.

Leonard S, Gault J, Hopkins J, Logel J, Vianzon R, Short M, Drebing C, Berger R, Venn D, Sirota P. et al., Association of promoter variants in the α7 nicotinic acetylcholine receptor subunit gene with an inhibitory deficit found in schizophrenia. *Arch Gen Psychiatry* 2002; 59: 1085-1096.

Lena C, Changeux J-P. Allosteric nicotinic receptors, human pathologies. *J Physiology* (Paris) 1998; 92: 63-74.

Lindstrom J. Nicotinic acetylcholine receptors in health and disease. *Molecular Neurobiology* 1997; 15: 193-222.

Liu Q-S, Kawai H, Berg DK. B-Amyloid peptide blocks the response of α7-containing nicotinic receptors on hippocampal neurons. *Proc Natl Acad Sci USA* 2001; 98: 4734-4739.

Long KD, Mastropaolo J, Rosse RB, Deutsch SI. Exogenously administered D-serine failed to potentiate the ability of MK-801 to antagonize electrically precipitated seizures in nonhandled control and stressed mice. *European Neuropsychopharmacology*, in the press.

Long KD, Mastropaolo J, Rosse RB, Manaye KF, Deutsch SI. Modulatory effects of D-serine and sarcosine on NMDA receptor-mediated neurotransmission are apparent after stress in the genetically inbred BALB/c mouse strain. *Brain Research Bulletin* 2006; 69: 626-630.

Maggouta F, Roberts SE, Dennis NR, Veltman MWM, Crolla JA. A supernumerary marker chromosome 15 tetrasomic for the Prader-Willi/Angelman syndrome critical region in a patient with a severe phenotype. *J Med Genet* 2003; 40:e84.

Mastropaolo J, Rosse RB, Deutsch SI. Anabasine, a selective nicotinic acetylcholine receptor agonist, antagonizes MK-801 –elicited mouse popping behavior, an animal model of schizophrenia. *Behavioural Brain Research* 2004; 153(2): 419-422.

Meguro M, Mitsuya K, Sui H, Shigenami K, Kugoh H, Nakao M, Oshimura M. Evidence for uniparental, paternal expression of the human $GABA_A$ receptor subunit genes, using microcell-mediated chromosome transfer. *Human Molecular Genetics* 1997; 6(12): 2127-2133.

Millan MJ. N-methyl-D-aspartate receptors as a target for improved antipsychotic agents: novel insights and clinical perspectives. *Psychopharmacology* 2005; 179: 30-53.

Nurmi EL, Dowd M, Tadevosyan-Leyfer O, Haines JL, Folstein SE, Sutcliffe JS. Exploratory subsetting of autism families based on savant skills improves evidence of genetic linkage to 15q11-q13. *J Am Acad Child & Adolescent Psychiatry* 2003; 42(7): 856-863.

Olsen RW. GABA. In: Davis KL, Charney D, Coyle JT, Nemeroff (eds). *Neuropsychopharmacology: The Fifth Generation of Progress*. Philadelphia: Lippincott Williams & Wilkins; 2002; pp 159-168.

Ranna M, Sinkkonen ST, Moykkynen T, Uusi-Oukari M, Korpi ER. Impact of ε and θ subunits on pharmacological properties of α3β1 $GABA_A$ receptors expressed in Xenopus oocytes. *BMC Pharmacology* (*http://www.biomedcentral.com/1471-2210/6/1*) 2006; 6:1.

Rosse RB, Schwartz BL, Zlotolow S, Banay-Schwartz M, Trinidad AC, Peace TD, Deutsch SI. Effects of a low-tryptophan diet as an adjuvant to conventional neuroleptic therapy in schizophrenia. *Clinical Neuropharmacology* 1992; 15(2): 129-141.

Rosse RB, Deutsch SI. Adjuvant galantamine administration improves negative symptoms in a patient with treatment-refractory schizophrenia. *Clinical Neuropharmacology* 2002; 25(5): 272-275.

Rudolph U, Crestani F, Benke D, Brunig I, Benson JA, Fritschy J-M, Martin JR, Bluethmann H, Mohler H. Benzodiazepine actions mediated by specific γ-aminobutyric $acid_A$ receptor subtypes. *Nature* 1999; 401: 796-800.

Schwartz BL, Hashtroudi S, Herting RL, Handerson H, Deutsch SI. Glycine prodrug facilitates memory retrieval in humans. *Neurology* 1991; 41: 1341-1343.

Schwartz BL, Hashtroudi S, Herting RL, Deutsch SI. The effects of milacemide on item and source memory. *Clinical Neuropharmacology* 1992; 15(2): 114-119.

Schwartz BL, Hashtroudi S, Herting RL, Schwartz P, Deutsch SI. D-Cycloserine enhances implicit memory in Alzheimer patients. *Neurology* 1996; 46: 420-424.

Sugiura C, Ogura K, Ueno M, Toyoshima M, Oka A. High-dose ethosuximide for epilepsy in Angelman syndrome: implications of $GABA_A$ receptor subunit. *Neurology* 2001; 57: 1518-1519.

Sutcliffe JS, Nurmi EL. Genetics of childhood disorders: XLVII. Autism, Part 6: Duplication and inherited susceptibility of chromosome 15q11-q13 genes in autism. *J Am Acad Child & Adolescent Psychiatry* 2003; 42(2): 253-256.

Ungaro P, Christian SL, Fantes JA, Mutirangura A, Black S, Reynolds J, Malcolm S, Dobyns WB, Ledbetter DH. Molecular characterization of four cases of intrachromosomal triplication of 15q11-q14. *J Med Genet* 2001; 38: 26-34.

Wang HY, Lee DHS, D'Andrea MR, et al. β-$Amyloid_{1\text{-}42}$ binds to α7 nicotinic acetylcholine receptor with high affinity. *J Biol Chem* 2000; 275: 5626-5632.

Weiland S, Bertrand D, Leonard S. Neuronal nicotinic acetylcholine receptors: from the gene to the disease. *Behavioural Brain Res* 2000; 113: 43-56.

Wisden W, Stephens DN. Towards better benzodiazepines. *Nature* 1999; 401: 751-752.

In: Focus on Mental Retardation Research
Editor: Marina I. Carson, pp. 29-47
ISBN: 978-1-60021-647-3

Chapter 2

SEARCHING FOR CAUSE: CONSIDERATION OF THE CO-OCCURRENCE OF MENTAL RETARDATION AND OTHER CONDITIONS

Laura L. Jelliffe-Pawlowski
California Department of Health Services, Genetic Disease Branch, Richmond, CA.

ABSTRACT

Mental retardation (MR) often occurs with other developmental disabilities (e.g. autism, cerebral palsy, epilepsy), yet historically, epidemiologic study of MR and of these other conditions has given little attention to examining co-occurrence as a strategy for revealing causal pathways and mechanisms. Co-occurrence of MR and other conditions may suggest alternative causes compared to the occurrence of MR in isolation. Failure to consider such co-occurrence may mask important within group differences and in turn, slow epidemiologic progress. Findings characterizing the prevalence of MR occurring in isolation and with these other conditions are presented as is our data and that of other investigators revealing differing patterns of epidemiologic risk when co-occurrence with other disabilities is considered. Data revealing potential causal pathways and mechanisms when other co-occurrence groupings such as co-occurrence with birth defects are discussed as are advances pointing to gene-environment interactions wherein better understanding and consideration of co-occurrence and phenotype have advanced identification of genetic causes of MR – including fragile X syndrome. Strategies for increasing commitment to the consideration of co-occurrence in epidemiologic studies of MR are outlined.

Mental retardation (MR), autism, cerebral palsy, and epilepsy often co-occur yet epidemiologic studies focused on MR or these other developmental disabilities rarely consider co-occurrence[1]. Ignoring such co-occurrence may, in part, be due to the complexity

[1] Zero of the four studies identified in PubMed (2006) as published January 2006 through June 2006 for "mental retard* and epidemiolog*" considered co-occurrence with autism, epilepsy and/or cerebral palsy in their analyses (Collier & Hogue, 2006; Trasande, Schechter, Haynes, & Landrigan, 2006; Chen, Schwarz,

related to disentangling and reporting on co-occurrence and the associated need for the use of larger samples if co-occurrence groupings are considered. While this tendency and the reasons behind it are perhaps understandable from a conceptual standpoint, evidence suggests that studies focused on MR and these other developmental disabilities that report risks but do not consider co-occurrence may slow epidemiologic progress by confusing whether findings apply to isolated versus co-occurring conditions. Data suggests that studies considering co-occurrence may be more likely to reveal potential causal pathways and mechanisms due to better characterization of patterns that appear to differ as a function of diagnostic group membership.

Co-occurrence of MR, Autism, Cerebral Palsy and Epilepsy

Although prevalence estimates differ, in general, if ranked by the number of children in a population with MR, autism, cerebral palsy and/or epilepsy, the number of children with MR would likely be the highest (approximately 5 to 15 per 1000) (Katusic et al., 1996; Murphy, Yeargin-Allsopp, Decoufle, & Drews, 1995; Fernell, 1998; Jelliffe-Pawlowski, Shaw, Nelson, & Harris, 2005; van Schrojenstein Lantman-de Valk HM et al., 2006), while the number of children with autism would likely be the lowest (approximately 0.4 to 4.0 per 1000) (Kirby, Canino, Brewster, & Pavin, 1995; Fombonne, Mazaubrun, Cans, & Grandjean, 1997; Bertrand et al., 2001; Croen, Grether, Hoogstrate, & Selvin, 2002). The prevalence of epilepsy is consistently found to be between 3 and 10 per 1000 (Kirby et al., 1995; Steffenburg, Hagberg, Viggedal, & Kyllerman, 1995; Larsson et al., 2006; Sun et al., 2006) and the prevalence of cerebral palsy between 2 and 4 per 1000 (Boyle et al., 1996; Nordmark, Hagglund, & Lagergren, 2001; Bhasin, Brocksen, Avchen, & Van Naarden, 2006).

More than half of all children with autism or cerebral palsy have MR (Fombonne et al., 1997; Boyle, 1997; Nordmark et al., 2001) and about a third of all children with epilepsy (Steffenburg et al., 1995). Studies reporting co-occurrence within MR groupings show that among children with mild MR (Intelligence Quotient (IQ) ≥ 50 and < 70) about 15% have autism (Fernell, 1996), about 6% have cerebral palsy (Murphy et al., 1995; Fernell, 1996), and about 10 to 15% have epilepsy (Murphy et al., 1995; Steffenburg et al., 1995; Christianson et al., 2002). Data suggests that approximately one fifth to one third of all children with mild MR have at least one of these other disabilities (Murphy et al., 1995;

Radcliffe, & Rogan, 2006; van Schrojenstein Lantman-de Valk HM et al., 2006). Of these studies, only Collier and Hogue (2006) reported rates of co-occurrence (they did not consider co-occurrence in any analyses). Two of the nine studies published during this time period found in a search for "autis* and epidemiolog*" considered co-occurrence with MR (Lord et al., 2006; Badawi et al., 2006). Seven did not consider co-occurrence (Gillberg, Cederlund, Lamberg, & Zeijlon, 2006; Lord et al., 2006; Wier, Yoshida, Odouli, Grether, & Croen, 2006; Palmer, Blanchard, Stein, Mandell, & Miller, 2006; Badawi et al., 2006; Centers for Disease Control and Prevention (CDC), 2006; Centers for Disease Control and Prevention (CDC), 2006; Koishi et al., 2006; Harrison, O'Hare, Campbell, Adamson, & McNeillage, 2006; Guerini et al., 2006). Two of the five studies published during this period and found in a search for "cerebral palsy and epidemiolog*" considered co-occurrence with MR (Dolk, Parkes, & Hill, 2006; Tang-Wai, Webster, & Shevell, 2006), three did not (Serdaroglu, Cansu, Ozkan, & Tezcan, 2006; Glinianaia et al., 2006; Collier et al., 2006). Four of the nine studies published during the first 6-months of 2006 and found in a PubMed search for "epilepsy and epidemiolog*" considered co-occurrence with MR (Hoie, Mykletun, Waaler, Skeidsvoll, & Sommerfelt, 2006; Devlin, Shepherd, Crawford, & Morrison, 2006; Larsson & Eeg-Olofsson, 2006; Oka et al., 2006), the other

Fernell, 1996; Jelliffe-Pawlowski, Shaw, Nelson, & Harris, 2003a; 2003b). Among children with severe MR (IQ < 50), more than 20% have autism (Steffenburg et al., 1995; Jelliffe-Pawlowski et al., 2005), 25 to 50% have cerebral palsy (Murphy et al., 1995; Steffenburg et al., 1995; Christianson et al., 2002; Jelliffe-Pawlowski et al., 2005), and 25 to 50% have epilepsy (Murphy et al., 1995; Steffenburg et al., 1995; Christianson et al., 2002; Jelliffe-Pawlowski et al., 2005). In our study examining risks for severe MR occurring in isolation or with these other disabilities among a sample of California children between the ages of seven and nine years of age, we found that 73.0% of children diagnosed with severe MR had autism, cerebral palsy or epilepsy (Jelliffe-Pawlowski et al., 2005). In their study of the administrative prevalence of MR among 10-year olds in Atlanta, Murphy and colleagues (1995) found that 45% of children with severe MR had one or more of these other disabilities. Figure 1 depicts the relative prevalence and co-occurrence of MR, autism, cerebral palsy and epilepsy based on the findings cited.

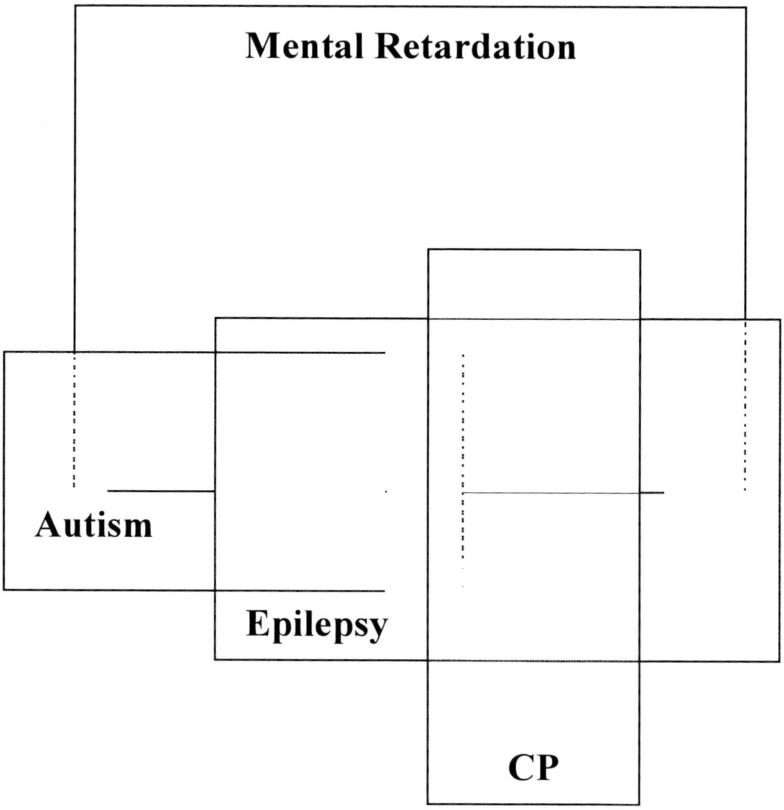

Figure 1. Relative prevalence and co-occurrence of target developmental disabilities.

five did not (Whitehead et al., 2006; Sun, Vestergaard, Pedersen, Christensen, & Olsen, 2006; Reading, Haynes, & Beach, 2006; Archer & Bunby, 2006; Ehrenstein et al., 2006).

CONSIDERING CO-OCCURRENCE AND RISK

The importance of considering co-occurrence is evident in epidemiologic studies examining risk factors for MR, autism, cerebral palsy, and epilepsy. Although studies considering co-occurrence are few, those that have considered co-occurrence have consistently found a different constellation of risk factors associated with isolated occurrence of the target disability (MR, autism, cerebral palsy, or epilepsy occurring without any other of these disabilities) than for co-occurrence groupings (Drews, Yeargin-Allsopp, Decoufle, & Murphy, 1995; Hultman, Sparen, & Cnattingius, 2002; Jelliffe-Pawlowski et al., 2005). With respect to findings on MR, among an Atlanta cohort of children, Drews and colleagues (1995) found that maternal education < 12 years or 12 years (compared to > 12 years), black race (compared to white), third or later birth order (compared to first), and male sex (compared to female) were significant risk factors for isolated mild MR (among this cohort those considered to have isolated MR did not have CP, epilepsy, hearing impairment, visual impairment, or any structural, chromosomal, or metabolic birth defect affecting the central nervous system). None of these factors were significant predictors of mild MR co-occurring with the other target conditions. Black race and < 12-years completed maternal education were found to be significant predictors of isolated severe MR. Male sex and maternal age ≥ 30 (compared to 20 –29 years) were significant predictors of severe MR co-occurring with the other target conditions.

Like the Atlanta researchers, in our study of California children we also noted a different grouping of risk factors for isolated compared to co-occurring severe MR (Jelliffe-Pawlowski et al., 2005). Preterm birth (< 37 completed weeks of gestation), low-birth-weight (LBW)(< 2500 grams), male sex, < 12-years completed years maternal education, and Mother born in Mexico (compared to the U.S.) were found to be significant predictors of isolated severe MR (where for this study, isolated was defined as not co-occurring with autism or another pervasive developmental disorder (PDD), cerebral palsy, or epilepsy). Only preterm birth and LBW were found to be significant predictors of severe MR co-occurring with cerebral palsy or epilepsy. Significant predictors of severe MR co-occurring with autism or a PDD included male sex, black race/ethnicity, and asian race/ethnicity. Table 1 includes some of the specific findings for the Atlanta and California studies.

Consideration of co-occurrence is of equal importance in studies of other developmental disabilities where research also suggests that consideration of co-occurrence has the potential to significantly alter the constellation of risk factors identified. For example, a recent epidemiologic study of autism in Sweden by Hultman and colleagues (2002) found that exclusion of children with MR or epilepsy from their analysis greatly changed their findings with respect to perinatal risk factors for autism. Prior to exclusions these researchers found numerous risk factors for autism including (among others) Apgar score > 6 (compared to < 6), Cesarean section (compared to vaginal birth), maternal age ≥ 35 (compared to 20 – 34), parity ≥ 4 (compared to 2-3), and preterm birth. Although some predictors like Apgar score remained predictive after exclusions, several factors including maternal age ≥ 35, parity ≥ 4, and preterm birth were not predictive after exclusions. Some factors like the presence of congenital malformations ("yes" compared to "no") were not predictive before but were found to be predictive after exclusions.

Table 1. Findings for selected factors: Atlanta and California studies considering co-occurrence with other developmental disabilities when evaluating risk factors for mental retardation (MR) (significant predictors are in bold)

	LBW[a]	Preterm Birth[b]	Economic Status[c]	Maternal Age[d]	Maternal Education[e]	Race[f]	Sex[g]
Drews et al., 1995							
Isolated Mild MR[h]							
Odds Ratio	n/a	n/a	1.5	0.8	**4.9**	**2.1**	**1.7**
(95% CI)			(0.9, 2.5)	(0.5, 1.2)	**(2.7, 8.7)**	**(1.4, 3.1)**	**(1.2, 2.3)**
Co-Occurring Mild MR[h]							
Odds Ratio	n/a	n/a	2.2	0.5	2.7	0.9	1.5
(95% CI			(0.9, 5.6)	(0.2, 1.3)	(1.0, 6.9)	(0.4, 1.7)	(0.9, 2.7)
Isolated Severe MR[h]							
Odds Ratio	n/a	n/a	0.7	1.3	**4.9**	**3.8**	1.5
(95% CI)			(0.3, 1.8)	(0.5, 3.3)	**(1.2, 19.9)**	**(1.5, 9.5)**	(0.8, 2.9)
Co-Occurring Severe MR[h]							
Odds Ratio	n/a	n/a	1.3	**2.0**	1.2	1.0	**1.7**
(95% CI			(0.6, 2.8)	**(1.1, 3.7)**	(0.6, 2.5)	(0.5, 1.7)	**(1.1, 2.8)**
Jelliffe-Pawlowski et al., 2005							
Isolated Severe MR[i]							
Relative Risk	**3.9**	**2.7**	n/a	0.8	**2.8**	2.0	**2.0**
(95% CI)	**(2.1, 7.4)**	**(1.4, 5.3)**		(0.3, 2.0)[j]	**(1.2, 6.2)**	(0.8, 5.4)	**(1.2, 3.3)**
Severe MR co-occurring with Cerebral Palsy							
Relative Risk	**9.9**	**4.3**	n/a	n/a	1.3	n/a	0.9
(95% CI)	**(4.1, 23.8)**	**(1.3, 13.6)**			(0.5, 3.8)		(0.4, 2.0)
Severe MR co-occurring with Epilepsy							
Relative Risk	**3.5**	**2.7**	n/a	1.2	1.6	3.2	0.9
(95% CI)	**(1.5, 7.9)**	**(1.2, 6.1)**		(0.4, 3.3)[j]	(0.7, 3.7)	(1.0, 10.3)	(0.5, 1.7)
Severe MR co-occurring with Autism or a PDD							
Relative Risk	2.3	n/a	n/a	2.1	0.7	**5.1**	**3.4**
(95% CI)	(0.8, 6.5)			(0.8, 5.6)[j]	(0.3, 1.5)	**(1.7, 15.5)**	**(1.5, 7.9)**

n/a Did not consider variable in analyses due to study design or cell frequency < 4.

[a] Birth weight < 2500 grams compared to ≥ 2500.

[b] < 37 completed weeks gestation compared to ≥ 37.

[c] "Low" economic status compared to "high" economic status based on census groupings.

[d] ≥ 30 years of age compared to 20 – 29.

[e] < 12 years completed education compared to > 12-years.

[f] Black race compared to white.

[g] Male gender compared to female.

[h] Defined as MR occurring with (co-occurring) or without (isolated) cerebral palsy, epilepsy, hearing impairment, visual impairment or structural, chromosomal, or metabolic birth defect affecting the central nervous system.

[I] Defined as MR occurring without autism or another Pervasive Developmental Disorder, cerebral palsy, or epilepsy.

[j] ≥ 35 years of age compared to 25 – 29.

Co-occurrence and Birth Defects

Few epidemiologic studies have examined the co-occurrence of MR and birth defects despite the potential of such investigations to reveal alternative cause(s) compared to when birth defects or MR occur in isolation. Studying co-occurrence with birth defects has the potential to narrow the timeframe of insult to the prenatal period for many children with MR and to specific prenatal time periods for children with MR and specific birth defects.

As Kirby (2002) points out, the reasons few studies consider the co-occurrence of MR and birth defects despite the promise of doing so is likely due to the fact that there a few surveillance programs for developmental disabilities for which there is also similar population-based tracking of birth defects. When both exist, he argues, it is then possible to link to birth certificates and in turn, calculate prevalence ratios.

Our study (Jelliffe-Pawlowski et al., 2003a; 2003b) and that of Decoufle and colleagues (Decoufle, Boyle, Paulozzi, & Lary, 2001) are examples of studies where population-based monitoring or population based service provision of both MR and birth defects was present and where linkage to birth certificates was used to calculate prevalence ratios. Our study examined the rate of isolated and co-occurring MR diagnosed by age 7 among a cohort of infants born in 1992 or 1993 in nonmilitary hospitals in the California Central Valley for whom information about the presence or absence of birth defects was recorded in the first year of life (n = 119,556). Decoufle and colleagues examined the rate of isolated and co-occurring MR diagnosed by age 3 to 10 years among a cohort of children born in 5 Georgia counties between 1981 and 1991 for whom information about the presence or absence of birth defects was recorded (n = 358,051).

Although our study (Jelliffe-Pawlowski et al., 2003a; 2003b) defined "Isolated MR" as MR occurring without Cerebral Palsy, epilepsy, autism or another Pervasive Developmental Disorder (PDD) and Decoufle and colleagues (Decoufle et al., 2001) defined "Isolated MR" as MR occurring without cerebral palsy, epilepsy, hearing impairment, visual impairment or structural, chromosomal, or metabolic birth defect affecting the central nervous system, the findings were consistent for both studies with respect to observing a significantly increased risk for MR among children born with any birth defect. As is evident in Table 2, both studies found that compared to children born without any birth defect, children born with one or more defect were at more than a four-fold increased risk for isolated mild-MR (prevalence ratios 4.7 and 28.7), at more than a twenty-fold increased risk for isolated severe-MR (prevalence ratios 21.8 and 90.3), at more than a five-fold increased risk for mild-MR co-occurring with another developmental disability (prevalence ratios 5.8 and 8.6), and at more than an eleven-fold increased risk for severe-MR co-occurring with another developmental disability (prevalence ratios 11.3 and 18.2). We suspect that our substantially higher observed risks compared to that of Decoufle and colleagues for the isolated groupings was due to their exclusion of children with structural, chromosomal or metabolic birth defects affecting the central nervous system from their isolated MR groupings. As such, their reported findings could be interpreted as observed risk for isolated MR among children with birth defects not including those related to the CNS.

Table 2. Prevalence of isolated and co-occurring mental retardation (MR) among children with one or more birth defect compared to children without any birth defect: Atlanta and California studies

	Isolated Mild-MR[a]		Mild-MR/ Other Disability		Isolated Severe-MR[a]		Severe-MR/ Other Disability	
	n/1000	Ratio[b] (95% CI)	n/1000	Ratio[b] (95% CI)	n/1000	Ratio[b] (95% CI)	n/1000	Ratio[b] (95% CI)
Decoufle et al., 2001								
No Birth Defect *(n = 348,909)*	3.7	Ref.	0.7	Ref.	0.7	Ref.	1.1	Ref.
One or More Birth Defect *(n=9,142)*	17.3	4.7 (4.0, 5.5)	3.8	5.8 (4.1, 8.3)	15.8	21.8 (17.8, 26.7)	12.1	11.3 (9.1, 13.9)
Jelliffe-Pawlowski et al., 2003								
No Birth Defect *(n = 117,219)*	1.1	Ref.	0.8	Ref.	0.3	Ref.	1.1	Ref.
One or More Birth Defect *(n=2337)*	32.5	28.7 (21.6, 38.0)	6.8	8.6 (5.1, 14.7)	30.8	90.3 (61.3, 132.9)	19.7	18.2 (13.0, 5.5)

[a] For the Atlanta sample (Decoufle et al., 2001) isolated MR is defined as MR occurring without cerebral palsy, epilepsy, hearing impairment, visual impairment or structural, chromosomal, or metabolic birth defect affecting the central nervous system. For the California sample (Jelliffe-Pawlowski et al., 2003) isolated MR is defined as MR occurring without autism or another Pervasive Developmental Disorder, cerebral palsy, or epilepsy.

[b] Prevalence of MR among individuals with one or more birth defect divided by the prevalence of MR among individuals without a major birth defect.

Tables 3 and 4 report some of the defect-specific findings from the California study which arguably, are more telling than the higher-order "defect" versus "no-defect" findings included in Table 2. These findings show that across category of defect, children with a defect are at increased risk for MR compared to children without any defect but also point to defect specific degrees of risk. As was expected, the findings show that those at the highest risk are children born with Down syndrome or another autosomal or sex chromosomal abnormality (prevalence ratios $\geq$ 35.0 across MR groupings) followed by Spina Bifida or other nervous system defect (prevalence ratios $\geq$ 24.2 across MR groupings). What was unexpected was the degree of risk posed by defects peripherally involved with the central nervous system or without a clear central nervous system link. For example, children with a musculoskeletal defect were at between a 29.7 and 69.0-fold increased risk for MR across groupings and children with a defect of the integument were at a between 24.2 and 70.9-fold increased risk for MR across groupings. Also illustrative were the percentages of children with birth defects diagnosed by 1-year who were later diagnosed with MR. For example, among this sample, 44.4% of children with an autosomal abnormality, and 19.2% of children with a sex chromosomal abnormality were diagnosed with MR by age 7. 14.1% of children with a musculoskeletal defect and 16.1% of children with a defect of the integument were diagnosed with MR by age 7. It is important to note that these findings were for children with these specified defects who did not have other known defects affecting the central nervous system.

Table 3. Prevalence of mild-MR among children with specific types of non-chromosomal birth defects[a] compared to the prevalence of mild-MR among children without any birth defect: California study (Jelliffe-Pawlowski et al., 2003a)

	Isolated Mild-MR			Mild-MR/ Other Disability		
	n/1000[b]	Ratio[c]	95% CI	n/1000[b]	Ratio[c]	95% CI
No Birth Defect *(n = 117219)*	1.1	Ref.		0.8	Ref.	
Spina Bifida *(n=29)*	103.4	91.2	29.0, 286.3	–	–	–
Other Nervous System *(n=232)*	34.5	30.4	14.9, 62.0	30.2	38.0	17.6, 82.0
Other Structural Defects:[d]						
Eye *(n=204)*	24.5	21.6	8.8, 52.8	24.5	30.9	12.6, 76.0
Ear, Face and Neck *(n=170)*	–	–	–	11.8	14.8	3.7, 60.2
Bulbus Cordis/ Cardiac Septal Closure *(n=163)*	6.1	5.4	0.8, 38.7	18.4	23.2	7.3, 73.2
Other Heart *(n=56)*	17.9	15.7	2.2, 112.6	71.4	90.0	33.1, 244.9
Circulatory System *(n=29)*	34.5	30.4	4.2, 217.3	34.5	43.5	6.1, 311.8
Respiratory System *(n=45)*	–	–	–	44.4	56.0	13.8,227.3
Cleft Palate and Cleft Lip *(n=105)*	28.6	25.2	8.0, 79.1	9.5	12.0	1.7, 86.1
Other Upper Alimentary Tract *(n=203)*	14.8	13.0	4.1, 40.9	4.9	6.2	0.9, 44.5
Other Digestive System *(n=98)*	10.2	9.0	1.3, 64.3	–	–	–
Genital Organs *(n=244)*	4.1	3.6	0.5, 25.8	–	–	–
Urinary System *(n=112)*	–	–	–	–	–	–
Musculoskeletal *(n=85)*	47.1	41.5	15.3, 112.1	23.5	29.7	7.3, 120.9
Limbs *(n=153)*	19.6	17.3	5.5, 54.3	–	–	–
Other Musculoskeletal *(n=90)*	11.1	9.8	1.4, 70.0	11.1	14.0	2.0, 100.5
Integument *(n=87)*	80.5	70.9	33.2, 151.6	23.0	29.0	7.1, 117.6
Other and Unspecified Anomalies *(n=13)*	–	–	–	–	–	–

[a] Excludes all children with Down syndrome or other identified chromosomal defects.
[b] Prevalence by birth defect group (survivors to 1-year, non-military births).
[c] Prevalence of severe-MR among individuals with specific birth defect divided by the prevalence of severe-MR among individuals without a major birth defect.
[d] Excludes children with nervous system defects, not mutually exclusive of other structural birth defects.

Table 4. Prevalence of severe-MR among children with specific non-chromosomal birth defects[a] compared to the prevalence of severe-MR among children without any birth defect: California study (Jelliffe-Pawlowski et al., 2003a; 2003b)

	Isolated Severe-MR			Severe-MR/ Other Disability		
	n/1000[b]	Ratio[c]	95% CI	n/1000[b]	Ratio[c]	95% CI
No Birth Defect *(n = 117219)*	0.3	Ref.		1.1	Ref.	
Spina Bifida *(n=29)*	–	–	–	34.5	31.8	4.4, 227.7
Other Nervous System *(n=232)*	30.2	88.4	39.6, 197.4	94.8	87.5	55.7, 137.6
Other Structural Defects:[d]						
Eye *(n=204)*	24.5	71.8	28.3, 182.0	73.5	67.9	39.7, 115.9
Ear, Face and Neck *(n=170)*	5.9	17.2	2.4, 125.4	5.9	5.4	0.8, 38.8
Bulbus Cordis/ Cardiac Septal Closure *(n=163)*	6.1	18.0	2.5, 130.8	12.3	11.3	2.8, 45.8
Other Heart *(n=56)*	–	–	–	35.7	33.0	8.2, 133.2
Circulatory System *(n=29)*	34.5	101.1	13.9, 735.0	69.0	63.7	15.7, 257.3
Respiratory System *(n=45)*	–	–	–	–	–	–
Cleft Palate and Cleft Lip *(n=105)*	9.5	27.9	3.8, 203.0	–	–	–
Other Upper Alimentary Tract *(n=203)*	9.9	28.9	7.0, 119.5	–	–	–
Other Digestive System *(n=98)*	–	–	–	20.4	18.8	4.7, 76.1
Genital Organs *(n=244)*	4.1	12.0	1.7, 87.4	12.3	11.3	3.6, 35.7
Urinary System *(n=112)*	–	–	–	–	–	–
Musculoskeletal *(n=85)*	23.5	69.0	16.7, 285.3	23.5	21.7	5.4, 87.8
Limbs *(n=153)*	13.1	38.3	9.3, 158.5	13.1	12.1	3.0, 48.8
Other Musculoskeletal *(n=90)*	11.1	32.6	4.5, 236.8	11.1	10.3	1.4, 73.4
Integument *(n=87)*	11.5	33.7	4.6, 245.0	23.0	21.2	5.2, 85.8
Other and Unspecified Anomalies *(n=13)*	76.9	225.4	31.0, 1639.7	–	–	–

[a] Excludes all children with Down syndrome or other identified chromosomal defects.

[b] Prevalence by birth defect group (survivors to 1-year, non-military births).

[c] Prevalence of severe-MR among individuals with specific birth defect divided by the prevalence of severe-MR among individuals without a major birth defect.

[d] Excludes children with nervous system defects, not mutually exclusive of other structural birth defects.

Table 5. Sample findings: Study by Weir and colleagues (2006) examining the rate of congenital anomalies among children with autism spectrum disorders (ASDs) and comparison children

	ASD (n = 417)		Comparison (n = 2067)		Adjusted Odds Ratio[a]	95% CI
	n =	%	n =	%		
One or more congenital anomaly	45	10.8	128	6.2	1.7	1.1, 2.4
Isolated anomaly	32	71.1[b]	99	77.3[b]	1.5	1.0, 2.3
Multiple anomalies	11	24.4[b]	24	18.8[b]	2.1	1.0, 4.5
Syndrome	2	4.4[b]	5	3.9[b]	–	–
Congenital anomaly by organ system:[c]						
Central nervous system	5	1.2	9	0.4	1.8	0.5, 5.7
Eye/ear/face/neck	2	0.5	1	0.1	–	–
Heart	13	3.1	39	1.9	1.5	0.7, 2.8
Respiratory System	4	1	10	0.5	–	–
Gastrointestinal	8	1.9	8	0.4	5.1	1.8, 14.1
Genito-urinary	12	2.9	33	1.6	1.6	0.8, 3.2
Musculoskeletal	13	3.1	32	1.6	1.8	0.9, 3.5
Integument	1	0.2	3	0.2	–	–

[a] Adjusted for plurality, birth order, gestational age, maternal age, maternal ethnicity, and maternal education.

[b] Reported percentage is percent of "one or more congenital anomaly" group.

[c] Each child represented once per organ system category.

Results do not consider the presence or absence of mental retardation in the ASD or comparison population.

As was suggested in the initial report of these findings (Jelliffe-Pawlowski et al., 2003a; 2003b), the observed relationships suggest a pathogenetic link between MR and birth defects. Such a relationship might be causal whereas a birth defect causes MR, may be temporal where a deleterious event or teratogen caused the birth defect and MR, may be genetic where a gene or genes caused both the birth defect and MR, or may be characterized by multiple causal pathways and mechanisms. Whatever the pathway or mechanism, understanding such relationships has the potential to further progress towards finding and addressing other causes of MR in addition to suggesting new in-roads for early intervention.

A recent study by Weir and colleagues (Wier et al., 2006) is illustrative with respect to demonstrating the importance of considering the co-occurrence of MR and other disabilities in studies of associations with other factors like birth defects and the risks associated with not considering such co-occurrence.

In their case-comparison study these researchers examined whether major congenital structural anomalies occurred more frequently among children diagnosed with an autism spectrum disorder (ASD) compared to children without an ASD diagnosis. They reported that children with an ASD were at a significantly increased risk for having had one or more birth defect and reported other defect-specific associations (adjusted odds ratios 1.7 – 5.1). These researchers did not consider MR status in their groupings or in their analyses and as such, given the substantial co-occurrence of MR and ASD's (e.g. 50% or more of those with autism have MR) (Fombonne et al., 1997; Boyle, 1997; Nordmark et al., 2001) and our findings and those of Decoufle and colleagues demonstrating a potent relationship between birth defects and MR, the reported relationship between birth defects and ASD's presented by these researchers is an uncertain one. As is demonstrated in Table 5 (adapted from Wier et al., 2006), these researchers report that 10.8% of children with an ASD had at least one or more congenital anomaly compared to 6.2% of comparison children. The associated significant adjusted odds ratio was 1.7 with a 95% confidence interval of 1.1 and 2.4. Comparison of results in Table 5 with those in Tables 3 and 4 show that many if not all findings reported by Wier may have been driven, at least in part, by MR status. Given the relatively small differences in percentages of ASD children with an anomaly compared to children without, it appears highly likely that children with an ASD and no MR may have demonstrated a different or non-existent relationship to birth defects compared to children with an ASD and MR. Consideration of MR status in this study would have avoided such speculation and perhaps, may have pointed to ASD specific patterns.

CO-OCCURRENCE AND THE DISCOVERY OF FRAGILE-X

Perhaps the most telling historical example of how consideration of co-occurrence in epidemiologic studies of MR can yield potent answers with respect to identifying cause is exemplified by the discovery of the fragile X mental retardation (FMR1) gene in 1991 (Verkerk et al., 1991; Yu et al., 1991; Oberle et al., 1991) and the subsequent sequencing of the FMR1 gene in 1993 (Snow et al., 1993). Sequencing of the FMR1 gene allowed for measurement of trinucleotide repeat patterns which has in turn been used for diagnosis of fragile X syndrome – the second most common cause of mental impairment after Down syndrome (Rousseau, Rouillard, Morel, Khandjian, & Morgan, 1995).

Discovery of the FMR1 gene and its subsequent sequencing grew out of the earlier discovery of a chromosome believed to be a marker for X-linked MR in some males (Lubs, 1969) and the identification of a connection between this X-linked pattern of MR and macro-orchidism (enlarged testes) (Escalante, Grunspun, & Frota-Pessoa, 1971; Cantu et al., 1976), low-set long ears, asymmetric facial features, prominent jaw (Lubs, Watson, Breg, & Lujan, 1984), and unusual behavior characterized by increased anxiety and disorganized hyperactivity (Mattei, Mattei, Aumeras, Auger, & Giraud, 1981).

Today, diagnosis of fragile X is accomplished via the analysis of unstable expanded repeats of the cytosine-cytosine-guanine (CCG) trinucleotide on the FMR1 gene. In the normal population the repeat is generally between 6 and 54 with an average of 30 whereas among those with the FMR1 premutation have between 43 and 200 repeats and those with full mutation have > 200 repeats (Fu et al., 1991). Repeat number is closely related to the capacity for producing the FMR1 protein – FMRP. This protein exists in nearly all neurons and appears to be a key component for learning and behavioral regulation (Devys, Lutz, Rouyer, Bellocq, & Mandel, 1993; Kooy et al., 1996). Individuals with the premutation generally have normal cognitive functioning but present with a number of other physical and behavioral characteristics including fragile X-associated tremor/ataxia syndrome (FXTAS) among men with the permutation (Hagerman & Hagerman, 2004b; Hagerman & Hagerman, 2004a). Males with the full mutation generally have fragile X syndrome which generally includes MR and the originally identified constellation of characteristics (e.g. low-set long ears, asymmetric facial features, prominent jaw, and unusual behavior). Males with fragile X syndrome also present with a host of other characteristics and diagnosis which include (among others), double jointed thumbs (53%), heart murmur or click (18%), seizures/epilepsy diagnosis (22%), and/or an autism diagnosis (20%) (Merenstein et al., 1996; Hagerman, 1996). Table 6 includes a list of medical problems encountered in ≥ 10% of males with the fragile X full-mutation (adapted from Hagerman, 1996).

Females also present with the permutation and the full mutation but are in general, more mildly affected (Hagerman, 1997). Ovarian failure occurs in about one third of women with the permutation (Hagerman et al., 2004b; Hagerman et al., 2004a) and fragile X syndrome occurs in about half of the females with the full mutation (compared to nearly all of males with the full mutation) (Maes, Fryns, Ghesquiere, & Borghgraef, 2000).

Identification of the FMR1 gene, its sequencing, and subsequent clarification of permutation and full mutation phenotypes has led to genetic counseling and earlier identification of affected individuals (Pandey, Phadke, & Mittal, 2004; 2002) which in turn, has led to progress with respect to prevention and early intervention. With respect to prevention, collection of family history data particularly with respect to developmental delay, ovarian failure and FXTAS has been a useful first step towards genetic testing of the FMR1 gene in potentially affected individuals and/or in couples considering pregnancy and/or prenatal testing (Wattendorf & Muenke, 2005). Whereas early intervention is concerned, data suggests that early intervention aimed at behavioral regulation can be of particular benefit to those with fragile X syndrome (Sobesky, 1996; Scharfenaker et al., 1996; Hills Epstein, Riley, & Sobesky, 2002) as are efforts aimed at addressing potentially serious co-morbid medical conditions (e.g. failure to thrive, mitral valve prolapse) (Bailey, Jr., 2004).

Table 6. Medical problems encountered in ≥ 10% of males with fragile X syndrome (adapted from Hagerman, 1996)

Problem	%
Apnea	10
Failure to thrive	15
Hernia	15
Motor tics	19
Autism	20
Orthopedic problems	21
Seizures	22
Myopia or hyperopia	22
Sinusitis	23
Persistent vomiting	31
Mitral valve prolapse	35
Strabismus	36
ADHD	80
Otitis media	85

LESSONS LEARNED: FRAGILE X

The pathway to the discovery of the genetic defect responsible for fragile X syndrome and progress resulting from its discovery exemplifies both the common co-occurrence between MR and other developmental disabilities as well as the utility of considering co-occurrence in epidemiologic studies of MR.

Initial discovery of the gene resulted from the description of a well-defined phenotype (Lubs, 1969; Escalante et al., 1971; Cantu et al., 1976; Lubs et al., 1984). Once discovered and sequenced, identification of the gene led to a much broader understanding of other phenotypes associated with the FRA1 premutation and full-mutation (Mattei et al., 1981; Hagerman, 1997; Hagerman et al., 2004b; Hagerman et al., 2004a), and as such, an etiologic explanation for a myriad of conditions – including MR, for thousands of families and individuals where no cause would have been identified. It is now known for example, that about 5.0% of children with MR and about 7 – 8% of those with autism have fragile X syndrome (see van Kernebeek and colleagues for review of diagnostic investigations of MR and fragile X (van Karnebeek, Jansweijer, Leenders, Offringa, & Hennekam, 2005) and Muhle and colleagues for a review of autism related genetic findings (Muhle, Trentacoste, & Rapin, 2004)). Findings with respect to the co-occurrence of MR, autism and fragile X syndrome has led to the argument that all children with MR and/or autism of unknown cause be screened for the FRA1 premutation and full mutation (Hagerman, 2007).

INCREASING COMMITMENT TO THE CONSIDERATION OF CO-OCCURRENCE

In general, epidemiologic studies focused on MR rely, at least in part, on clinical records related to provision of health care to children with MR (e.g. Murphy et al., 1995; Kirby et al., 1995; Rantakallio & von Wendt, 1986; and Jelliffe-Pawlowski et al., 2005). As such, increasing commitment to the consideration of co-occurrence in study design and analyses likely needs to include increased commitment to consideration of co-occurrence by clinicians – particularly with respect to child-specific diagnosis. It can certainly be argued that when a child-specific diagnostic evaluation is lacking, any epidemiologic research where that child is included as a member of the study group will also be lacking it its ability to appropriately categorize, include, and exclude children. It is also of great importance to recognize that with a through diagnostic evaluation comes the potential for increased and/or better focused treatment options, increased support system building for affected children and their families, and, where an etiology is identified, greater potential for understanding reoccurrence risks and short and long-term prognoses.

The research reviewed in the present chapter suggests that not only should children with MR be systematically and consistently evaluated for co-occurrence with autism, cerebral palsy, epilepsy, but they should also be evaluated for having any known birth defects including chromosomal abnormalities. It is also likely that children with MR, their families, the clinicians and service providers treating them, and in turn, the researchers who are utilizing the data related to these children would benefit greatly from consistently applied diagnostic evaluations that include detailed dysmorphologic evaluations (beyond identification of known birth defects), metabolic evaluations for identification of conditions like phenylketonuria, and neurologic evaluations that including EEG and neuroimaging in all instances where symptoms suggest an etiology that is potentially neurologic (e.g. where seizures are present or there is abnormal brain size).

In their rigorous review of 219 diagnostic studies of MR published over a thirty year period (all of whom met strict inclusion criteria), Van karnebeek and colleagues (van Karnebeek et al., 2005) found that the greatest diagnostic yield (percent of individuals with MR for whom a diagnostic evaluation yielded an additional diagnosis possibly related to cause) was for dysmorphologic evaluations (39-81%) and neurological evaluations (42.9%) followed by cytogenetic evaluations (9.5%), fragile X screening (5.4%), and subtelomeric evaluations (4.4%). At a minimum, these results argue that all children with MR of unknown cause should receive dysmorphologic evaluations and complete genetic testing and that children with MR and seizures or other significant neurological symptoms (e.g. abnormal brain size), should receive detailed neurological evaluations. It seems likely that if such practices were consistently applied and data related to their findings was consistently recorded, that consideration of co-occurrence in downstream epidemiologic studies might result.

Of course, even with better and more consistent clinical evaluations of children with MR, increased consideration of co-occurrence will require a considerably increased commitment to such a pursuit by investigators and their peers and, to a larger extent, an increased commitment to these principles by healthcare, governmental and funding agencies. As was pointed out by Kirby in his 2002 paper (in which he also argued for the importance of considering co-occurrence in studies of developmental disabilities), appropriate consideration of co-occurrence of developmental disabilities and birth defects requires population-based surveillance of both. Such surveillance is rare – likely due to associated costs but also, increasingly, due to privacy concerns. Kirby rightly points out that it is up to the public health surveillance community to demonstrate that epidemiologic progress with respect to MR and other developmental disabilities requires simultaneous surveillance of often co-occurring conditions and that such progress outweighs privacy concerns.

Regardless of whether significant progress is made with respect to consistent and through diagnoses of children with MR or with respect to better surveillance systems (changes that perhaps would provide the greatest push towards increasing consideration of co-occurrence), investigators can certainly increase their own consideration of co-occurrence. Suggestions for doing so include: 1) Remaining up to date on epidemiologic research for commonly co-occurring conditions; 2) Increasing within study efforts to collect complete clinical profiles; 3) Increased commitment to co-occurrence considerations in analyses; 4) Report of co-occurrence statistics regardless of whether or not there is complete ascertainment of specific clinical subgroups or enough data to allow for analyses by specific subgroup. There are, of course, many other strategies investigators might adopt to increase their own consideration of co-occurrence in epidemiologic studies of MR and other developmental disabilities. Implementation only requires that they be convinced of the importance and utility of doing so.

REFERENCES

Delayed diagnosis of fragile x syndrome - United States, 1990-1999 (2002). *Morbidity and Mortality Weekly Report, 51,* 740-742.

PubMed (2006). National Library of Medicine [On-line]. Available: www.ncbi.nlm.gov.

Archer, J. & Bunby, R. (2006). Epilepsy in Indigenous and non-Indigenous people in Far North Queensland. *The Medical Journal of Australia, 184,* 607-610.

Badawi, N., Dixon, G., Felix, J. F., Keogh, J. M., Petterson, B., Stanley, F. J. et al. (2006). Autism following a history of newborn encephalopathy: more than a coincidence? *Developmental Medicine and Child Neurology, 48,* 85-89.

Bailey, D. B., Jr. (2004). Newborn screening for fragile X syndrome. *Mental Retardation and Developmental Disabilities Research Reviews, 10,* 3-10.

Bertrand, J., Mars, A., Boyle, C., Bove, F., Yeargin-Allsopp, M., & Decoufle, P. (2001). Prevalence of autism in a United States population: the Brick Township, New Jersey, investigation. *Pediatrics, 108,* 1155-1161.

Bhasin, T. K., Brocksen, S., Avchen, R. N., & Van Naarden, B. K. (2006). Prevalence of four developmental disabilities among children aged 8 years--Metropolitan Atlanta Developmental Disabilities Surveillance Program, 1996 and 2000. *Morbidity and Mortality Weekly Report, 55,* 1-9.

Boyle, C. A. (1997). Surveillance of development disabilities with an emphasis on special studies. *Reproductive Toxicology, 11,* 271-274.

Boyle, C. A., Yeargin-Allsopp, M., Doernberg, N. S., Holmgreen, P., Murphy, C. C., & Schendel, D. E. (1996). Prevalence of selected developmental disabilities in children 3-10 years of age: The metropolitan Atlanta developmental disabilities surveillance program, 1991. *Morbidity and Mortality Weekly Report, 45,* 1-14.

Cantu, J. M., Scaglia, H. E., Medina, M., Gonzalez-Diddi, M., Morato, T., Moreno, M. E. et al. (1976). Inherited congenital normofunctional testicular hyperplasia and mental deficiency. *Human Genetics, 33,* 23-33.

Centers for Disease Control and Prevention (CDC) (2006). Mental health in the United States: parental report of diagnosed autism in children aged 4-17 years--United States, 2003-2004. *Morbidity and Mortality Weekly Report, 55,* 481-486.

Chen, A., Schwarz, D., Radcliffe, J., & Rogan, W. J. (2006). Maternal IQ, child IQ, behavior, and achievement in urban 5-7 year olds. *Pediatric Research, 59,* 471-477.

Christianson, A. L., Zwane, M. E., Manga, P., Rosen, E., Venter, A., Downs, D. et al. (2002). Children with intellectual disability in rural South Africa: prevalence and associated disability. *Journal of Intellectual Disability Research, 46,* 179-186.

Collier, S. A. & Hogue, C. J. (2006). Modifiable risk factors for low birth weight and their effect on cerebral palsy and mental retardation. *Maternal and Child Health Journal, 11,* 65-71.

Croen, L. A., Grether, J. K., Hoogstrate, J., & Selvin, S. (2002). The changing prevalence of autism in California. *Journal of Autism and Developmental Disorders, 32,* 207-215.

Decoufle, P., Boyle, C. A., Paulozzi, L. J., & Lary, J. M. (2001). Increased risk for developmental disabilities in children who have major birth defects: a population-based study. *Pediatrics, 108,* 728-733.

Devlin, L. A., Shepherd, C. H., Crawford, H., & Morrison, P. J. (2006). Tuberous sclerosis complex: clinical features, diagnosis, and prevalence within Northern Ireland. *Developmental Medicine and Child Neurology, 48,* 495-499.

Devys, D., Lutz, Y., Rouyer, N., Bellocq, J. P., & Mandel, J. L. (1993). The FMR-1 protein is cytoplasmic, most abundant in neurons and appears normal in carriers of a fragile X premutation. *Nature Genetics, 4,* 335-340.

Dolk, H., Parkes, J., & Hill, N. (2006). Trends in the prevalence of cerebral palsy in Northern Ireland, 1981-1997. *Developmental Medicine and Child Neurology, 48,* 406-412.

Drews, C. D., Yeargin-Allsopp, M., Decoufle, P., & Murphy, C. C. (1995). Variation in the Influence of selected sociodemographic risk factors for mental retardation. *American Journal of Public Health, 85,* 329-334.

Ehrenstein, V., Sorensen, H. T., Pedersen, L., Larsen, H., Holsteen, V., & Rothman, K. J. (2006). Apgar score and hospitalization for epilepsy in childhood: a registry-based cohort study. *BMC Public Health, 6,* 23.

Escalante, J. A., Grunspun, H., & Frota-Pessoa, O. (1971). Severe sex-linked mental retardation. *Journal of Medical Genetics, 19,* 137-140.

Fernell, E. (1996). Mild mental retardation in schoolchildren in a Swedish suburban municipality: prevalence and diagnostic aspects. *Acta Paediatrica, 85,* 584-588.

Fernell, E. (1998). Aetiological factors and prevalence of severe mental retardation in children in a Swedish municipality; the possible role of consanguinity. *Developmental Medicine and Child Neurology, 40,* 608-611.

Fombonne, E., Mazaubrun, C. D., Cans, C., & Grandjean, H. (1997). Autism and associated medical disorders in a French epidemiological survey. *Journal of the American Academy of Child and Adolescent Psychiatry, 36,* 1516-1569.

Fu, Y. H., Kuhl, D. P., Pizzuti, A., Pieretti, M., Sutcliffe, J. S., Richards, S. et al. (1991). Variation of the CGG repeat at the fragile X site results in genetic instability: resolution of the Sherman paradox. *Cell, 67,* 1047-1058.

Gillberg, C., Cederlund, M., Lamberg, K., & Zeijlon, L. (2006). Brief report: "the autism epidemic". The registered prevalence of autism in a Swedish urban area. *Journal of Autism and Developmental Disorders, 36,* 429-435.

Glinianaia, S. V., Jarvis, S., Topp, M., Guillem, P., Platt, M. J., Pearce, M. S. et al. (2006). Intrauterine growth and cerebral palsy in twins: a European multicenter study. *Twin Research and Human Genetics, 9,* 460-466.

Guerini, F. R., Manca, S., Sotgiu, S., Tremolada, S., Zanzottera, M., Agliardi, C. et al. (2006). A family based linkage analysis of HLA and 5-HTTLPR gene polymorphisms in Sardinian children with autism spectrum disorder. *Human Immunology, 67,* 108-117.

Hagerman, P. J. & Hagerman, R. J. (2004a). Correction: The fragile-X premutation: a maturing perspective. *American Journal of Human Genetics, 75,* 352.

Hagerman, P. J. & Hagerman, R. J. (2004b). The fragile-X premutation: a maturing perspective. *American Journal of Human Genetics, 74,* 805-816.

Hagerman, R. J. (1996). Physical and behavioural phenotype. In R.J.Hagerman & A. Cronister (Eds.), *Fragile-X syndrome: diagnosis, treatment and research* (pp. 3-87). Baltimore: The Johns Hopkins University Press.

Hagerman, R. J. (1997). Fragile X syndrome. Molecular and clinical insights and treatment issues. *The Western Journal of Medicine, 166,* 129-137.

Hagerman, R. J. (2007). How do the behaviors seen in persons with fragile X relate to those seen in autism. The National Fragile X Foundation [On-line]. Available: www.fragilex.org/html/autism.htm

Harrison, M. J., O'Hare, A. E., Campbell, H., Adamson, A., & McNeillage, J. (2006). Prevalence of autistic spectrum disorders in Lothian, Scotland: an estimate using the "capture-recapture" technique. *Archives of Disease in Childhood, 91,* 16-19.

Hills Epstein, J. L., Riley, K., & Sobesky, W. E. (2002). The treatment of emotional and behavioural problems. In R.J.Hagerman & P. J. Hagerman (Eds.), *Fragile X syndrome* (pp. 339-362). Baltimore: The Johns Hopkins University Press.

Hoie, B., Mykletun, A., Waaler, P. E., Skeidsvoll, H., & Sommerfelt, K. (2006). Executive functions and seizure-related factors in children with epilepsy in Western Norway. *Developmental Medicine and Child Neurology, 48,* 519-525.

Hultman, C. M., Sparen, P., & Cnattingius, S. (2002). Perinatal risk factors for infantile autism. *Epidemiology, 13,* 417-423.

Jelliffe-Pawlowski, L. L., Shaw, G. M., Nelson, V., & Harris, J. A. (2003). Risk of mental retardation among children born with birth defects. *Archives of Pediatrics & Adolescent Medicine, 157,* 545-550.

Jelliffe-Pawlowski, L. L., Shaw, G. M., Nelson, V., & Harris, J. A. (2003). Correction: Risk of mental retardation among children born with birth defects. *Archives of Pediatrics & Adolescent Medicine, 158,* 332.

Jelliffe-Pawlowski, L. L., Shaw, G. M., Nelson, V., & Harris, J. A. (2005). Risks for severe mental retardation occurring in isolation and with other developmental disabilities. *American Journal of Medical Genetics Part A, 136,* 152-157.

Katusic, S. K., Colligan, R. C., Beard, C. M., O'Fallon, W. M., Bergstralh, E. J., Jacobsen, S. J. et al. (1996). Mental retardation in a birth cohort, 1976-1980, Rochester, Minnesota. *American Journal of Mental Retardation, 100,* 335-344.

Kirby, R. S. (2002). Co-occurrence of developmental disabilities with birth defects. *Mental Retardation and Developmental Disabilities, 8,* 182-187.

Kirby, R. S., Canino, C. U., Brewster, M. A., & Pavin, M. (1995). Early childhood surveillance of developmental disorders by birth defects surveillance system: methods, prevalence comparisons, and mortality patterns. *Developmental and Behavioral Pediatrics, 16,* 318-326.

Koishi, S., Yamamoto, K., Matsumoto, H., Koishi, S., Enseki, Y., Oya, A. et al. (2006). Serotonin transporter gene promoter polymorphism and autism: a family-based genetic association study in Japanese population. *Brain Development, 28,* 257-260.

Kooy, R. F., D'Hooge, R., Reyniers, E., Bakker, C. E., Nagels, G., De Boulle, K. et al. (1996). Transgenic mouse model for the fragile X syndrome. *American Journal of Medical Genetics, 64,* 241-245.

Larsson, K. & Eeg-Olofsson, O. (2006). A population based study of epilepsy in children from a Swedish county. *European Journal of Paediatric Neurology, 10,* 107-113.

Lord, C., Risi, S., DiLavore, P. S., Shulman, C., Thurm, A., & Pickles, A. (2006). Autism from 2 to 9 years of age. *Archives of General Psychiatry, 63,* 694-701.

Lubs, H. A. (1969). A marker X chromosome. *American Journal of Human Genetics, 21,* 231-244.

Lubs, H. A., Watson, M., Breg, R., & Lujan, E. (1984). Restudy of the original marker X family. *American Journal of Medical Genetics, 17,* 133-144.

Maes, B., Fryns, J. P., Ghesquiere, P., & Borghgraef, M. (2000). Phenotypic checklist to screen for fragile X syndrome in people with mental retardation. *Mental Retardation, 38,* 207-215.

Mattei, J. F., Mattei, M. G., Aumeras, C., Auger, M., & Giraud, F. (1981). X-linked mental retardation with the fragile X. A study of 15 families. *Human Genetics, 59,* 281-289.

Merenstein, S. A., Sobesky, W. E., Taylor, A. K., Riddle, J. E., Tran, H. X., & Hagerman, R. J. (1996). Molecular-clinical correlations in males with an expanded FMR1 mutation. *American Journal of Medical Genetics, 64,* 388-394.

Muhle, R., Trentacoste, S. V., & Rapin, I. (2004). The genetics of autism. *Pediatrics, 113,* e472-e486.

Murphy, C. C., Yeargin-Allsopp, M., Decoufle, P., & Drews, C. D. (1995). The administrative prevalence of mental retardation in 10-year-old children in metropolitan Atlanta, 1985-1987. *American Journal of Public Health, 85,* 319-323.

Nordmark, E., Hagglund, G., & Lagergren, J. (2001). Cerebral palsy in southern Sweden I. Prevalence and clinical features. *Acta Paediatrica, 90,* 1271-1276.

Oberle, I., Rousseau, F., Heitz, D., Kretz, C., Devys, D., Hanauer, A. et al. (1991). Instability of a 550-base pair DNA segment and abnormal methylation in fragile X syndrome. *Science, 252,* 1097-1102.

Oka, E., Ohtsuka, Y., Yoshinaga, H., Murakami, N., Kobayashi, K., & Ogino, T. (2006). Prevalence of childhood epilepsy and distribution of epileptic syndromes: a population-based survey in Okayama, Japan. *Epilepsia, 47,* 626-630.

Palmer, R. F., Blanchard, S., Stein, Z., Mandell, D., & Miller, C. (2006). Environmental mercury release, special education rates, and autism disorder: an ecological study of Texas. *Health & Place, 12,* 203-209.

Pandey, U. B., Phadke, S. R., & Mittal, B. (2004). Molecular diagnosis and genetic counseling for fragile X mental retardation. *Neurology India, 52,* 36-42.

Rantakallio, P. & von Wendt, L. (1986). Mental retardation and subnormality in a birth cohort of 12,000 children in Northern Finland. *American Journal of Mental Deficiency, 90,* 380-387.

Reading, R., Haynes, R., & Beach, R. (2006). Deprivation and incidence of epilepsy in children. *Seizure, 15,* 190-193.

Rousseau, F., Rouillard, P., Morel, M. L., Khandjian, E. W., & Morgan, K. (1995). Prevalence of carriers of premutation-size alleles of the FMRI gene--and implications for the population genetics of the fragile X syndrome. *American Journal of Human Genetics, 57,* 1006-1018.

Scharfenaker, S., O'Conner, R., Stackhouse, T., Braden, M., Hickman, L., & Gray, K. (1996). An integrated approach to intervention. In R.J.Haggerman & A. Cronister (Eds.), *Fragile X syndrome: diagnosis, treatment, and research* (pp. 349-411). Baltimore: The Johns Hopkins University Press.

Serdaroglu, A., Cansu, A., Ozkan, S., & Tezcan, S. (2006). Prevalence of cerebral palsy in Turkish children between the ages of 2 and 16 years. *Developmental Medicine and Child Neurology, 48,* 413-416.

Snow, K., Doud, L. K., Hagerman, R., Pergolizzi, R. G., Erster, S. H., & Thibodeau, S. N. (1993). Analysis of a CGG sequence at the FMR-1 locus in fragile X families and in the general population. *American Journal of Human Genetics, 53,* 1217-1228.

Sobesky, W. E. (1996). The treatment of emotional and behavioral problems. In R.J.Hagerman & A. Cronister (Eds.), *Fragile X syndrome: diagnosis, treatment, and research* (pp. 332-348). Baltimore: The Johns Hopkins University Press.

Steffenburg, U., Hagberg, G., Viggedal, G., & Kyllerman, M. (1995). Active epilepsy in mentally retarded children. I. Prevalence and additional neuro-impairments. *Acta Paediatrica, 84,* 1147-1152.

Sun, Y., Vestergaard, M., Pedersen, C. B., Christensen, J., & Olsen, J. (2006). Apgar scores and long-term risk of epilepsy. *Epidemiology, 17,* 296-301.

Tang-Wai, R., Webster, R. I., & Shevell, M. I. (2006). A clinical and etiologic profile of spastic diplegia. *Pediatric Neurology, 34,* 212-218.

Trasande, L., Schechter, C. B., Haynes, K. A., & Landrigan, P. J. (2006). Mental retardation and prenatal methylmercury toxicity. *American Journal of Industrial Medicine, 49,* 153-158.

van Karnebeek, C. D., Jansweijer, M. C., Leenders, A. G., Offringa, M., & Hennekam, R. C. (2005). Diagnostic investigations in individuals with mental retardation: a systematic literature review of their usefulness. *European Journal of Human Genetics, 13,* 6-25.

van Schrojenstein Lantman-de Valk HM, Wullink, M., van den, A. M., Heurn-Nijsten, E. W., Metsemakers, J. F., & Dinant, G. J. (2006). The prevalence of intellectual disability in Limburg, the Netherlands. *Journal of Intellectual Disability Research, 50,* 61-68.

Verkerk, A. J., Pieretti, M., Sutcliffe, J. S., Fu, Y. H., Kuhl, D. P., Pizzuti, A. et al. (1991). Identification of a gene (FMR-1) containing a CGG repeat coincident with a breakpoint cluster region exhibiting length variation in fragile X syndrome. *Cell, 65,* 905-914.

Wattendorf, D. J. & Muenke, M. (2005). Diagnosis and management of fragile X syndrome. *American Family Physician, 72,* 111-113.

Whitehead, E., Dodds, L., Joseph, K. S., Gordon, K. E., Wood, E., Allen, A. C. et al. (2006). Relation of pregnancy and neonatal factors to subsequent development of childhood epilepsy: a population-based cohort study. *Pediatrics, 117,* 1298-1306.

Wier, M. L., Yoshida, C. K., Odouli, R., Grether, J. K., & Croen, L. A. (2006). Congenital anomalies associated with autism spectrum disorders. *Developmental Medicine and Child Neurology, 48,* 500-507.

Yu, S., Pritchard, M., Kremer, E., Lynch, M., Nancarrow, J., Baker, E. et al. (1991). Fragile X genotype characterized by an unstable region of DNA. *Science, 252,* 1179-1181.

In: Focus on Mental Retardation Research
Editor: Marina I. Carson, pp. 49-76
ISBN: 978-1-60021-647-3

Chapter 3

GENOMIC IMPRINTING AND MENTAL RETARDATION: ANGELMAN AND PRADER-WILLI SYNDROMES

A. K. Thomson[1], E. J. Glasson[1,2] and A. H. Bittles[1,3]
[1]School of Exercise, Biomedical and Health Sciences, Edith Cowan University, Western Australia
[2]School of Population Health, University of Western Australia
[3]Centre for Comparative Genomics, Murdoch University, Western Australia

ABSTRACT

Genomic imprinting is a prime example of epigenetic change leading to variable gene expression. Angelman syndrome (AS) and Prader-Willi syndrome (PWS) are disorders associated with failure of genomic imprinting at the same locus but exhibiting different clinical presentations. The loss of maternal imprint at the chr15q11-q13 locus leads to AS, while lack of paternal patterning results in PWS. Individuals with AS exhibit severe to profound mental retardation (MR) in combination with epilepsy, abnormal EEG patterns, movement disorders, inappropriate smiling or laughter, a happy demeanor, minimal speech, and an easily excitable personality. People with PWS typically present with mild MR, behavior problems, hypotonia, hyperphagia and obesity, and delayed or incomplete sexual development.

Comprehensive clinical and laboratory studies have been undertaken into the medical profiles and life experiences of patient cohorts with AS (n = 34) and PWS (n = 46) in Western Australia. The members of the study cohorts ranged in age from 0.9 years to 48.3 years, with a mean age of 21.2 years. A majority of the group were mentally retarded with only four of the 80 individuals exhibiting IQ levels greater than 84 points which is regarded as the borderline for MR. The results clearly indicated age-specific comorbidities, and specialist care needs were associated with both AS and PWS.

Although the oldest member of the cohorts was under 50 years, it seems probable that people with these disorders will live to significantly older ages in the future. In turn, this will require greater attention to the health, residential and social requirements both of individuals with AS and PWS, and their family carers. Further investigations into the specific etiologies, underlying genetic mechanisms and age- and condition-dependent morbidities that are associated with each syndrome should enable the provision of better care regimes.

Genomic Imprinting: An Example of Epigenetic Modification

Studies conducted in both developing and developed countries have indicated that 22-58% cases of mental retardation (MR) result from congenital or genetic defects [1-4]. While the most common such disorder is Down syndrome, there are also a number of conditions which are produced by epigenetic mechanisms, with Angelman syndrome and Prader-Willi syndrome well characterized examples of the phenomenon.

Epigenetic modification literally refers to changes that occur 'outside' the gene, and although the nucleotide sequence is unchanged the pattern of gene expression is altered [5-8]. A number of epigenetic processes have been identified, including chromatin modifications, at least four different patterns of X-chromosome dosage compensation [9], RNA silencing [10,11], and stochastic interactions. However, to date the most thoroughly studied epigenetic process is genomic imprinting, which involves the differential expression of alleles in both the developing zygote and the mature organism dependent on the parent of origin [12,13]. An online catalogue of imprinted genes which have been identified to date is available at http://igc.otago.ac.nz/home.html

Effects of Imprinting

Genomic imprinting has been described as an elegant solution to the conflict of interest that is presumed to exist in reproduction between the paternal and maternal genomes [14]. The role of the paternal genome is to increase the fitness of progeny, irrespective of maternal cost. In contrast, the objective of the maternal genome is to ensure that offspring fitness is maintained while preventing the over-use of maternal resources [15]. The profile of paternally and maternally imprinted genes found throughout the genome is thus likely to represent a compromise between these two factors, especially as many genes that are known to be imprinted influence pre- or postnatal growth [12,15-17]. Generally, paternally-expressed genes promote embryonic and fetal growth while maternal expression tends to reduce the levels of maternal resources available to the developing offspring [18]. It has also been suggested that the paternal and maternal genomes complement each other, thus preventing the possibility of asexual reproduction. Under this scenario, gene dosage reduction may be another function of the imprinting process [19,20]. Yet another theory suggests that imprinting is a means of silencing parasitic retrotransposons which could otherwise damage the host genome or interfere with normal transcription processes [21].

The importance of the contribution of both parents to normal development is demonstrated by the production of modified mouse embryos. Androgenetic embryos, containing paternal genes only, exhibit reduced fetal growth but a very high growth rate of extra-embryonic tissues (placenta and amnion). Conversely, gynogenetic embryos that have only a maternal gene contribution show normal fetal growth but greatly reduced extra-embryonic growth. In neither case is the embryo viable to term [12,19].

Gene expression from a single allele may be confined to specific tissues [22,23], or the effect may be specific to particular stages of development [22,24]. In general, the imprint takes the form of hypermethylation of cytosine-rich regions at specific loci on the chromosome to be silenced, thus limiting expression to the allele from the other parent.

Failure of Imprinting

Loss of effective imprinting can be due to one or more of three possible situations:

1. Deletion or loss of a portion of either the paternal or maternal chromosome which includes the relevant gene or genes;
2. Uniparental disomy (UPD), i.e., the inheritance of two chromosomes from one parent and none from the other. The effect of UPD on gene expression can vary greatly, depending on the normal role of each allele at that locus. UPD has usually no influence on the expression of genes that are not imprinted, although there are cases where a recessive allele is 'unmasked' due to the presence of two copies from one parent, instead of one from each parent [22]. Any imprinted gene which is hypermethylated on both alleles due to UPD will not be expressed, i.e., nullisomy, but it would be expected that imprinted genes which are non-methylated on both alleles will both be expressed, leading to diploid overdose [25]. In cases where there is phenotypic variation between patients with either a deletion or UPD, it is possible that the difference results from a gene dosage effect;
3. Deletion or substitution within the imprinting centre (IC) that leads to failure to reset the correct imprint during gamete production [26-28]. The maternally-inherited chromosomes in males must be reset with the paternal pattern before being passed on to offspring, and the reverse occurs in females. This process is governed by a *cis*-acting element, the IC, which is responsible for setting the correct configuration [22].

Angelman Syndrome and Prader-Willi Syndrome: The Disease Phenotypes

Angelman Syndrome

Angelman syndrome (AS) was first described in 1965, with the phenotype characterized as a combination of severe mental retardation or learning disability, seizures with a specific electroencephalogram (EEG) pattern, absent speech, jerky ataxic movements, and a generally happy sociable disposition [29]. The first laboratory diagnostic tests for AS were introduced in 1987 [30] and further studies into the syndrome resulted in the publication in 1995 of consensus diagnostic criteria, with an update in 2006 [31,32]. Techniques are now available for the identification of all the known genetic defects associated with the disorder [33,34].

All people diagnosed with AS exhibit symptoms of mental retardation (MR), usually within the severe to profound range with measured IQ levels and adaptive behavior assessments of <40 [30,35-37]. The disease phenotype includes epilepsy and seizures, an abnormal EEG pattern, movement disorder, inappropriate smiling or laughter, a happy demeanor, minimal speech, and an easily excitable personality [32,36,38-40]. A significant proportion of AS individuals also suffer from night-time settling problems, and reduced need for sleep or abnormal sleep/wake cycles [27,30,36,39,41]. Another common feature of the disorder is hypertonicity of the limbs, generally found in conjunction with truncal hypotonia. This can lead to joint contractures and a stooping posture as individuals become older, and may have a detrimental effect on their mobility [27,30,35]. Autistic behaviors are also commonly reported in AS patients [42], as are a fascination for water, reflective surfaces, and balloons [30,32,36,37,39], although the significance of these preoccupations is unknown.

Prader-Willi Syndrome

Prader-Willi syndrome (PWS) was first described by Prader, Labhart and Willi in 1956 [43], and is characterized by mental retardation or learning disabilities, behavior problems, hyperphagia and obesity, and delayed or incomplete sexual development [43,44]. The genetic basis of PWS was identified in the 1980s, with consensus diagnostic criteria published by Holm *et al.* in 1993 [45]. More recent research has produced additional information on the wide range of phenotypic variation found in people diagnosed with PWS. For this reason it has been suggested that the existing clinical criteria may need to be revised, and that specific features of PWS should be differentially weighted as diagnostic tools at different stages of life [46]. For example, during infancy, hypotonia and feeding difficulties are the most reliable indicators of the syndrome [47], and it is only after the first two or three years of life that hyperphagia, global developmental delay and obesity become prominent diagnostic traits [46,48].

Mild to moderate MR is present in a majority of cases with associated learning difficulties, although 27-40% of people with PWS function at low average or borderline intelligence levels and 7-19% of individuals are severely mentally retarded [27,44,49-51]. Specific facial features, which include doliocephaly (a relatively long head), almond-shaped eyes, small bifrontal diameter, a thin upper lip in a small mouth, and/or down-turned corners of the mouth, are often present [45,47]. Osteopoenia or osteoporosis occur in a majority of PWS adults [52]. Although hypogonadism is a common finding in PWS and generally results in infertility, there have been two reports of children born to women with genetically-confirmed PWS [53,54].

Most PWS patients are reduced in stature when compared to other family members and growth hormone (GH) treatment has been used to increase the growth velocities of PWS children with partial success [55-57]. This therapy can also minimize the development of the characteristic facies associated with the syndrome, improve respiratory and muscle function, alleviate sleep problems, and reduce depressive symptoms, especially in older children and adults [58-61]. Among the secondary morbidities associated with the obesity usually found in people with PWS are limited mobility, cardio-pulmonary disease, leg ulcers, and diabetes mellitus, any or all of which can lead to increased hospitalization and earlier death [52,62,63]. Daytime sleepiness and skin-picking are reported in many PWS cases [51,64-69], and people with PWS are prone to the development of psychoses and other mental disturbances in adulthood, especially those with UPD or moderate to severe MR [65,70-74].

The Role of Imprinting Failure in the Development of Angelman Syndrome and Prader-Willi Syndrome

Angelman and Prader-Willi syndromes both result from failure of imprinting or gene mutation within the same region of chr15q11-q13. In general, if the affected chromosome is maternally derived then AS occurs, whereas PWS results if the paternal chromosome is altered. Usually there is no obvious gender bias in either syndrome, although more boys than girls are identified with PWS before adolescence, possibly due to obvious male hypogonadism as opposed to the more subtle phenotypic changes in prepubescent girls [75].

The most frequent origin of AS is deletion of a section of the maternally-derived chr15q11-q13 region [26,37]. An imprinting centre (IC) is located in chr15q11-q13 [76], and mutations in this region are found in 2-10% of individuals with AS [26,77-79]. A similar proportion of AS patients have a paternal UPD15 [26,77,78], and point mutations within the *UBE3A* gene on the maternal chromosome at 15q11-q13 have been reported in 4-14% of people with AS [26,37,77,78]. However, as many as 15% of the patients clinically diagnosed with AS have none of these specific genetic abnormalities [32,37].

A majority of people with PWS have a similar deletion to that found in AS, in this case in the paternal chr15q11-q13 [80]. Maternal UPD15 accounts for almost a third of people with PWS [80], and mutations within the IC are present in a small proportion of PWS cases, including most families in which there have been two or more affected individuals. Unlike AS, there is no single gene that produces the phenotype, rather the disorder is regarded as a contiguous gene syndrome [81]. Fewer than 1% of patients with the PWS phenotype lack any of these three major forms of chr15q11-q13 defect.

Angelman and Prader-Willi Syndromes in Western Australia

Western Australia (WA) has an area of more than one million square miles (2.5 million square kilometers), and is home to 2.1 million people. Approximately 70% of the population live in cities, 22% in regional districts, and 8% are resident in rural and remote areas of the state [82]. The Disability Services Commission (DSC) of WA has been the primary support organization responsible for providing services to residents with MR since 1952. Any individual referred to DSC has information stored in their electronic client database, which by June 2003 contained diagnostic and demographic information on over 15,000 persons.

Clients are referred to DSC for initial assessment from a variety of sources around the state, including hospitals, educators, specialist physicians and general practitioners, although referrals also are accepted from family members on behalf of people with MR. At the time of registration, clients are assessed in terms of their needs, with advice offered on disability-related services for which they are eligible. Further details regarding the data available from DSC and statistics on some of the more common MR-associated syndromes can be found in a number of published papers [83-89]. One study using DSC data covering the period 1983 to 1992 estimated that there were 14.3 persons with MR born per 1000 births, with a majority (10.6/1000) having IQ and adaptive behavior scores within the range of 41-69 points [90].

Western Australian Population Health Datasets

Western Australia has a number of population-based health data sets that are available for use in approved health research projects, including inpatient hospitalizations, midwife notifications and cancer notifications [91]. Records for the same individuals that appear within and between these data sets are linked regularly by the WA Data Linkage Unit using extensive data linkage methodologies [91]. The population data sets can potentially be linked to other stand-alone data sets via probabilistic matching and extensive clerical review, using demographic details such as names, addresses and dates of birth, to an accuracy of ~99% [91,92]. Health information for all AS and PWS cases identified in the DSC client files was extracted from the WA Hospital Morbidity Data System, Death Registry, Mental Health Information System, and the Cancer Registry, with data linkage performed by the WA Data Linkage Unit. In this way a comprehensive individual health profile could be constructed for each AS or PWS patient.

Patient Profiles

The basic patient profiles of people with a recorded diagnosis of Angelman syndrome or Prader-Willi syndrome identified via the DSC database are shown in Table 1.

Significantly fewer young children were diagnosed with AS than PWS (Figure 1), which is probably indicative of the more subtle clinical signs of AS in infancy. There also were very few individuals with either disorder who were over 40 years of age, which may be indicative of the impact of comorbidities. However, as AS and PWS were described as disease entities quite recently, and with the underlying mechanisms defined only within the last twenty years, in the early years of the DSC client registry some individuals with AS and PWS may have been recruited but with no specific diagnosis recorded.

Table 1. Characteristics of the study cohort (n=80)

		AS	PWS	Total
Diagnosis: (number of individuals)		34	46	80
Gender: number (%)	Male	15 (44.0)	23 (50.0)	38 (47.5)
	Female	19 (56.0)	23 (50.0)	42 (52.5)
Mean age, in years (range)		21.6 (6.5-36.6)	21.0 (0.9-48.3)	
Deceased: (number of individuals)		2	6	8

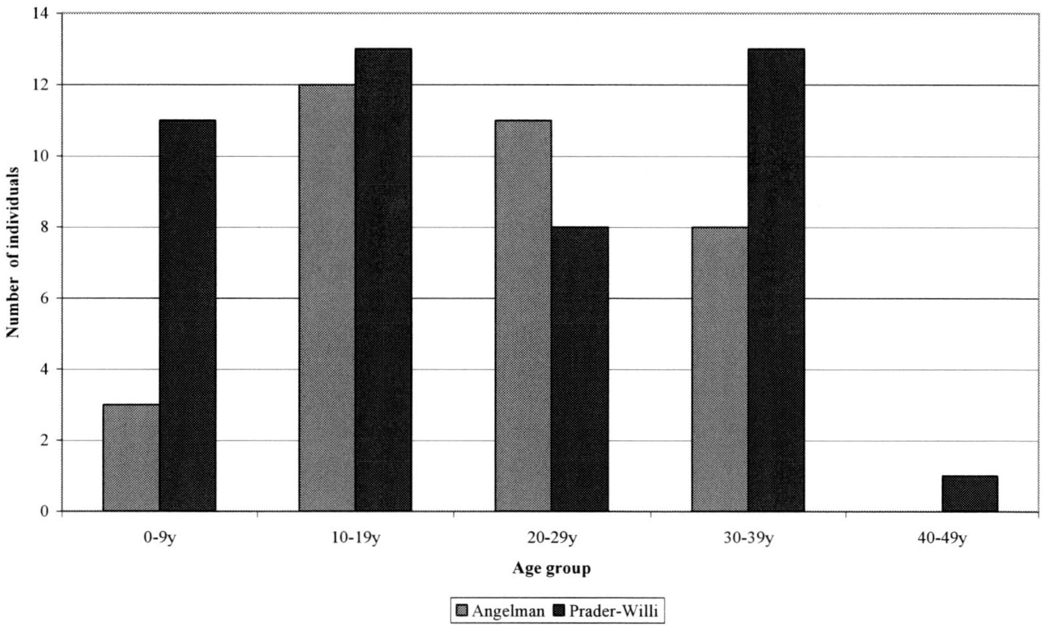

Figure 1. Age groups of the study cohort (n=80).

Lifestyle Characteristics

Of the 32 living AS cases, 20 resided at home, nine were resident in group homes or hostels, and one each lived in foster care, in an independent home, and with adoptive parents. The mean age of AS individuals in private residences was significantly lower than those in supported accommodation (20.2 years vs 27.9 years). The majority of people were registered within the Perth metropolitan region, with fewer than 10% living in rural areas.

Twenty-eight PWS patients lived at home and six were resident in supported accommodation. Once again, there was a significant difference between the mean ages of individuals living at home and those in residential care (20.2 years vs 32.6 years). No place of residence was recorded for six individuals, and the remaining six people were deceased. The Perth metropolitan region was home to 70.0% of living PWS individuals, with a further 17.5% living in rural and remote regional locations throughout Western Australia. The place of residence for the remaining five individuals was unspecified.

Prevalence and Age at Diagnosis

The birth prevalence of Angelman syndrome in the cohort was approximately 1:40,000 live births, and for Prader-Willi syndrome it was 1:29,500. These figures may be underestimates, since only individuals who were registered with DSC were included in the study. Internationally, the prevalence rates for the two disorders have ranged from 1:10,000 [93] to 1:76,574 [94]. However, as noted by Õiglane-Shlik *et al.* [95], there are major dissimilarities in both the methodologies adopted and the study populations recruited, which makes meaningful comparisons extremely problematic. The Estonian study group [95] reported a significantly lower birth prevalence for AS than for PWS, but as their cohort was restricted to individuals with a genetically confirmed diagnosis, the true prevalence of AS in the community may have been under-estimated.

The mean age at diagnosis for AS patients was 5.8 years (range, 1-27 years), while that for PWS was 5.3 years, with 34.8% diagnosed before the age of one year. Within the subset of 35 individuals with PWS registered at DSC prior to 1998 the mean age at diagnosis was 6.6 years (range, 0.2-17.0 years), whereas the 11 individuals who were recruited after 1998 had a mean age at diagnosis of 1.1 years (range, 0.1-6.0 years). Thus it is apparent that diagnosis at earlier ages has become more frequent given the advances in the clinical description and genetic determination of the disorders over the last twenty-five years [32,44-46,78,96-98].

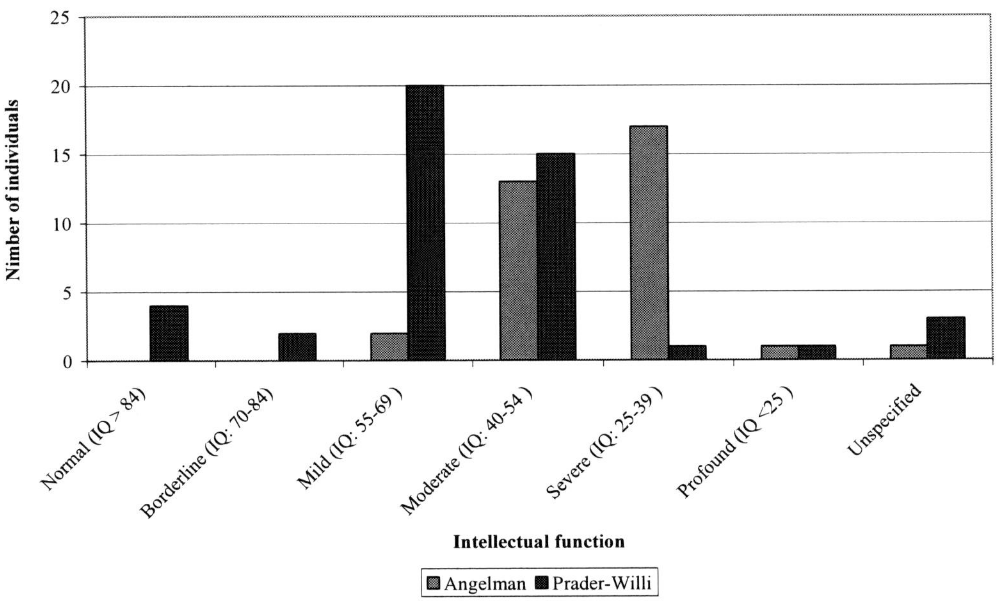

Figure 2. Levels of intellectual function of the study group (n=80).

Clinical Presentation

The level of intellectual function of the study group varied from 'low average' to profoundly handicapped, with 4.4% not having been formally tested due to their youth or for other reasons. The range of IQ scores reported for the cohort are shown in Figure 2.

Angelman Syndrome

Developmental motor delay was not universally evident, as indicated by the lower boundary of the sitting/walking range which fell within the parameters for the general population (Table 2). There was a significant gender difference in the mean ages at which children could walk: males (3.5 years; range, 1.1-9.0 years) versus females (5.2 years; range,

2.2-9.0 years). Three females aged 21 years, 6 years, and 6.5 years (deceased) had never walked, while two males aged 11.8 years and 12.8 years (deceased) were reported as non-ambulant.

All patients with AS had delay and/or inadequacy of speech, and a majority had only managed to acquire a few words. Ataxia and inappropriate laughter were present in most cases. Microcephaly was diagnosed in 44% of individuals, although the requisite information was available on too few cases for statistical comparisons to be made. A large proportion of persons had experienced seizures, with 26% suffering frequent episodes. In addition, 82% of individuals had at least one abnormal EEG reading, with only three people never having been tested.

Table 2. The comparative clinical profile of Angelman syndrome cases in Western Australia and internationally

Characteristic	Western Australia	International	References
Developmental delay: (n = 29; n = 28)	sit = 1.4yr walk = 4.4yr*	sit = 1.0-1.7yr walk = 2.8-6.0yr	[35,177-179]
Absent/minimal speech (n = 34)	82% (delayed; 18%)	70-100%	[35,97,179]
Ataxia (n = 34)	91%	79-100%	[35,97,177]
Behavior (n = 34)	77%	77-100%	[36,177,179]
Microcephaly (n = 20)	44%	44-93%	[97,178,179]
Epilepsy (n = 34)	88%	79-88%	[30,35,40]
Abnormal EEG (n = 27)	82%	82-100%	[35,40,179]
Feeding difficulties (n = 25)	41%	21-77%	[97,179]
Strabismus (n = 27)	47%	21-57%	[179,180]
Hypopigmentation (n = 17)	35%	0-64%	[178,179]
Hypotonia (n = 34)	79%	48-85%	[97,181]
Scoliosis (> 15y: n = 23)	56%	25-70%	[27,30,178]
Obesity (n = 34)	38%	15-50%	[30,178,179]

* Five individuals had never walked.

A number of additional clinical characteristics were frequently reported within the AS cohort, e.g., strabismus in 47% of patients and hypopigmentation in 35%, but information on these characteristics was unavailable in a significant number of cases. Although most people with AS had been hypotonic at birth, half of the group were regarded as hyperactive. Some 38% of AS patients were obese, in comparison to international studies that report up to 60% obesity in individuals with MR [99-101]. Skin picking, a self-injurious habit usually associated with PWS, also was reported in seven AS patients, mainly older individuals. Scoliosis was present in 33% of all individuals with AS, and in more than half of those more than 15 years old (Table 2). Three males with AS had either undescended testes or a small penis.

Prader-Willi Syndrome

As indicated in Table 3, a majority of PWS individuals had hypotonia, infantile feeding problems, and rapid weight gain at an early age, followed by obesity. Hyperphagia was less frequently described (61%). Unfortunately, reporting of the characteristic facial features was poor, with over 90% of case files lacking details of this feature. Hypogonadism and/or cryptorchidism were present in 67% of PWS patients: in 91% of males of all ages and 58% of females over 15 years. All of the adult female patients with a confirmed gene deletion had absent or delayed menses, but menstrual dysfunction was reported in only 30% of females of similar age without an identified deletion. Motor developmental delay was present in 20/46 cases, but a further 18 persons reached the sitting and walking milestones at ages comparable to the general population.

Table 3. The comparative clinical profile of Prader-Willi syndrome cases in Western Australia and internationally

Characteristic	Western Australia	International	References
Hypotonia (n = 46)	96%	83-100%	[48,182,183]
Feeding difficulties (n = 43)	85%	81-100%	[182,183]
Weight gain (n = 46)	87%	73-93%	[46,48]
Hypogonadism (n = 15; n = 19)	male = 91% female = 58%	male = 94-100% female = 60-100%	[48,182]
Developmental delay (n = 34; n = 39)	sit = 1.0yr walk = 2.6yr	sit = 1.0yr walk = 2.0-2.4yr	[182]
Hyperphagia (n=33)	85%	66-90%	[48,183]
Short stature (n = 39)	72%	48-83%	[183]
Hypopigmentation (n = 20)	75%	33-57%	[48]
Eye abnormalities (n = 35)	66%	58-77%	[48,183]
Speech defects (n = 45)	85%	79-90%	[48,63]
Scoliosis (n = 30)	37%	32-75%	[48]
Epilepsy (n = 46)	29%	14-46%	[63,183]

Over half of the patients (57%) had exhibited the temper tantrums and violent outbursts characteristically associated with PWS, although these behaviors previously have been reported in 70-88% of cases [73,80,102]. An estimated 72% of patients were short in stature compared to family members, but only four individuals had received growth hormone therapy. Ocular abnormalities were reported by 66% of patients, and 85% of people with PWS suffered from delayed speech development and/or articulation defects (Table 3).

Scoliosis was reported in 11 of the 30 PWS cases aged 15 years or more, and two individuals had received corrective surgery for the condition, but younger members of the cohort had not developed the disorder. Osteoporosis or osteopenia was identified only in a single female, aged 32 years, compared to 75% of adults aged 19-36yr with PWS in Sweden [52]. A Danish study reported significantly lower bone mineral densities in PWS individuals than in obese controls [103].

At least one episode of epilepsy or convulsions was reported for 28.3% of people with PWS (Table 3), which is similar to the rates observed for MR in general [63,104]. Of the 13 persons who had an epileptic episode, five showed a deletion in chr15q11-q13, one was diagnosed as UPD15, four had never been tested, and four had no specific genetic mechanism identified. Diabetes was reported in four adults, with no data available for the other 30 adult members of the PWS cohort.

Laboratory Findings

The laboratory findings obtained with both sets of patients are summarized in Table 4. A majority of the study cohort had received some form of genetic testing, although fewer patients had been assessed using the most recent investigative techniques, such as mutation detection in the IC region of chr15q11-q13. As expected, a genetic deletion had been more frequently diagnosed than any other causative mechanism.

Table 4. Proportion of cases given diagnostic testing for Angelman syndrome (n = 34) and Prader-Willi syndrome (n = 46)

		AS	PWS
Type of molecular tests used: (% tested)	Karyotype/banding	23.5	30.5
	FISH	11.8	17.4
	Methylation	55.9	36.9
	Unknown/no test	11.8	15.2
Molecular test results: (% of those tested)	Deletion	33.3	43.6
	Uniparental disomy	6.7	10.2
	Positive (not specified)	6.7	15.4
	Inconclusive	10.0	7.7
	No abnormality detected	43.3	23.1

Hospital Admissions

Individuals with AS had been admitted to hospital on a total of 301 occasions between 1970 and 2003, with an average of 8.8 (SD = 8.6) inpatient episodes per person. As shown in Table 5, epilepsy and/or seizures were the most common primary reasons for admission, followed by gastrointestinal tract disorders, holiday or respite care, dental care, and respiratory tract disorders. The grounds for the remaining admissions were varied, including eye abnormalities, burns, and congenital deformities. Four of 34 people with AS (age range 10.3-30.4 years) had no recorded hospital admissions, and no diagnosis of cancer had been reported among the AS cohort.

More than half of the individuals with AS were hospitalized one or more times for dental work, and almost as many had been admitted with a diagnosis of epilepsy. A further 12 individuals were hospitalized for failure to thrive or developmental delay (Table 5). It is notable that admission for dental work was over-represented in patients with severe or profound mental retardation (62% of dental admissions), even though this group comprised only 52% of the AS population. Individuals with severe intellectual limitations often do not tolerate medical procedures such as filling or scaling of teeth without use of sedation or general anesthesia [105,106].

Table 5. Total hospital admissions for the Angelman syndrome cohort (1970-2003)

Reason for admission	Number of admitted individuals	Total number of admissions (% of total admissions)
Epilepsy	16	43 (14.3)
Gastrointestinal disorders	10	39 (13.0)
Holiday care	1	34 (11.3)
Dental	18	29 (9.6)
Respiratory disorders	10	26 (8.6)
Otitis media	7	15 (5.0)
Skin disorders	4	15 (5.0)
Open wound, various sites	8	13 (4.3)
Failure to thrive/feeding difficulties	12	12 (4.0)
Foreign body inserted, various sites	5	9 (3.0)
Congenital anomaly	5	8 (2.7)
Urinary tract disorders	4	6 (2.0)
Fractured bone ± complications	4	5 (1.7)
Other causes (various)		47 (15.6)

Adapted from Thomson *et al.* (2006) [88].

As shown in Table 6, people with PWS had been hospitalized on a total of 328 occasions (mean admissions, 7.4; SD, 6.9), with respiratory tract infections accounting for the largest number of admissions, followed by breathing difficulties, dental care, undescended testes, gastrointestinal disorders, and unspecified congenital anomalies. A large and varied number of additional diagnoses were listed in the patients' files as reasons for their admission to hospital, including cellulitis, musculoskeletal disorders, and ingestion of toxic substances. However, six of 46 PWS patients (age range 0.9-39.1 years) had no record of hospitalization.

Table 6. Total hospital admissions for the Prader-Willi syndrome cohort (1970-2003)

Reason for admission	Number of admitted individuals	Total number of admissions (% of total admissions)
Respiratory infections	17	25 (7.6)
Breathing difficulties	14	24 (7.3)
Dental	14	21 (6.4)
Undescended testes	9	19 (5.8)
Congenital anomaly	10	18 (5.5)
Gastrointestinal disorders	8	18 (5.5)
Fractured bone ± complications	8	16 (4.9)
Epilepsy	9	15 (4.6)
Urinary tract disorders	9	11 (3.4)
Failure to thrive/feeding difficulties	6	11 (3.4)
Otitis media	4	11 (3.4)
Skin disorders	4	5 (1.5)
Foreign body inserted, various sites	2	2 (0.6)
Open wound, various sites	1	2 (0.6)
Other causes (various)		130 (39.5)

Adapted from Thomson *et al.* (2006) [89].

Some 37% of hospitalized PWS patients suffered from at least one respiratory infection, and 14 individuals had been admitted to hospital for dental work or with breathing difficulties (Table 6). Thick saliva is often reported in individuals with PWS and this trait may increase the development of dental problems in this population. Cardiovascular problems were not recorded as the primary reason for admission for any adult with PWS, which was a rather unexpected finding in a population which tends to be morbidly obese, although the oldest member of the PWS cohort was not yet 50 years old. Three individuals with PWS had been diagnosed with carcinoma over the years 1970-2003, all of whom were treated successfully. One patient had a benign endocrine tumor, another had a malignant melanoma removed at 16 years of age, and the third person had a thyroidectomy for malignancy at age 35 years [89].

In a sub-study conducted in the four years from 1998-2001, PWS patients were over five times more likely to be admitted to hospital than members of the general population [107,108], whereas admissions for individuals with AS occurred at similar rates to the wider community (Figure 3). However, AS patients in the age range 5-14 years were hospitalized at greater rates and for longer periods than either people with PWS or the general population of comparable age (Figures 3 & 4), which may be indicative of the increased rates of seizure activity in younger pre-pubertal AS patients. There was no appreciable difference between the hospitalization rates for people with AS, or for the general population when assessed by gender, with the exception of females of reproductive age (15-34 years) in the general population who had admission rates almost double those of males of similar age, due to admissions for childbirth and the complications of pregnancy [107,108].

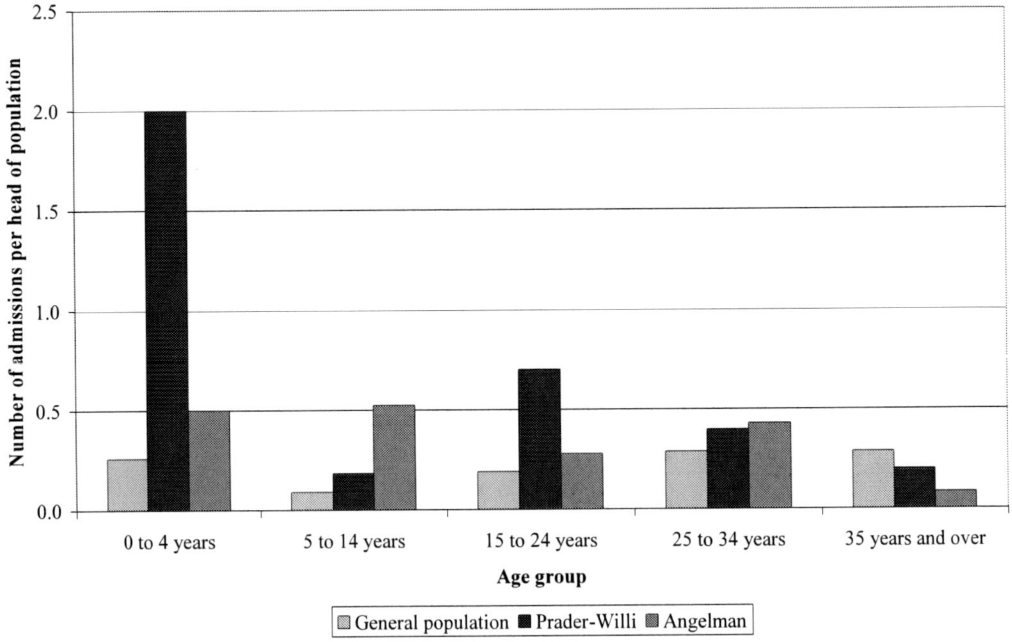

Figure 3. Comparison of hospital admissions per head of population between the study cohort and the general population (1998-2001).

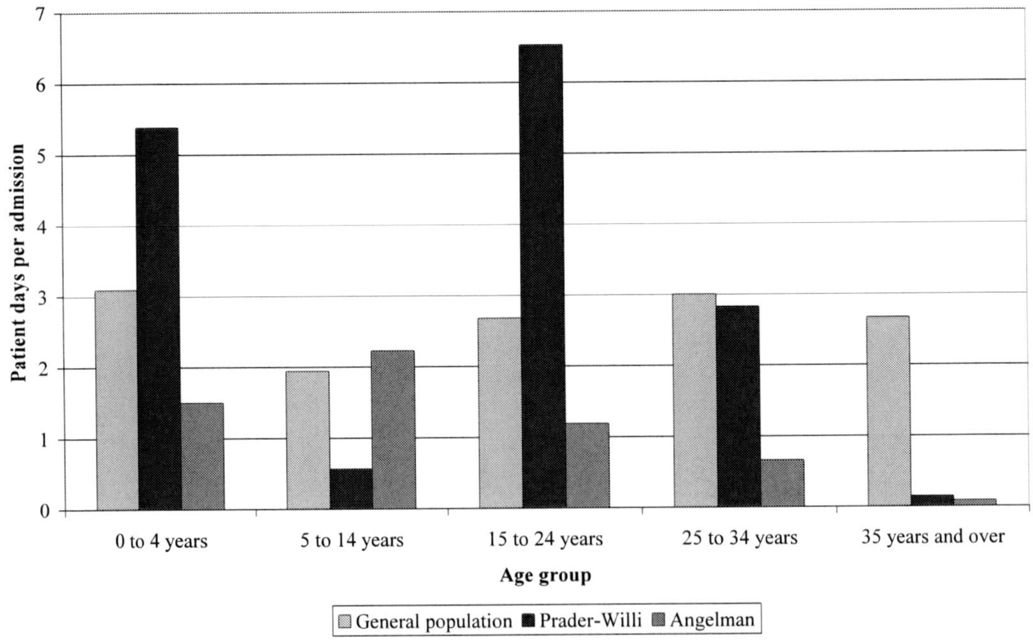

Figure 4. Comparison of the mean patient days per admission between members of the study group and the general population (1998-2001).

The highest rates of admission for patients with PWS were in those younger than five years and 15-24 years of age, and their hospital stay was typically longer in duration (Figures 3 & 4). Infants with PWS exhibit a range of health problems that may require frequent hospitalization, including hypotonia, poor suckling, and hypogonadism. Among children with PWS who were less than five years old, males were 4.4 times and females were 3.4 times more likely to be admitted to hospital than members of the general population, and almost half the boys with PWS had been treated for undescended testes.

Older children and adults with PWS are often obese because of their compulsive eating habits, with a resultant increased requirement for clinical care (Figures 3 & 4). With the exception of the adolescent years when their epilepsy is often difficult to control, the medical conditions associated with AS are less acute in persons of 15 years and above, as indicated by their comparatively lower use of hospital-based care.

The apparent reduction in hospital admissions for the study cohort after the age of 25 years may be an artifact of the small target population size, or reflect the increased mortality rates among some individuals with the conditions. Alternatively, it could be that the parents/carers of people with AS and PWS become more proficient at coping with health issues at home and have less need of hospital care for their charges. In addition, as women with MR rarely reproduce, hospital admissions for pregnancy and childbirth are very uncommon in this group.

Three individuals with AS and six of the PWS cohort were admitted to psychiatric units for periods of up to 96 days on the grounds of developmental delay, MR, epilepsy or, in one case, non-organic psychosis. Three other AS patients attended psychiatric outpatient clinics on two, six and eighteen occasions respectively. The diagnoses reported for these persons were severe MR, microcephalus, and 'psychosocial circumstances (unemployment)'. One individual with PWS attended group therapy sessions for mixed disturbance of conduct and emotions over a period of nine years, at an average of 10 visits per month. Further outpatient visits to psychiatric units were made by three persons. The total number of visits per person ranged from 3 to 12 with MR, developmental delay and disturbance of conduct recorded as the main grounds for attendance.

Mortality

There had been two deaths within the group of 34 AS patients. One person died of *status epilepticus* at the age of 12.8 years, and the other patient died of pneumonia aged 6.5 years. Of the six deceased PWS patients, aged 2.3 years to 36.5 years, two died from cardiac arrest/myocardial infarction, one from pneumonia, with no cause of death recorded in the remaining three cases. Mortality rates for this cohort could not be calculated given the small number of deceased persons.

Epilepsy at any time of life increases the relative risk of death for any person, irrespective of the level of MR of the individual [109]. However, over the last half century there has been a decrease in the proportion of people with MR who die from *status epilepticus*, because of the improved medication regimes to control seizures [110,111]. This is reflected in the scarcity of deaths from epilepsy in the AS cohort from Western Australia even though a majority of individuals have experienced seizure activity.

Respiratory complaints are regarded as significant primary causes of death among individuals with MR, as are diseases of the circulatory system [110,112-116]. One person with PWS and one with AS from the WA study cohort had died of pneumonia, and two PWS individuals died from cardiovascular failure.

DISCUSSION

People with mental retardation are living significantly longer than in the past [84,116-118], and in developed countries individuals with mild MR now have a median life expectancy of 74 years [84], and even severe MR only decreases life expectancy by 20% or less [109,113,119]. Members of the study cohort were all less than 50 years old, which would seem to indicate that people with AS or PWS do not have life expectancies that match those of people with other forms of MR. However, both disorders have been quite recently described and defined, and it is at least possible that there are numbers of older people with AS and PWS in Western Australia who have never been specifically diagnosed with the conditions. Reports from other developed countries have included individuals with PWS up to 71 years old, some of whom were not diagnosed with the disorder until mid-life [27,120-123].

An extended lifespan may fail to be translated into disease-free old age. The development of chronic disease states can be predicted by many factors, including low educational attainment, female gender, low income, reduced access to health services, paucity of close personal contacts, and restricted levels of physical activity [124,125]. People with MR frequently fall into two or more of these categories, and so they are expected to apply to individuals with AS and PWS [126-128]. Children with PWS and AS tend to have increased health needs compared to the general population, and indications are that adults also require substantial amounts of medical assistance [63,129,130]. Individuals with AS may continue to have epileptic seizures throughout life, and often become less mobile due to a combination of ataxia, scoliosis, and obesity [88]. People with either AS or PWS frequently suffer from respiratory and gastrointestinal disorders. Since older PWS patients are generally obese, they may display all the attendant health problems, including cardiovascular disease and greatly reduced mobility [88,89].

In general, people with MR may be inadequately treated by health systems which concentrate on provision of care only when requested [131-134]. Individuals with MR or their carers may fail to recognize symptoms that would be of concern to others, or they may be unable to adequately articulate their concerns, especially if they have minimal speech capabilities, as in AS [116,135-137]. Another problem is 'diagnostic overshadowing', where physical or behavioral symptoms are attributed to MR, rather than being recognized as separate comorbid disorders [138]. Obstacles to adequate health care access for people with MR have been increased by the transition from institutional living to community-based residence over the last few decades. Although health care in large institutions was reported to be sub-optimal in the past [110], physicians attached to the facilities were responsible for the health of residents and many had extensive experience in providing clinical care to patients with MR. Currently, in developed countries people with MR who live in the community may not have a regular medical attendant, or may be referred to a medical practitioner untrained in the specific health problems and communication difficulties that they exhibit [139-141]. Over a decade ago, an examination of individuals with MR in North Sydney, Australia, indicated that more than half of their health problems were inadequately managed, and that a large percentage of these problems had not been diagnosed prior to the study [142]. These findings have subsequently been confirmed in other countries [143-145].

In common with members of the wider community, the health care needs and phenotypic profiles of people with AS and PWS vary with increasing age. These changes have significant implications with regard to their support requirements and the resultant economic costs [146]. In addition, ageing parental carers, who may have been under considerable stress for many years, require increasing levels of support to fulfill their caring role [147-150]. An indication of the level of psychological stress, and the resultant biological burden faced by the long-term carers of people with MR, was provided by a study of premature ageing exhibited at the cellular level by women caring for chronically ill children [151]. There seems little doubt that similar findings would apply to the carers of those with MR, which raises important questions as to how carers can best be assisted to continue in that role in an effective manner, especially if their health is already impaired [152]. In some countries there also may be potential difficulties associated with the provision of appropriate life and health insurance cover for the carers of people with MR. Different stressors and types of resources have been found to modify psychological stress, especially factors in the social environment [153], and a study examining the physical and emotional effects of the caring role on the family members of the Western Australian PWS and AS cohort is in progress.

In many cases, older parents are no longer physically capable of providing the necessary level of care and support for their adult child at home, and assistance with the transition to out-of-home living for the affected individual and their parents may be necessary [154-156]. Older members of the AS and PWS study cohort in Western Australia were more likely to be living away from the family home [88,89]. The term 'launching' was used by Blacher *et al.* (1999) to describe the normal course of young adults leaving the parental home, and this process is likely to become more common as families acknowledge the benefit to the young adult with MR of moving from home and taking further steps along the path to an independent lifestyle [157,158].

Out-of-home placement for people with MR can take the form of a group home, larger-scale residential setting, or independent living with minimal support. There are reports from the U.S.A. and Australia of insufficient places in supported accommodation [156,159,160], and the cost of residential accommodation differs according to the type of facility and the intellectual and behavioral characteristics of the individual [161,162]. In developed countries there is increased emphasis on normalization and inclusion, encouraging participation in the wider community through employment, leisure and residence [163-167]. However, employment in the open market for people with MR is often confined to manual, unskilled work, with fewer hours and lower pay rates than the general population [168,169], which may contribute to financial difficulties. It is envisaged that there will be an increased need for supported employment opportunities in adulthood for people with PWS. There are specific requirements for the suitable placement of an individual with PWS, as some of the behavioral characteristics, such as food obsession, insistence on sameness, and temper tantrums, need effective management to enable a successful working life [170]. Due to the communication difficulties exhibited by many individuals with AS they are less suited to work outside sheltered workshops. Indeed, the combination of ataxia, epilepsy and minimal speech abilities may make it extremely difficult for such people to successfully undertake any employment without considerable amounts of assistance and supervision.

Although AS and PWS both result from small deletions or point mutations in a defined region of a single chromosome, they have markedly different clinical and morbidity profiles. There is evidence that some imprinted genes affect the regulation of interactions between the placenta and the fetus during embryogenesis and therefore loss of expression of one or more of these imprinted genes could be responsible for the development of disease phenotypes [17,171]. Disruption of the normal placental-fetal interactions has been implicated in the later development of MR in individuals without a recognized etiology for that condition [172], and failure of imprinting may be responsible for the distinctive behavioral and cognitive profiles exhibited by individuals with AS and PWS [17]. Dysregulation of gene suppression is implicated in some cancers, and in other human diseases, such as Angelman, Prader-Willi, and Beckwith-Wiedemann syndromes [12,173-176]. Ongoing studies should greatly assist in providing detailed information on genotype-phenotype correlations, and the role of epigenetic changes in the development of these and other disorders [176].

REFERENCES

[1] Stromme P. Aetiology in severe and mild mental retardation: a population-based study of Norwegian children. *Dev Med Child Neurol.* 2000 Feb;42(2):76-86.

[2] Yaqoob M, Bashir A, Zaman S, Ferngren H, Von Dobeln U, Gustavson KH. Mild intellectual disability in children in Lahore, Pakistan: aetiology and risk factors. *J Intellect Disabil Res.* 2004 Oct;48(Pt 7):663-71.

[3] Lantigua-Cruz A, Mora F, Arechaederra M, Rojas I, Morales E, Rodríguez H, *et al.* Etiological Characterization of 512 Severely Mentally Retarded Institutionalized Patients in Havana. *Comm Genet.* 1999;2(4):184-9.

[4] Arvio M, Sillanpaa M. Prevalence, aetiology and comorbidity of severe and profound intellectual disability in Finland. *J Intellect Disabil Res.* 2003 Feb;47(Pt 2):108-12.

[5] Kelly TL, Trasler JM. Reproductive epigenetics. *Clin Genet.* 2004 Apr;65(4):247-60.

[6] Reik W, Dean W, Walter J. Epigenetic reprogramming in mammalian development. *Science.* 2001 Aug 10;293(5532):1089-93.

[7] Wu C, Morris JR. Genes, genetics, and epigenetics: a correspondence. *Science.* 2001 Aug 10;293(5532):1103-5.

[8] Jones PA, Takai D. The role of DNA methylation in mammalian epigenetics. *Science.* 2001 Aug 10;293(5532):1068-70.

[9] Park Y, Kuroda MI. Epigenetic aspects of X-chromosome dosage compensation. *Science.* 2001 Aug 10;293(5532):1083-5.

[10] Matzke M, Matzke AJ, Kooter JM. RNA: guiding gene silencing. *Science.* 2001 Aug 10;293(5532):1080-3.

[11] Rougeulle C, Heard E. Antisense RNA in imprinting: spreading silence through Air. *Trends Genet.* 2002 Sep;18(9):434-7.

[12] Falls JG, Pulford DJ, Wylie AA, Jirtle RL. Genomic imprinting: implications for human disease. *Am J Pathol.* 1999 Mar;154(3):635-47.

[13] Morison IM, Ramsay JP, Spencer HG. A census of mammalian imprinting. *Trends Genet.* 2005 Aug;21(8):457-65.

[14] Haig D, Wilkins JF. Genomic imprinting, sibling solidairity and the logic of collective action. *Philos Trans R Soc Lond.* 2000 Nov 29;355(1403):1593-7.

[15] Haig D, Wharton R. Prader-Willi syndrome and the evolution of human childhood. *Am J Hum Biol.* 2003 May-Jun;15(3):320-9.

[16] Maher ER, Afnan M, Barratt CL. Epigenetic risks related to assisted reproductive technologies: epigenetics, imprinting, ART and icebergs? *Hum Reprod.* 2003 Dec;18(12):2508-11.

[17] Miozzo M, Simoni G. The role of imprinted genes in fetal growth. *Biol Neonate.* 2002;81(4):217-28.

[18] Ferguson-Smith AC, Surani MA. Imprinting and the epigenetic asymmetry between parental genomes. *Science.* 2001 Aug 10;293(5532):1086-9.

[19] Greally JM, State MW. Genetics of childhood disorders: XIII. Genomic imprinting: the indelible mark of the gamete. *J Am Acad Child Adolesc Psychiatr.* 2000 Apr;39(4):532-5.

[20] Beaudet AL, Jiang YH. A rheostat model for a rapid and reversible form of imprinting-dependent evolution. *Am J Hum Genet.* 2002 Jun;70(6):1389-97.

[21] Bestor TH. Cytosine methylation mediates sexual conflict. *Trends Genet.* 2003 Apr;19(4):185-90.

[22] Hitchins MP, Moore GE. Genomic imprinting in fetal growth and development. *Expert Rev Molec Med.* 2002 9 May 2004 [cited 9 May 2004]; Available from: http://www.expertreviews.org/0200457Xh.htm

[23] Albrecht U, Sutcliffe JS, Cattanach BM, Beechey CV, Armstrong D, Eichele G, *et al.* Imprinted expression of the murine Angelman syndrome gene, *Ube3a*, in hippocampal and Purkinje neurons. *Nat Genet.* 1997;17:75-8.

[24] Davies SM. Developmental regulation of genomic imprinting of the IGF2 gene in human liver. *Cancer Res.* 1994 May 15;54(10):2560-2.

[25] Smith A. Why is there no diploid overdose effect in Prader-Willi syndrome due to uniparental disomy? *Acta Genet Med Gemellol (Roma).* 1996;45(1-2):179-89.

[26] Jiang Y-h, Lev-Lehman E, Bressler J, Tsai T-F, Beaudet AL. Neurogenetics '99; Genetics of Angelman syndrome. *Am J Hum Genet.* 1999 June 7;65:1-6.

[27] Clayton-Smith J. Angelman syndrome: evolution of the phenotype in adolescents and adults. *Dev Med Child Neurol.* 2001;43:476-80.

[28] Everman DB, Cassidy SB. Genetics of childhood disorders: XII. Genomic imprinting: breaking the rules. *J Am Acad Child Adolesc Psychiatr.* 2000 Mar;39(3):386-9.

[29] Angelman H. 'Puppet' children. A report on three cases. *Dev Med Child Neurol..* 1965;7:681-8.

[30] Clayton-Smith J, Laan L. Angelman syndrome: a review of the clinical and genetic aspects. *J Med Genet.* 2003 Feb;40(2):87-95.

[31] Williams CA, Angelman H, Clayton-Smith J, Driscoll DJ, Hendrickson JE, Knoll JH, *et al.* Angelman syndrome: consensus for diagnostic criteria. Angelman Syndrome Foundation. *Am J Med Genet.* 1995 Mar 27;56(2):237-8.

[32] Williams CA, Beaudet AL, Clayton-Smith J, Knoll JH, Kyllerman M, Laan LA, *et al.* Angelman syndrome 2005: updated consensus for diagnostic criteria. *Am J Med Genet.* 2006 Mar 1;140A(5):413-8.

[33] Runte M, Kroisel PM, Gillessen-Kaesbach G, Varon R, Horn D, Cohen MY, *et al.* SNURF-SNRPN and UBE3A transcript levels in patients with Angelman syndrome. *Hum Genet.* 2004 May 2004;114(6):553.

[34] Ohta T, Buiting K, Kokkonen H, McCandless S, Heeger S, Leisti H, *et al.* Molecular mechanism of Angelman syndrome in two large families involves an imprinting mutation. *Am J Hum Genet.* 1999 Feb;64(2):385-96.

[35] Beckung E, Steffenburg S, Kyllerman M. Motor impairments, neurological signs, and developmental level in individuals with Angelman syndrome. *Dev Med Child Neurol.* 2004 Apr;46(4):239-43.

[36] Berry RJ, Leitner RP, Clarke AR, Einfeld SL. Behavioral aspects of Angelman syndrome: a case control study. *Am J Med Genet.* 2005 Jan 1;132A(1):8-12.

[37] Didden R, Korzilius H, Kamphuis A, Sturmey P, Lancioni G, Curfs LM. Preferences in individuals with Angelman syndrome assessed by a modified Choice Assessment Scale. *J Intellect Disabil Res*. 2006 Jan;50(Pt 1):54-60.

[38] Laan LA, van Haeringen A, Brouwer OF. Angelman syndrome: a review of clinical and genetic aspects. *Clin Neurol Neurosurg.* 1999 Sep;101(3):161-70.

[39] Horsler K, Oliver C. The behavioural phenotype of Angelman syndrome. *J Intellect Disabil Res.* 2006;50(1):33-53.

[40] Valente KD, Andrade JQ, Grossmann RM, Kok F, Fridman C, Koiffmann CP, *et al.* Angelman syndrome: difficulties in EEG pattern recognition and possible misinterpretations. *Epilepsia.* 2003 Aug;44(8):1051-63.

[41] Didden R, Korzilius H, Smits MG, Curfs LM. Sleep problems in individuals with Angelman syndrome. *Am J Ment Retard.* 2004 Jul;109(4):275-84.

[42] Peters S, Beaudet A, Madduri N, Bacino C. Autism in Angelman syndrome: implications for autism research. *Clin Genet.* 2004 December 01, 2004;66(6):530-6.

[43] Prader A, Labhart A, Willi H. Ein syndrom von adipositas, kleinwuchs, kryptorchismus, und oligophrenie nach myatonieartigem Zustand im Neugeborenalter. *Schweizerische Medizinische Wochenschrift.* 1956;86:1260-1.

[44] State MW, Dykens EM. Genetics of childhood disorders: XV. Prader-Willi syndrome: genes, brain, and behavior. *J Am Acad Child Adolesc Psychiatr.* 2000 Jun;39(6):797-800.

[45] Holm VA, Cassidy SB, Butler MG, Hanchett JM, Greenswag LR, Whitman BY, *et al.* Prader-Willi syndrome: consensus diagnostic criteria. *Pediatr.* 1993 Feb;91(2):398-402.

[46] Gunay-Aygun M, Schwartz S, Heeger S, O'Riordan MA, Cassidy SB. The changing purpose of Prader-Willi syndrome clinical diagnostic criteria and proposed revised criteria. *Pediatr.* 2001 Nov;108(5):E92.

[47] Õiglane-Shlik E, Žordania R, Varendi H, Antson A, Magi ML, Tasa G, *et al.* The neonatal phenotype of Prader-Willi syndrome. *Am J Med Genet.* 2006 Jun 1;140A(11):1241-4.

[48] Whittington J, Holland A, Webb T, Butler J, Clarke D, Boer H. Relationship between clinical and genetic diagnosis of Prader-Willi syndrome. *J Med Genet.* 2002 Dec;39(12):926-32.

[49] Einfeld SL, Smith A, Durvasula S, Florio T, Tonge BJ. Behavior and emotional disturbance in Prader-Willi syndrome. *Am J Med Genet.* 1999 Jan 15;82(2):123-7.

[50] Cassidy SB, Schwartz S. Prader-Willi and Angelman syndromes. Disorders of genomic imprinting. *Med.* 1998 Mar;77(2):140-51.

[51] Clarke DJ, Boer H, Whittington J, Holland A, Butler J, Webb T. Prader-Willi syndrome, compulsive and ritualistic behaviours: the first population-based survey. *Br J Psychiatr.* 2002 Apr;180:358-62.

[52] Hoybye C, Hilding A, Jacobsson H, Thoren M. Metabolic profile and body composition in adults with Prader-Willi syndrome and severe obesity. *J Clin Endocrinol Metabol.* 2002 Aug;87(8):3590-7.

[53] Akefeldt A, Tornhage CJ, Gillberg C. A woman with Prader-Willi syndrome gives birth to a healthy baby girl. *Dev Med Child Neurol.* 1999 Nov;41(11):789-90.

[54] Schulze A, Mogensen H, Hamborg-Petersen B, Graem N, Ostergaard JR, Brondum-Nielsen K. Fertility in Prader-Willi syndrome: a case report with Angelman syndrome in the offspring. *Acta Paed.* 2001 Apr;90(4):455-9.

[55] Myers SE, Carrel AL, Whitman BY, Allen DB. Physical effects of growth hormone treatment in children with Prader-Willi syndrome. *Acta Paed (Suppl).* 1999 Dec;88(433):112-4.

[56] Carrel AL, Myers SE, Whitman BY, Allen DB. Benefits of long-term GH therapy in Prader-Willi syndrome: a 4-year study. *J Clin Endocrinol Metabol.* 2002 Apr;87(4):1581-5.

[57] Lindgren AC, Ritzen EM. Five years of growth hormone treatment in children with Prader-Willi syndrome. Swedish National Growth Hormone Advisory Group. *Acta Paed (Suppl).* 1999 Dec;88(433):109-11.

[58] Whitman BY, Myers S, Carrel A, Allen D. The behavioral impact of growth hormone treatment for children and adolescents with Prader-Willi syndrome: a 2-year, controlled study. *Pediatr.* 2002 Feb;109(2):E35.

[59] Hoybye C, Hilding A, Jacobsson H, Thoren M. Growth hormone treatment improves body composition in adults with Prader-Willi syndrome. *Clin Endocrinol.* 2003 May;58(5):653-61.

[60] Haqq AM, Stadler DD, Jackson RH, Rosenfeld RG, Purnell JQ, LaFranchi SH. Effects of growth hormone on pulmonary function, sleep quality, behavior, cognition, growth velocity, body composition, and resting energy expenditure in Prader-Willi syndrome. *J Clin Endocrinol Metabol.* 2003 May;88(5):2206-12.

[61] Hoybye C, Thoren M, Bohm B. Cognitive, emotional, physical and social effects of growth hormone treatment in adults with Prader-Willi syndrome. *J Intellect Disabil Res.* 2005;49(Pt 4):245-52.

[62] Goldberg DL, Garrett CL, Van Riper C, Warzak WJ. Coping with Prader-Willi syndrome. *J Am Diet Assoc.* 2002 Apr;102(4):537-42.

[63] Butler JV, Whittington JE, Holland AJ, Boer H, Clarke D, Webb T. Prevalence of, and risk factors for, physical ill-health in people with Prader-Willi syndrome: a population-based study. *Dev Med Child Neurol.* 2002 Apr;44(4):248-55.

[64] Butler J, Whittington J, Holland A, Boer H, Clarke D, Webb T. Prevalence of, and risk factors for, physical ill-health in people with Prader-Willi syndrome: a population-based study. *Dev Med Child Neurol.* 2002;44:248-55.

[65] Descheemaeker MJ, Vogels A, Govers V, Borghgraef M, Willekens D, Swillen A, *et al.* Prader-Willi syndrome: new insights in the behavioural and psychiatric spectrum. *J Intellect Disabil Res.* 2002 Jan;46(Pt 1):41-50.

[66] Wigren M, Heimann M. Excessive picking in Prader-Willi syndrome: a pilot study of phenomenological aspects and comorbid symptoms. *Intl J Disabil Dev Edu.* 2001;48(2):129-42.
[67] Greaves N, Prince E, Evans DW, Charman T. Repetitive and ritualistic behaviour in children with Prader-Willi syndrome and children with autism. *J Intellect Disabil Res.* 2005;50(2):92-100.
[68] Milner KM, Craig EE, Thompson RJ, Veltman MW, Thomas NS, Roberts S, *et al.* Prader-Willi syndrome: intellectual abilities and behavioural features by genetic subtype. *J Child Psychol Psychia.* 2005 Oct;46(10):1089-96.
[69] Dimitropoulos A, Blackford J, Walden T, Thompson T. Compulsive behavior in Prader-Willi syndrome: examining severity in early childhood. *Res Dev Disabil.* 2006 Mar-Apr;27(2):190-202.
[70] Boer H, Holland A, Whittington J, Butler J, Webb T, Clarke D. Psychotic illness in people with Prader Willi syndrome due to chromosome 15 maternal uniparental disomy. *Lancet.* 2002 Jan 12;359(9301):135-6.
[71] Verhoeven WM, Tuinier S, Curfs LM. Prader-Willi syndrome: cycloid psychosis in a genetic subtype? *Acta Neuropsychiatr.* 2003;15:32-7.
[72] Vogels A, De Hert M, Descheemaeker MJ, Govers V, Devriendt K, Legius E, *et al.* Psychotic disorders in Prader-Willi syndrome. *Am J Med Genet.* 2004 Jun 15;127A(3):238-43.
[73] Steinhausen HC, Eiholzer U, Hauffa BP, Malin Z. Behavioural and emotional disturbances in people with Prader-Willi Syndrome. *J Intellect Disabil Res.* 2004 Jan;48(1):47-52.
[74] Varela MC, Kok F, Setian N, Kim CA, Koiffmann CP. Impact of molecular mechanisms, including deletion size, on Prader-Willi syndrome phenotype: study of 75 patients. *Clin Genet.* 2005;67(1):47-52.
[75] Smith A, Egan J, Ridley G, Haan E, Montgomery P, Williams K, *et al.* Birth prevalence of Prader-Willi syndrome in Australia. *Arch Dis Child.* 2003 Mar;88(3):263-4.
[76] Farber C, Dittrich B, Buiting K, Horsthemke B. The chromosome 15 imprinting centre (IC) region has undergone multiple duplication events and contains an upstream exon of SNRPN that is deleted in all Angelman syndrome patients with an IC microdeletion. *Hum Mol Genet.* 1999 Feb;8(2):337-43.
[77] Williams CA, Lossie A, Driscoll D. Angelman syndrome: mimicking conditions and phenotypes. *Am J Med Genet.* 2001 Jun 1;101(1):59-64.
[78] Lossie AC, Whitney MM, Amidon D, Dong HJ, Chen P, Theriaque D, *et al.* Distinct phenotypes distinguish the molecular classes of Angelman syndrome. *J Med Genet.* 2001 Dec;38(12):834-45.
[79] Buiting K, Gross S, Lich C, Gillessen-Kaesbach G, el-Maarri O, Horsthemke B. Epimutations in Prader-Willi and Angelman syndromes: a molecular study of 136 patients with an imprinting defect. *Am J Hum Genet.* 2003 Mar;72(3):571-7.
[80] Cassidy SB, Dykens E, Williams CA. Prader-Willi and Angelman syndromes: sister imprinted disorders. *Am J Med Genet.* 2000 Summer;97(2):136-46.
[81] Johnstone KA, DuBose AJ, Futtner CR, Elmore MD, Brannan CI, Resnick JL. A human imprinting centre demonstrates conserved acquisition but diverged maintenance

of imprinting in a mouse model for Angelman syndrome imprinting defects. *Hum Mol Genet*. 2006;15(3):393.

[82] Australian Bureau of Statistics. National Regional Profile: #5 Western Australia. *Canberra: Australian Bureau of Statistics;* 2004. Report No.: Cat. No. 1379.0.55.001.

[83] Bittles AH, Glasson EJ. Clinical, social, and ethical implications of changing life expectancy in Down syndrome. *Dev Med Child Neurol.* 2004 Apr;46(4):282-6.

[84] Bittles AH, Petterson BA, Sullivan SG, Hussain R, Glasson EJ, Montgomery PD. The influence of intellectual disability on life expectancy. *J Gerontol.* 2002 Jul;57(7):M470-2.

[85] Glasson EJ, Sullivan SG, Hussain R, Bittles AH. An assessment of intellectual disability among Aboriginal Australians. *J Intellect Disabil Res.* 2005;49(Pt 8):626-34.

[86] Glasson EJ, Sullivan SG, Hussain R, Petterson BA, Montgomery PD, Bittles AH. The changing survival profile of people with Down's syndrome: implications for genetic counselling. *Clin Genet.* 2002 Nov;62(5):390-3.

[87] Glasson EJ, Sullivan SG, Hussain R, Petterson BA, Montgomery PD, Bittles AH. Comparative survival advantage of males with Down syndrome. *Am J Hum Biol.* 2003;15:192-5.

[88] Thomson AK, Glasson EJ, Bittles AH. A long-term population-based clinical and morbidity profile of Angelman syndrome in Western Australia: 1953-2003. *Disabil Rehab.* 2006;28(5):299-305.

[89] Thomson AK, Glasson EJ, Bittles AH. A long-term population-based clinical and morbidity review of Prader-Willi syndrome in Western Australia. *J Intellect Disabil Res.* 2006 January 2006;50(1):69-78.

[90] Leonard H, Petterson B, Bower C, Sanders R. Prevalence of intellectual disability in Western Australia. *Paediatr Perinat Epidem.* 2003 Jan;17(1):58-67.

[91] Holman CD, Bass AJ, Rouse IL, Hobbs MS. Population-based linkage of health records in Western Australia: development of a health services research linked database. *ANZ J Pub Health.* 1999;23(5):453-9.

[92] Kelman CW, Bass AJ, Holman CD. Research use of linked health data--a best practice protocol. *ANZ J Pub Health.* 2002;26(3):251-5.

[93] Petersen MB, Brondum-Nielsen K, Hansen LK, Wulff K. Clinical, cytogenetic, and molecular diagnosis of Angelman syndrome: estimated prevalence rate in a Danish county. *Am J Med Genet.* 1995 Jun 19;60(3):261-2.

[94] Vogels A, Van Den Ende J, Keymolen K, Mortier G, Devriendt K, Legius E, *et al.* Minimum prevalence, birth incidence and cause of death for Prader-Willi syndrome in Flanders. *Eur J Hum Genet.* 2004 Mar;12(3):238-40.

[95] Õiglane-Shlik E, Talvik T, Žordania R, Põder H, Kahre T, Raukas E, *et al.* Prevalence of Angelman syndrome and Prader-Willi syndrome in Estonian children: Sister syndromes not equally represented. *Am J Med Genet.* 2006 Sep 15;140A(18):1936-43.

[96] Jiang Y, Lev-Lehman E, Bressler J, Tsai TF, Beaudet AL. Genetics of Angelman syndrome. *Am J Hum Genet.* 1999 Jul;65(1):1-6.

[97] Varela MC, Kok F, Otto PA, Koiffmann CP. Phenotypic variability in Angelman syndrome: comparison among different deletion classes and between deletion and UPD subjects. *Eur J Hum Genet.* 2004 Dec;12(12):987-92.

[98] Runte M, Farber C, Lich C, Zeschnigk M, Buchholz T, Smith A, *et al.* Comprehensive methylation analysis in typical and atypical PWS and AS patients with normal biparental chromosomes 15. *Eur J Hum Genet.* 2001 Jul;9(7):519-26.

[99] Emerson E. Underweight, obesity and exercise among adults with intellectual disabilities in supported accommodation in Northern England. *J Intellect Disabil Res.* 2005 Feb;49(Pt 2):134-43.

[100] Rimmer JH, Yamaki K. Obesity and intellectual disability. *Ment Retard Dev Disabil Res Rev.* 2006;12(1):22-7.

[101] Marshall D, McConkey R, Moore G. Obesity in people with intellectual disabilities: the impact of nurse-led health screenings and health promotion activities. *J Adv Nurs.* 2003 Jan;41(2):147-53.

[102] Holland AJ, Whittington JE, Butler J, Webb T, Boer H, Clarke D. Behavioural phenotypes associated with specific genetic disorders: evidence from a population-based study of people with Prader-Willi syndrome. *Psychol Med.* 2003 Jan;33(1):141-53.

[103] Vestergaard P, Kristensen K, Bruun JM, Ostergaard JR, Heickendorff L, Mosekilde L, *et al.* Reduced bone mineral density and increased bone turnover in Prader-Willi syndrome compared with controls matched for sex and body mass index--a cross-sectional study. *J Pediatr.* 2004 May;144(5):614-9.

[104] Lewis JN, Tonge BJ, Mowat DR, Einfeld SL, Siddons HM, Rees VW. Epilepsy and associated psychopathology in young people with intellectual disability. *J Paediatr Child Health.* 2000 Apr;36(2):172-5.

[105] Balogh RS, Hunter D, Ouellette-Kuntz H. Hospital utilization among persons with an intellectual disability, Ontario, Canada, 1995-2001. *J Appl Res Intellect Disabil.* 2005;18:181-90.

[106] Miyawaki T, Kohjitani A, Maeda S, Egusa M, Mori T, Higuchi H, *et al.* Intravenous sedation for dental patients with intellectual disability. *J Intellect Disabil Res.* 2004 Nov;48(Pt 8):764-8.

[107] Australian Institute of Health and Welfare (AIHW). Australian Hospital Statistics 2000-01: *Canberra: AIHW*; 2002. AIHW Cat. No. HSE-20.

[108] Australian Institute of Health and Welfare (AIHW). Australian Hospital Statistics 2003-04: *Canberra: AIHW*; 2005. AIHW Cat. No. HSE 37.

[109] Patja K, Iivanainen M, Vesala H, Oksanen H, Ruoppila I. Life expectancy of people with intellectual disability: a 35-year follow-up study. *J Intellect Disabil Res.* 2000 Oct;44(Pt 5):591-9.

[110] Chaney RH, Eyman RK. Patterns in mortality over 60 years among persons with mental retardation in a residential facility. *Ment Retard.* 2000 Jun;38(3):289-93.

[111] O'Callaghan FJ, Osborne JP, Martyn CN. Epilepsy related mortality. *Arch Dis Child.* 2004 Aug;89(8):705-7.

[112] Beange H, Lennox N. Physical aspects of health in the learning disabled. *Curr Op Psychiatr.* 1998 Sept;11(5):531-4.

[113] Patja K, Molsa P, Iivanainen M. Cause-specific mortality of people with intellectual disability in a population-based, 35-year follow-up study. *J Intellect Disabil Res.* 2001 Feb;45(Pt 1):30-40.

[114] Strauss D, Cable W, Shavelle R. Causes of excess mortality in cerebral palsy. *Dev Med Child Neurol.* 1999 Sep;41(9):580-5.

[115] Reddihough DS, Baikie G, Walstab JE. Cerebral palsy in Victoria, Australia: mortality and causes of death. *J Paed Child Health.* 2001 Apr;37(2):183-6.
[116] Janicki MP, Dalton AJ, Henderson CM, Davidson PW. Mortality and morbidity among older adults with intellectual disability: health services considerations. *Disabil Rehab.* 1999 May-Jun;21(5-6):284-94.
[117] Hogg J, Lucchino R, Wang K, Janicki M. Healthy ageing - adults with intellectual disabilities: ageing and social policy. *J Appl Res Intellect Disabil.* 2001;14(3):229-55.
[118] Gustavson K-H, Umb-Carlsson O, Sonnander K. A follow-up study of mortality, health conditions and associated disabilities of people with intellectual disabilities in a Swedish county. *J Intellect Disabil Res.* 2005;49(12):905-14.
[119] Sutherland G, Couch MA, Iacono T. Health issues for adults with developmental disability. *Res Dev Disabil.* 2002 Nov-Dec;23(6):422-45.
[120] Laan LA, den Boer AT, Hennekam RC, Renier WO, Brouwer OF. Angelman syndrome in adulthood. *Am J Med Genet.* 1996 Dec 18;66(3):356-60.
[121] Laurance BM, Brito A, Wilkinson J. Prader-Willi Syndrome after age 15 years. *Arch Dis Child.* 1981 Mar;56(3):181-6.
[122] Greenswag LR. Adults with Prader-Willi syndrome: a survey of 232 cases. *Dev Med Child Neurol.* 1987;29(2):145-52.
[123] Carpenter PK. Prader-Willi syndrome in old age. *J Intellect Disabil Res.* 1994 Oct;38(Pt 5):529-31.
[124] Walsh PN. Ageing and mental retardation. *Curr Op Psychiatr.* 2002;15:509-14.
[125] Leveille SG, Guralnik JM, Ferrucci L, Langlois JA. Aging successfully until death in old age: opportunities for increasing active life expectancy. *Am J Epidem.* 1999 Apr 1;149(7):654-64.
[126] Temple VA, Walkley JW. Physical activity of adults with intellectual disability. *J Intellect Dev Disabil.* 2003;28(4):342-52.
[127] Holland AJ. Ageing and learning disability. *Br J Psychiatr.* 2000 Jan;176:26-31.
[128] Stanish HI, Temple VA, Frey GC. Health-promoting physical activity of adults with mental retardation. *Ment Retard Dev Disabil Res Rev.* 2006;12(1):13-21.
[129] Clayton-Smith J. Clinical research on Angelman syndrome in the United Kingdom: observations on 82 affected individuals. *Am J Med Genet.* 1993 Apr 1;46(1):12-5.
[130] Leitner RP, Smith A. An Angelman syndrome clinic: report on 24 patients. *J Paediatr Child Health.* 1996 Apr;32(2):94-8.
[131] Leeder SR, Dominello A. Health, equity and intellectual disability. *J Appl Res Intellect Disabil.* 2005;18:97-100.
[132] Melville C. Discrimination and health inequalities experienced by disabled people. *Med Edu.* 2005 Feb;39(2):124-6.
[133] Walsh KK, Kastner TA. Quality of health care for people with developmental disabilities: the challenge of managed care. *Ment Retard.* 1999 Feb;37(1):1-15.
[134] Melville CA, Finlayson J, Cooper SA, Allan L, Robinson N, Burns E, *et al.* Enhancing primary health care services for adults with intellectual disabilities. *J Intellect Disabil Res.* 2005 Mar;49(Pt 3):190-8.
[135] Hogg J. Essential healthcare for people with learning disabilities: barriers and opportunities. *J R Soc Med.* 2001 Jul;94(7):333-6.
[136] Lunsky Y, Reiss S. Health needs of women with mental retardation and developmental disabilities. *Am Psychol.* 1998 Mar;53(3):319.

[137] Evenhuis HM. Medical aspects of ageing in a population with intellectual disability: III. Mobility, internal conditions and cancer. *J Intellect Disabil Res.* 1997 Feb;41(Pt 1):8-18.

[138] NSW Council for Intellectual Disability. Health and People with Intellectual Disability. Position Paper 2004 [cited 21-07-2006]; Available from: http://www.nswcid.org.au/systemic/position/health.html

[139] Iacono T, Johnson H. Patients with disabilities and complex communication needs. The GP consultation. *Aust Fam Phys.* 2004 Aug;33(8):585-9.

[140] Lennox N, Eastgate G. Adults with intellectual disability and the GP. *Aust Fam Phys.* 2004 Aug;33(8):601-6.

[141] Lennox NG, Diggens J, Ugoni A. Health care for people with an intellectual disability: General Practitioners' attitudes, and provision of care. *J Intellect Dev Disabil.* 2000;25(2):127-33.

[142] Beange H, McElduff A, Baker W. Medical disorders of adults with mental retardation: a population study. *Am J Ment Retard.* 1995 May;99(6):595-604.

[143] Timehin C, Timehin E. Prevalence of hearing impairment in a community population of adults with learning disability: access to audiology and impact on behaviour. *Br J Learn Disabil.* 2004;32:128-32.

[144] Lewis MA, Lewis CE, Leake B, King BH, Lindemann R. The quality of health care for adults with developmental disabilities. *Public Health Reports.* 2002 Mar-Apr;117(2):174-84.

[145] Parish SL, Saville AW. Women with cognitive limitations living in the community: evidence of disability-based disparities in health care. *Ment Retard.* 2006 Aug;44(4):249-59.

[146] Haveman MJ, van Berkum G, Reijnders R, Heller T. Differences in service needs, time demands, and caregiving burden among parents of persons with mental retardation across the life cycle. *Fam Relat.* 1997;46(4):417-25.

[147] Hodapp RM, Fidler DJ, Smith AC. Stress and coping in families of children with Smith-Magenis syndrome. *J Intellect Disabil Res.* 1998 Oct;42(Pt 5):331-40.

[148] Hodapp RM, Dykens EM, Masino LL. Families of children with Prader-Willi syndrome: stress-support and relations to child characteristics. *J Autism Dev Disord.* 1997 Feb;27(1):11-24.

[149] Dyson LL. Fathers and mothers of school-age children with developmental disabilities: parental stress, family functioning, and social support. *Am J Ment Retard.* 1997 Nov;102(3):267-79.

[150] Freedman RI, Griffiths D, Krauss MW, Seltzer MM. Patterns of respite use by aging mothers of adults with mental retardation. *Ment Retard.* 1999 Apr;37(2):93-103.

[151] Epel ES, Blackburn EH, Lin J, Dhabhar FS, Adler NE, Morrow JD, *et al.* Accelerated telomere shortening in response to life stress. *Proc Natl Acad Sci U S A.* 2004 Dec 7;101(49):17312-5.

[152] Chen SC, Ryan-Henry S, Heller T, Chen EH. Health status of mothers of adults with intellectual disability. *J Intellect Disabil Res.* 2001 Oct;45(Pt 5):439-49.

[153] Ensel WM, Lin N. The life stress paradigm and psychological distress. *J Health Soc Behav.* 1991 Dec;32(4):321-41.

[154] Bigby C, Ozanne E, Gordon M. Facilitating transition: elements of successful case management practices for older parents of adults with intellectual disability. *J Gerontol Soc Work.* 2002;37(3/4):25-43.

[155] Llewellyn G, Dunn P, Fante M, Turnbull L, Grace R. Family factors influencing out-of-home placement decisions. *J Intellect Disabil Res.* 1999 Jun;43(Pt 3):219-33.

[156] Heller T, Caldwell J. Supporting aging caregivers and adults with developmental disabilities in future planning. *Ment Retard.* 2006 Jun;44(3):189-202.

[157] Blacher J, Baker BL, Feinfield KA. Leaving or launching? Continuing family involvement with children and adolescents in placement. *Am J Ment Retard.* 1999 Sep;104(5):452-65.

[158] Duvdevany I, Ben-Zur H, Ambar A. Self-determination and mental retardation: is there an association with living arrangement and lifestyle satisfaction? *Ment Retard.* 2002 Oct;40(5):379-89.

[159] Young L, Ashman AF. Deinstitutionalization for older adults with severe mental retardation: results from Australia. *Am J Ment Retard.* 2004 Sep;109(5):397-412.

[160] Lakin KC, Prouty R, Polister B, Coucouvanis K. Selected changes in residential service systems over a quarter century, 1977-2002. *Ment Retard.* 2003 Aug;41(4):303-6.

[161] Hallam A, Knapp M, Jarbrink K, Netten A, Emerson E, Robertson J, *et al.* Costs of village community, residential campus and dispersed housing provision for people with intellectual disability. *J Intellect Disabil Res.* 2002 Jun;46(Pt 5):394-404.

[162] Knapp M, Comas-Herrera A, Astin J, Beecham J, Pendaries C. Intellectual disability, challenging behaviour and cost in care accommodation: what are the links? *Health Soc Care Comm.* 2005 Jul;13(4):297-306.

[163] Fillary R, Pernice R. Workplace culture analysis where people with intellectual disabilities work: a case study approach. *J Intellect Dev Disabil.* 2005 September;30(3):176-80.

[164] Young L, Sigafoos J, Suttie J, Ashman A, Grevell P. Deinstitutionalisation of persons with intellectual disabilities: a review of Australian studies. *J Intellect Dev Disabil.* 1998;23(2):155-70.

[165] Cinamon RG, Gifsh L. Conceptions of Work Among Adolescents and Young Adults With Mental Retardation. *Career Dev Q.* 2004 Mar 2004;52(3):212.

[166] Aspray TJ, Francis RM, Tyrer SP, Quilliam SJ. Patients with learning disability in the community. *Br Med J.* 1999 Feb 20;318(7182):476-7.

[167] Duvdevany I, Arar E. Leisure activities, friendships, and quality of life of persons with intellectual disability: foster homes vs community residential settings. *Int J Rehab Res.* 2004 Dec;27(4):289-96.

[168] Taanila A, Rantakallio P, Koiranen M, von Wendt L, Jarvelin MR. How do persons with intellectual disability manage in the open labour markets? A follow-up of the Northern Finland 1966 Birth Cohort. *J Intellect Disabil Res.* 2005 Mar;49(Pt 3):218-27.

[169] Reid PM, Bray A. Paid work and intellectual disability. *J Intellect Dev Disabil.* 1997;22(2):87-96.

[170] Wadsworth JS, McBrien DM, Harper DC. Vocational guidance and employment of persons with a diagnosis of Prader-Willi syndrome. *J Rehab.* 2003;69(1):15-21.

[171] Haig D. Intragenomic politics. *Cytogenet Genome Res.* 2006;113(1-4):68-74.

[172] Isles AR, Humby T. Modes of imprinted gene action in learning disability. *J Intellect Disabil Res.* 2006 May;50(Pt 5):318-25.

[173] Belinsky SA, Nikula KJ, Palmisano WA, Michels R, Saccomanno G, Gabrielson E, *et al.* Aberrant methylation of p16(INK4a) is an early event in lung cancer and a potential biomarker for early diagnosis. *Proc Natl Acad Sci U S A.* 1998 Sep 29;95(20):11891-6.

[174] DeBaun MR, Niemitz EL, Feinberg AP. Association of in vitro fertilization with Beckwith-Wiedemann syndrome and epigenetic alterations of LIT1 and H19. *Am J Hum Genet.* 2003 Jan;72(1):156-60.

[175] Gilchrist D, Glerum DM, Wevrick R. Deconstructing Mendel: new paradigms in genetic mechanisms. *Clin Investigat Med.* 2000 Jun;23(3):188-98.

[176] Horsthemke B. Epimutations in human disease. *Curr Top Microbiol Immunol.* 2006;310:45-59.

[177] Laan LA, v Haeringen A, Brouwer OF. Angelman syndrome: a review of clinical and genetic aspects. *Clin Neurol Neurosurg.* 1999 Sep;101(3):161-70.

[178] Moncla A, Malzac P, Livet MO, Voelckel MA, Mancini J, Delaroziere JC, *et al.* Angelman syndrome resulting from UBE3A mutations in 14 patients from eight families: clinical manifestations and genetic counselling. *J Med Genet.* 1999 Jul;36(7):554-60.

[179] Moncla A, Malzac P, Voelckel MA, Auquier P, Girardot L, Mattei MG, *et al.* Phenotype-genotype correlation in 20 deletion and 20 non-deletion Angelman syndrome patients. *Eur J Hum Genet.* 1999 Feb-Mar;7(2):131-9.

[180] Sandanam T, Beange H, Robson L, Woolnough H, Buchholz T, Smith A. Manifestations in institutionalised adults with Angelman syndrome due to deletion. *Am J Med Genet.* 1997 Jun 27;70(4):415-20.

[181] Smith A, Wiles C, Haan E, McGill J, Wallace G, Dixon J, *et al.* Clinical features in 27 patients with Angelman syndrome resulting from DNA deletion. *J Med Genet.* 1996 Feb;33(2):107-12.

[182] Webb T, Whittington J, Clarke D, Boer H, Butler J, Holland A. A study of the influence of different genotypes on the physical and behavioral phenotypes of children and adults ascertained clinically as having PWS. *Clin Genet.* 2002 Oct;62(4):273-81.

[183] Fridman C, Varela MC, Kok F, Setian N, Koiffmann CP. Prader-Willi syndrome: genetic tests and clinical findings. *Genet Test.* 2000;4(4):387-92.

In: Focus on Mental Retardation Research
Editor: Marina I. Carson, pp. 77-134
ISBN: 978-1-60021-647-3

Chapter 4

MOLECULAR MECHANISMS OF MENTAL RETARDATION IN DOWN SYNDROME

Rachidi Mohammed [*,1,2] ***and Lopes Carmela*** [1,2]
[1]Laboratory of Genetic dysregulation models: Trisomy 21 and Hyperhomocysteinemia, EA 3508, University Paris 7-Denis Diderot, Paris, France.
[2]University of French Polynesia, Dept of Sciences, Tahiti, French Polynesia.

ABSTRACT

Mental Retardation (MR) is a cognitive impairment affecting 3% of global population, characterized by subnormal intellectual functioning and impaired behavior. A large percent of individuals with mental deficiency have a significant chromosomal abnormality. Of these, Down syndrome (DS) is the major genetic cause of MR and contributes to about 30% of all moderate-to-severe cases of MR. This invalidating aspect of DS has hard impacts in public health and poses significant challenges for clinicians and scientists.

MR caused by trisomy 21 is mainly a consequence of brain developmental alterations in neurogenesis determined directly from the overexpression of the human chromosome 21 (HC21) gene products or indirectly from the interaction of these HC21 gene products with the whole genome, transcriptome and proteome. The Human genome project has delivered the complete DNA sequence allowing the HC21 gene identification. Molecular studies have been conducted to elucidate how trisomy 21 affects expression of these genes, by mRNA or protein quantifications. Gene dosage effect was found for some genes, but not for others for which there may be additional regulatory factors that override a mere gene dosage effect.

Actually, some genes are considered candidate genes for MR: *SIM2*, *DOPEY2* and *DYRK1A,* localized in the Down syndrome Critical Region 1 (DCR-1), and *SOD1*, *S100b* and *DSCR1,* localized outside the DCR-1. These candidate genes are overexpressed in the

* Corresponding Author: Dr. Rachidi Mohammed, BP 130228, Punaauia, Tahiti, French Polynesia.
E-mail address: mrachidi2@yahoo.fr

trisomic human and transgenic mouse brains, indicating their contribution in the pathogenesis of neurological alterations and MR in DS.

Two opposing hypotheses have been advanced to explain the molecular mechanism of the MR phenotype: "gene dosage effect" and "amplified developmental instability". According to the first hypothesis, the DS critical region DCR-1 was defined as the minimal interval of HC21 carrying a subset of triplicated dosage-sensitive genes directly responsible for this phenotype. The second hypothesis claims that dosage imbalance of hundreds of HC21 genes determine a non-specific genomic transcriptional regulation. This global disruption of the gene expression balance in pathways regulating brain development alters the normal developmental homeostasis and determines MR.

The MR may results from neurodevelopmental and biochemical primary alterations in the brain determined by the presence of 3 copies of HC21 genes. We hypothesize a global molecular mechanism in which dosage-dependent genes, expressed 1.5 fold the normal level as a direct consequence of the 1.5 gene dosage, could directly determine primary phenotypes in trisomic brain. Contrarily, some of these dosage-dependent genes could modulate the expression of target genes on the chromosome 21 or the others. The modulation of the target gene expression could be different of 1.5 fold up-regulation or could be down-regulated, determining a secondary gene dosage effect. In parallel, all or some HC21 genes showing expression changes, could participate to the amplified developmental instability of the genome in DS, determining a general gene expression disequilibrium that could also be responsible of primary phenotypes in the brain and participate to pathogenesis of MR.

Actually, the first molecular pathway for MR in DS is elucidated and involves two HC21 dosage-sensitive genes: DYRK1A and DSCR1. Both participate to the control of NFAT phosphorylation, determining converging effects on NFAT-depending gene activation pathways.

Drug treatment identifications for MR in DS need understanding of the molecular mechanisms underlying this cognitive phenotype. In this golden period for DS research, with the development of animal and molecular models, and new techniques for transcriptional regulation, we could hope to rescue the basic molecular defects giving rise to MR.

I. Introduction

a. Trisomy 21 or Down Syndrome

The first descriptions of the Trisomy 21 phenotype were by Esquirol (1838), Séguin (1846) and by Down (1866).

It took more than a century to discover the extra-chromosomal origin of the pathology commonly called Down syndrome or Trisomy 21 (Lejeune et al., 1958; 1959).

Trisomy 21 or Down syndrome is the most common autosomal trisomy, with an incidence of 1 in 700-800 live births, in comparison with other trisomies such as Trisomy 18 (1:3500) or Trisomy 13 (1:7000). However, its frequency is much higher at conception, given that up to 75% and 50% of Down syndrome fetuses identified during the first and second trimester, respectively, are lost before term (Morris et al., 1999; Spencer, 2001), while trisomy for some other autosomes nearly always resulting in prenatal loss (Hassold and Hunt,

2001). The relatively high frequency of postnatal survival for trisomy 21 is thought to be principally a function of the small number of genes on human chromosome 21, the smallest and the least gene-dense of the autosomes.

The most common origin of Trisomy 21 was a chromosomal non-disjunction during meiosis, more frequently in woman than in man. Moreover, the occurrence of the disorder increases significantly with advancing maternal age (Connor and Ferguson-Smith, 1997).

Down syndrome is characterized by complex phenotype affecting many different organs and tissues. It involves dysmorphic features, which collectively constitute its distinctive physical phenotype, endocardiac and immunological defects, haematological and endocrinal alterations, and hypotonia. Trisomy 21 is also a risk factor for a number of diseases. For example, it is among the leading causes of congenital heart diseases, some forms of which occur in about 50% of individuals with Down syndrome (Ferencz et al., 1989). The incidence of childhood onset leukemia and Hirschsprung disease are both significantly elevated in individuals with Trisomy 21, and metabolic disorders are also observed including a higher frequency of diabetes and obesity (Puffenberger et al, 1994; Epstein, 1995; Cohen, 1999).

Not all predisposing conditions caused by Trisomy 21 have a negative impact. Individuals with Down syndrome have reduced frequencies of solid tumors (Hasle, 2001; Yang et al., 2002) and have a lower incidence of atherosclerosis as well (Murdoch et al., 1977; Yla-Herttuala et al., 1989). Characterization of these effects could indicate approaches to reduce cancer incidence or cardiovascular disease in all people.

Neuropathology (mental retardation, increased occurrence of Alzheimer's disease), neuroanatomical and neurotransmitter alterations (Wisniewski and Bobinski, 1991; Epstein, 1995; Schneider et al., 1997; Risser et al., 1997) were also observed. Globally, more than one hundred clinical traits have been observed in Down syndrome, but high inter-individual differences characterize these patients (Antonarakis et al., 2004). For example, only about half of children with Down syndrome are born with congenital heart disease (Freeman et al., 1998). A few features occur to some degree in every individual with Trisomy 21, including characteristic facial dysmorphology, neurological alterations, and the histopathology of Alzheimer disease, which is present by the fourth decade.

b. Neuropathology in Down Syndrome and Mental Retardation

Mental retardation affects about 2% of global population. This condition was characterized by subnormal intellectual functioning, retardation and slowing down of the psychomotor development, decrease in learning capacity and impaired adaptive behaviour that become manifest during developmental years (Ohr and Fagen, 1994). A large percent of individuals with mental deficiency have a significant chromosomal abnormality.

Therefore, Down syndrome is the most frequent genetic non-heritable cause of mental retardation and contributes to about 30% of all moderate-to-severe cases of mental retardation (Lejeune, 1990; Stoll et al., 1990; Pulsifer, 1996), and has large individual and socio-economic consequences (Nicolaidis and Petersen, 1998).

All Down syndrome individuals are characterized by several neurological and behavioral phenotypes (Table 1), intensity of which can change in the different subjects. Overall, individuals with Down syndrome have invariably low intelligence quotient (IQ) and cognitive impairment, though the severity is highly variable (Nadel, 2003), and the mental retardation remains the invariable hallmark of this disorder and its more invalidating pathological aspect with a hard impact in the public health, also considering the increase of life expectancy of Down syndrome patients. The average IQ score for Down syndrome patients is around 50, with individual values ranging from 30 to 70 (Chapman and Hesketh, 2000; Vicari, 2004; 2006). The early infancy was characterized by a delayed cognitive development, leading to mild to moderate mental retardation. The IQ decreases in the first decade of life and, in the adolescent years, the cognitive function reaches a plateau that continues into adulthood (Brown et al., 1990).

The decline in cognitive performance that occurs in the adult life of Down syndrome patients has been interpreted as the consequence of accelerated aging which is very often, but non always, present in Down syndrome (Devenny et al., 1996; Lott and Head, 2005). It is known that the principal default responsible for mental retardation concerns the short-term memory rather than the learning process (Hulme and Mackenzie, 1992). Long-term memory deficits also characterize Down syndrome patients (Hodapp et al., 1999; Brown et al., 2003; Clark and Wilson, 2003).

It is known that maintaining spatial map requires intact long-term memory skills. Spatial long-term memory has been tested using a human version of the Morris water maze task used for rodents, in which animals used contextual cues in the environment to remember the location of a hidden platform. In the human test, a computer-generated virtual circular arena that had distinct objects on the walls that the child could use as a special map to orient himself to find a target hidden on the floor of the arena (Thomas et al., 2001). The results exhibit decline with age on measures of long-term memory, providing behavioral evidence of hippocampal dysfunction by adolescence (Carlesimo et al., 1997; Hyde and Crnic, 2001), consistent with the structural magnetic resonance imaging (MRI) finding of reduced hippocampal volumes in a small sample of adolescents with Down syndrome (Jernigan et al., 1993).

Learning can be complicated by a counterproductive style that includes avoidance strategies when faced with cognitive challenges (Wishart, 1995). Psychometric examinations of Down syndrome patients have shown that not all skills are affected in all persons or to the same extent (Crnic and Pennington, 2000; Krinsky-McHale et al., 2002; Laws, 2002; Pennington et al., 2003; Brown et al., 2003; Clark and Wilson, 2003; Vicari, 2006). Although all domains of development follow the usual sequence, a deficiency in language production relative to other areas of development often causes substantial impairment, and speech and articulation are also particularly affected. (Chapman et al., 1998). The forms of learning that depend on the hippocampus are particularly affected, and there is also evidence for impairment of prefrontal cortex and cerebellar function (Nadel, 2003).

In addition, Down syndrome children show continuous but gradual improvement in mental age throughout childhood. The IQ generally decline from early in the first year to late childhood (Hodapp and Zigler, 1990). Consequently, early implementation of special education programs results in improved cognitive abilities in Down syndrome individuals (Connolly et al., 1993). Children with Down syndrome have more behavioural and psychiatric problems than other children, but fewer than other individuals with mental retardation.

Table 1. Major Neurological and Behavioral Phenotypes in Down Syndrome

Down syndrome Neurological and Behavioral phenotypes	References
Altered neurogenesis, neuronal differentiation, myeliniztion and synaptogenesis	Coyle et al., 1986; Becker et al., 1991; Bahn et al., 2002
Early onset of Alzeimer disease-like neurohistopathology (fourth decade) Notable clinical signs and symtoms of Alzeimer disease	Dalton and Crapper-McLachlan, 1986
Hypoplasia of the hippocampus and cortex, larger parahippocampal gyrus	Weis et al., 1991; Wang et al., 1992; Raz et al., 1995; Teipel et al., 2003; Teipel et Hampel, 2006
Smaller cerebellum, reduced volume of Lobules VI to VIII	Jernigan et al., 1993; Raz et al., 1995; Aylward et al., 1997
Third ventricle enlargement	Schimmel et al., 2006
Retarded and disorganized fetal cortical lamination	Golden and Hyman, 1994
Neurodegeneration of basal forebrain cholinergic neurons BFCN	Yates et al., 1983; Casanova et al., 1985
Fetal microglial cells outnumber astroglial cells	Wierzba-Bobrowicz et al., 1999
Shortened basilar dendrites, decreased number of spines with altered morphology and defective several cortical layering	Marin-Padilla, 1976; Takashima et al., 1981; Becker et al., 1986; Takashima et al., 1994; Schmidt-Sidor et al., 1990
Delayed myelinization, fewer neurons, lower neuronal density, abnormal synaptic connection and spine length	Wisniewski and Schmidt-Sidor et al., 1989; Wisniewski, 1990
Neurotransmitter alterations with decrease of the choline acetyl-transferase, histidine decarboxylase, serotonine and glutamate	Wisniewski and Bobinski, 1991; Schneider et al., 1997; Risser et al., 1997
Low intelligence quotient (IQ) and cognitive impairment	Brown et al., 1990; Nadel, 2003
Long-term memory deficits	Hodapp et al., 1999; Brown et al., 2003; Clark and Wilson, 2003
Deficiency in language production, speech and articulation	Chapman et al., 1998
Impairment of prefrontal cortex and cerebellar function	Nadel, 2003
More behavioural and psychiatric problems than other children; Increased prevalence of depression	Collacot et al., 1998

Adults with Down syndrome can have a similar prevalence of psychiatric problems to other people with intellectual disability. A raised frequency of psychiatric problems is also related to the increased prevalence of depression in people with Down syndrome. However, they seem to be protected from some psychiatric disorders such as personality disorder, schizophrenia and anxiety (Collacot et al., 1998).

The relationship between mental retardation and the trisomic condition of Down syndrome is complex. Changes in the neuropathology, neurochemistry, neurophysiology, and neuropharmacology of Down syndrome brains indicate that there is probably abnormal development and maintenance of central nervous system structure and function. It is widely accepted that mental retardation caused by Trisomy 21 is mainly a consequence of brain developmental alterations in neurogenesis, neuronal differentiation, myelination and synaptogenesis (Coyle et al., 1986; Becker et al., 1991; Bahn et al., 2002).

The central nervous system is affected in Down syndrome, resulting in neurological phenotypes. An early onset of an Alzheimer disease-like neurohistopathology was systematically observed by the fourth decade. Clinical signs and symptoms of Alzheimer's disease are noted in 75% of such individuals over 60 years of age (Dalton and Crapper-McLachlan, 1986).

It is well known that hippocampal formation is critical for certain aspects of spatial cognition, including spatial learning (Black et al., 1977). The hippocampus is also assumed to play a broader role in learning about the contexts within animals and people experience events (Nadel and Willner, 1980), and hence to be essential to episodic memory (Milner et al., 1998). The hippocampal formation includes the entorhinal cortex in addition to the proper hippocampal structures. The entorhinal cortex directly exchanges projections with hippocampal pyramidal cells and the adjacent anatomically related perirhinal cortex. All these structures are part of the medial temporal-lobe system working as control center of the memory circuits (Milner et al., 1998). Thus, alterations observed in this region could be the origin of mental retardation in trisomic patients, but the altered cortical layer and cerebellum also may participate to cognitive and behavioral phenotypes in Down syndrome (Funahashi et al., 2004).

Morphological abnormalities start to be apparent in brains of newborns and older infants with DS, involving hypoplasia of the hippocampus and cortex, larger parahippocampal gyrus (Weis et al., 1991; Wang et al., 1992; Raz et al., 1995; Teipel et al., 2003; Teipel and Hampel, 2006), and third ventricle enlargement (Schimmel et al., 2006). Cerebellum also appeared smaller than average cerebellar volume in persons with Down syndrome (Jernigan et al., 1993; Raz et al., 1995; Aylward et al., 1997), and more particularly it shows a relative reduction in volume of lobules VI to VIII of subjects with Down syndrome, without any appreciable differences in other regions of the cerebellar vermis.

Stereological cell counting techniques revealed that the second phase of cortical development and the emergence of lamination are both delayed and disorganized in fetal Down syndrome brain (Golden and Hyman 1994).

Young persons with Down syndrome appear to be born with a normal septohippocampal cholinergic system (Kish et al., 1989), but an aging-dependent neurodegeneration of the Basal Forebrain Cholinergic Neurons (BFCN) was observed (Yates et al., 1983, Casanova et al., 1985). Because BFCN provide the major cholinergic input to the hippocampus and neocortex, the degeneration of these neurons may have functional consequences at level of cholinergic receptors. These dysfunctions could produce additional learning and memory deficits in older individuals with Down syndrome (Yates et al., 1983) and could be an outgrowth of the Alzheimer disease in these patients.

In addition, although the emergence and morphology of microglial cells appear not to differ from those in normal fetuses, microglial cells outnumber astroglial cells in fetal Down syndrome brain (Wierzba-Bobrowicz et al. 1999). They have shortened basilar dendrites, a decreased number of spines with altered morphology and defective cortical layering in several cortical areas (Marin-Padilla, 1976; Takashima et al., 1981; Becker et al., 1986; Schmidt-Sidor et al., 1990; Takashima et al., 1994). In addition, relatively delayed myelination, fewer neurons, lower neuronal density and distribution, abnormal synaptic connection and spine length have been revealed (Wisniewski and Schmidt-Sidor, 1989; Wisniewski, 1990). A series of biochemical alterations also occurs in fetal Down syndrome brain, which could serve as substrates for the morphological changes (Engidawork and Lubec, 2003), which involve a decrease of the choline acetyltransferase and histidine decarboxylase activities and also a decrease of serotonine, histamine, and glutamate levels (Wisniewski and Bobinski, 1991; Schneider et al., 1997; Risser et al., 1997).

Individuals with Down syndrome exhibit disturbances in the dynamics of movement production and postural control that are thought to have a significant impact in delaying their motor skill acquisition. The origin of these deficits has been attributed initially to hypotonia, but cerebellar abnormalities may be responsible for this motor impairment (Shumway-Cook and Woollacott, 1985).

II. Molecular Genetics of Down Syndrome

In most cases, Down syndrome results of an extracopy of chromosome 21 in all cells of the afflicted individuals (Lejeune et al., 1959). The most commonly accepted hypothesis for the molecular origin of Down syndrome is that the extra human chromosome 21 genes contribute to Down syndrome phenotypes (Antonarakis, 1998). Consequently, the Down syndrome may be considered as a multifactorial disease with an unusual etiology. In fact, this pathology results neither from a gene deletion, point mutation, chimerism, transposable element insertion, or triple repeat expansion, but rather from the overdosage of genes on chromosome 21 and that could be responsible for the complex phenotype in Down syndrome patients.

In some rare cases accounting for no more than 1% of living trisomic persons, Down syndrome results from a partial trisomy 21 showing variable phenotypes depending to triplicated region. Clinical, cytogenetic and molecular analysis of such patients allowed narrowing a region of chromosomal 21, called Down syndrome Chromosomal Region-1 (DCR-1), at 21q22.2 sub-band, on the distal part of the long arm, containing probe D21S55, and flanked by probes D21S17 and ERG (Rahmani et al., 1989; Delabar et al., 1993; Crété et al., 1993; Korenberg et al., 1994). The duplication of the DCR-1 region is associated with the expression of many features of the disease, including short stature, joint hyperlaxity, hypotonia, skeletal abnormalities, and several morphological anomalies of the face, hand and foot, and contributes significantly to the mental retardation (Rahmani et al., 1989; Delabar et al., 1993; Korenberg et al., 1994).

Since the number of genes involved in Down syndrome pathogenesis remains undetermined, candidate genes for this pathology should be searched on the whole chromosome 21, and more particularly in the DCR-1 region. As a first step in gene identification, extensive efforts have been carried out to construct transcriptional maps, using exon trapping and cDNA selection methods, of the whole human chromosome 21 (Lucente et al. 1995; Yaspo et al., 1995; Chen et al., 1996) and particularly of the critical region DCR-1 allowing identification of 27 potential units, eight of which were known genes (Dahmane et al., 1998).

The completion of the human chromosome 21 sequence (Hattori et al., 2000), its transcriptional activity analysis (Kapranov et al., 2002), and the frequent update of the genomic sequence allowed identification of more than 350 gene in the whole chromosome 21 (Gardiner et al., 2003). But, the complete list is still not complete, and in addition, non coding protein RNAs and microRNAs will be described in the next years (Kampa et al., 2004).

a. Down Syndrome as a Gene Expression Disease

A fundamental question of genetic research in human diseases is to precisely define their specific phenotypes. This is a particularly important in Down syndrome or trisomy 21, which results from complex genetic effects on different tissues and functions during development. Moreover, these primary phenotypes, at cellular level, may have cumulative and interactive effects to produce final evident phenotypes in a given individual with trisomy 21. Other crucial question is to identify genes involved in Down syndrome phenotypes and their individual role in phenotype determination.

Primary and Secondary Gene Effects

The principal difficulty to identify candidate genes for Down syndrome depends of its unusual etiology, determined by the presence in Down syndrome patients of three copies of all or some genes located on chromosome 21 in all or some cells. This 1.5-fold increase in the dosage of genes on the trisomic chromosome 21 may determine a primary effect on gene expression consisting in a 1.5 fold increase of expression level.

Genes on the trisomic chromosome 21 coding transcription factors, scaffold proteins and other proteins that can directly or indirectly influence gene expression, could produce a secondary genome-wide transcriptional downstream misregulation. This secondary effect of the chromosomal imbalance, which may consist in gene overexpression different than 1.5 fold, and also in down-regulation, is complex and highly variable in the different cells and during lifespan. Moreover, the secondary effect can concern genes located on both chromosome 21 and the other chromosomes (Epstein, 1986; 1988; FitzPatrick, 2005). On chromosome 21, gene expression may be regulated by dosage compensation or other mechanisms such that only a subset of those genes is expressed at the expected 1.5 fold.

The indirect effects on genes located on other chromosomes are widely used in antenatal screening programs for trisomy 21, which detect abnormal levels of fetal proteins in maternal serum. Although, the genes encoding alpha fetoprotein and chorionic gonadotrophin map to 4q11–13 and 19q13, respectively, the level of alpha fetoprotein is reduced (Newby et al., 1997) while human chorionic gonadotrophin is increased (Aitken et al., 1993), in trisomy 21. Moreover, the effects of three copies of a gene may be even more complex at the protein level, as additional regulatory points are introduced, such as post-translational modifications that can alter the function or stability of the protein. Consequently, the presence of an extra gene does not necessarily lead to a gain of function.

It appears that the global effect of the gene over-dosage can produce complex effects by direct and indirect mechanisms to produce a specific and morbid effect on development and on adult functions. However, to explain the highly variable phenotypes in trisomic adults directly with the presence of three copies of individual genes appears to be simplistic. The initial genetic insult determines a trisomy-induced alteration of the phenotype in one cell can cause concomitant changes in gene expression in downstream cells. The changes in secondarily affected cells are undoubtedly a result of aneuploidy, but could represent a perfectly normal response, in terms of gene expression, to the signals received from the first, directly affected cell. Particularly in the brain, the mere presence of the chromosomal imbalance determines misexpression and interaction of genes/proteins that play crucial roles in neuromorphogenesis and neurogenic cascades. The developmental error caused by trisomy 21 during neural patterning and signal transduction pathways may lead to defective functioning neuronal circuitry and could be the biological mechanism responsible for the pathogenesis of mental retardation in Down syndrome.

The various Down syndrome phenotypes may be determined directly from the overexpression of human chromosome 21 gene products or indirectly from the interaction of these human chromosome 21 gene products with the whole genome, transcriptome and proteome. Two opposing hypotheses have been advanced to explain the molecular mechanisms of the Down syndrome pathogenesis, the gene dosage effect hypothesis and the amplified developmental instability hypothesis (Epstein, 1986; Pritchard and Kola, 1999).

Gene Dosage Effect Hypothesis

The first hypothesis, the "gene dosage effect hypothesis", holds that the phenotype is a direct result of the cumulative effects of the imbalance of the individual gene located on the triplicated chromosome or chromosomal region. In this hypothesis, the simplest model for gene action in Down syndrome is a single dosage-sensitive gene that acts by itself to produce a phenotype, independently of other genes.

According to this "dosage-sensitive genes" hypothesis, a subset of genes on a triplicated chromosome is directly responsible for particular pathological traits associated with trisomy 21. Consequently, the Down syndrome Critical Region 1, DCR-1, was defined as a minimal interval of chromosome 21 that carries the dosage-sensitive genes necessary and sufficient for generation of the typical features seen in Down syndrome individuals (Rahmani et al., 1989; Korenberg et al., 1990; 1994; Delabar et al., 1993). Several phenotypes of Down syndrome have been found also in transgenic mice engineered to express high levels of human chromosome 21 genes or their mouse orthologs. Interestingly, the observations of cardiac pathology, malformation of cerebellum with reduced granular cell density, the deficit of cognitive functions, or characteristic craniofacial dysmorphism, observed both in Down syndrome individuals and in mouse models, were in accord with the "dosage-sensitive gene" hypothesis.

However, it seems unlikely that some aspects of the Down syndrome phenotypes that show high variability and derive from changes in structures that are the product of a long span of development reflect the effects of a single dosage-sensitive gene. In addition, the attempts to delineate a unique Down syndrome critical region more precisely and to map the individual loci responsible for particular complex traits mostly failed (Korenberg et al., 1994), also considering the high variability observed in individual phenotypes. In addition, in a mouse model carrying three copy of lonely the DCR-1 minimal region, the typical cranio-facial dysmorphism was not observed (Olson et al., 2004a).

Amplified Developmental Instability Hypothesis

In contrast, the second hypothesis, "the amplified developmental instability hypothesis", claims that dosage imbalance of the hundreds of genes on chromosome 21 determines a non-specific disturbance of genomic regulation and expression. This global disruption of the correct balance of gene expression in pathways regulating development alters the normal developmental homeostasis and determines most manifestations of Down syndrome (Shapiro, 1983; 1997; Pritchard and Kola, 1999).

According to this hypothesis, features observed in Down syndrome also occur at large frequency albeit much lower in other trisomies and in the normal population. Also, the significantly increased individual variability among those with trisomy 21, as compared with euploid individuals, supports this hypothesis.

These two hypotheses are not necessarily mutually exclusive. It is possible that single genes may be involved in specific Down syndrome phenotypes, while some other Down syndrome phenotypes may be due to disturbances in gene dosage balance as a result of the extra chromosomal material (Antonarakis, 2001).

Other Gene Mechanisms in Trisomy 21

In addition to these two general hypotheses, other gene mechanisms, concerning the triplicated genes of the chromosome 21, alone or in combination with diploid genes on other chromosomes, could participate to determine specific Down syndrome phenotypes.

In the model of "interacting-genes of major effect", additive effects of multiple dosage-sensitive genes are hypothesized. The effects of multiple dosage-sensitive genes might be amplified (or attenuated) when they occur within the same biochemical pathway (Gardiner et al., 2004).

In the model of "heteroallelic disequilibrium", variation in the Down syndrome phenotype could also be due to heterogenic presence of different alleles of the chromosome 21. These allele differences can be responsible of additional variability of gene expression depending of gain- or loss-of-function of the alleles and of their relative ratio. Moreover, in the case of chromosome 21 gene products acting on genes on other chromosomes, their effect also can be different depending of the 2 allele combinations of the target genes.

In the model of "small effect genes", an individual triplicated gene might have no sufficient effect on other genes to result in a significant impact on phenotype (Shapiro, 1983; Prichard and Kola, 1999). This model is based on the comparison of quantifiable phenotypes in two animal models: Ts65Dn mice show behavioral, structural, and functional brain phenotypes, dysmorphology of the skull, and gene expression patterns that are similar but attenuated in Ts1Cje, carrying a reduced trisomic region with fewer triplicated genes (Richtsmeier et al., 2002; Kleschevnikov et al., 2004; Olson et al., 2004b; Siarey et al., 2005; Potier et al., 2006).

We have seen that most of the features that occur frequently in Down syndrome are variable in severity (expressivity) and, except for a few characteristic phenotypes, in frequency (penetrance). Moreover, none of the commonly described Down syndrome phenotypes are unique to Down syndrome or other chromosome abnormalities but also may occur in euploid individuals (Epstein, 2001). The increased frequency of these phenotypes in Down syndrome, including Alzheimer disease, suggests that predisposing "modifier genes" result in an observable phenotype by a threshold effect in trisomy 21.

b. Variation of Gene Expression in Down Syndrome

As a consequence of the particular etiology of Down syndrome, expression studies of genes in normal and Down syndrome patients are necessary to identify candidate genes and to evaluate gene contribution to the phenotypes.

Identification of gene expression pattern, obtained by Northern blot, RT-PCR, and in situ or whole-mount hybridization, allows selection of chromosome 21 genes potentially involved in a given Down syndrome phenotype. Therefore, a gene expressed in developing and/or adult brain could be selected as a candidate gene for mental retardation, particularly whether its transcription is restricted to key regions for cognitive functions, such as the hippocampal formation, the cortex and the cerebellum.

The "in vitro" techniques (Northern blot and RT-PCR) appear advantageous because of their rapidity and high sensibility (RT-PCR) and thus, their possibility to be applied to large-scale approach (Dahmane et al., 1998; Reymond et al., 2002). But their limitation remains their application to whole tissues, constituted of several cell types. Consequently, these techniques give global transcriptional information that, particularly for complex tissues, such as the brain, could supply large variations due to sample variation. This limitation was particularly influent for gene having a very restricted expression pattern.

In contrast, the in situ hybridization techniques have the advantage to allow detailed gene expression pattern analysis at cellular level. The identification of cell types expressing the studied gene supplies fundamental information to help understanding of gene function. In particular, studies of complete expression pattern in the brain of genes localized in the critical region DCR-1, such as *TPRD*, *SIM2*, *DOPEY2* and *DYRK1A*, during brain development in mouse (Dahmane et al., 1995; Rahmani et al., 1998; Lopes et al., 1999; 2003) and human (Rachidi et al., 2000; 2005a; 2006) appear particularly interesting to identify candidate genes for mental retardation in Down syndrome.

Although these techniques are more complex and time consuming than the in vitro ones, they have also been used in large-scale approach, to establish an expression atlas of the chromosome 21 genes (Gitton et al., 2002; Reymond et al., 2002; http://www.tigem.it/ch21exp/; http://chr21.molgen.mpg.de/hsa21/).

The two "in vitro" techniques, Northern blot and RT-PCR, give quantitative (real time RT-PCR) or semi-quantitative findings, which are very interesting in comparative analyses between normal and trisomic tissues (Table 2). In addition, some improved protocols of the in situ hybridization techniques have been obtained allowing expression level quantification to study expression variation in trisomic brains compared to normal ones (Lopes et al., 2003; Rachidi et al., 2005b) (Table 2).

Table 2. Expression variations of genes involved in brain development and function

Genes	Expression changes	References
ADAMTS1	+ (RNA, Protein)	Saran et al., 2003; Lyle et al. 2004; Miguel et al., 2005
APP	+	Epstein, 2001; Lyle et al. 2004
BACE2	+	Lyle et al. 2004
BACH1	+	Lyle et al. 2004
COL6A1	+	Mao et al., 2005

Table 2. (Continued)

Genes	Expression changes	References
DSCR1	+	Fuentes et al., 2000; Amano et al., 2004 Lyle et al. 2004; Dauphinot et al., 2005
Ets2	+	Saran et al., 2003; Lyle et al. 2004; Dauphinot et al., 2005
GART	+	Saran et al., 2003; Lyle et al. 2004; Dauphinot et al., 2005
GRIK1	-	Saran et al., 2003
HMGN1	+ (RNA, Protein)	Epstein, 2001; Saran et al., 2003; Amano et al., 2004; Lyle et al. 2004; Dauphinot et al., 2005
Ifnar2	+	Chrast et al., 2000a; Saran et al., 2003; Lyle et al. 2004
Ifnar1	+	Saran et al., 2003; Dauphinot et al., 2005
Ifngr2	+	Chrast et al., 2000a; Saran et al., 2003; Amano et al., 2004; Lyle et al. 2004; Mao et al., 2005
Intersectin	+	Pucharcos et al., 1999; Amano et al., 2004; Lyle et al. 2004
OLIG1	+	Lyle et al. 2004
OLIG2	+	Lyle et al. 2004
PCP4	+	Saran et al., 2003; Amano et al., 2004; Lyle et al. 2004
S100b	+ (RNA, Protein)	Griffin et al., 1998; Epstein, 2001;
SOD1	+ (RNA, Protein)	de Haan et al., 1997; Saran et al., 2003; Lyle et al. 2004; Kadota et al., 2004; Mao et al., 2005
Synaptojanin	+ (RNA, Protein)	Arai et al., 2002; Lyle et al. 2004
DCR-1 genes		
CBR1	+	Saran et al., 2003; Amano et al., 2004; Lyle et al. 2004
CBR3	+	Lyle et al. 2004
CLDN14	+	Lyle et al. 2004
DOPEY2	+	Lopes et al., 2003; Lyle et al. 2004; Rachidi et al., 2005b
DSCR3	+	Saran et al., 2003; Amano et al., 2004; Lyle et al. 2004; Mao et al., 2005; Dauphinot et al., 2005
DYRK1A	+	Guimera et al., 1999; Saran et al., 2003; Lyle et al. 2004
ERG	+	Lyle et al. 2004
HLCS	+	Lyle et al. 2004
KCNJ6/GIRK2	+	Lyle et al. 2004; Harashima et al., 2006
KCNJ15	+	Lyle et al. 2004
MORC3	+	Lyle et al. 2004
PIGP/DSCR5	+ (RNA, Protein)	Amano et al., 2004; Lyle et al. 2004; Ferrando-Miguel et al., 2004
SIM2	+	Vialard et al., 2000; Lyle et al. 2004
TTC3	+	Saran et al., 2003; Amano et al., 2004; Lyle et al. 2004

In the last years, the human genome sequencing project delivered the complete DNA sequence of our species (Lander et al., 2001; Venter et al., 2001; International Human Genome Sequencing Consortium, 2004) and in particular of the chromosome 21 (Hattori et al., 2000). Numerous data mining tools allowed gene identification, prediction, annotation and precise localization. The availability of these data promises breakthroughs in understanding of human pathologies. Important progresses could be particularly expected in regard to multifactorial pathologies, determined by interactions of a variable number of genes and characterized by complex phenotypes. Between the multifactorial pathologies, Down syndrome had beneficed of these advances, with the identification of the chromosome 21 genes, in particular in the critical region DCR-1.

In this way, whole-genome approaches (transcriptome) have been used in different groups to study gene expression variations in trisomic tissues compared to the euploid ones (Chrast et al., 2000a; FitzPatrick et al., 2002; Saran et al., 2003; Mao et al., 2003; 2005; Amano et al., 2004; Wang et al., 2004; Lyle et al., 2004; Kahlem et al., 2004). These works used microarrays or Serial Analysis of Gene Expression (SAGE), and comparisons between euploid and trisomic tissues have been performed using human tissues or cell lines, and also mouse trisomic model tissues and their non-trisomic littermates. Transcriptome studies of brain, cerebellum or neuronal cell lines appeared particularly abundant, considering the major interest in understanding of the mechanisms involved in mental retardation pathogenesis in Down syndrome (Chrast et al., 2000a; Mao et al., 2003; 2005; Saran et al., 2003; Amano et al., 2004; Kahlem et al., 2004; Dauphinot et al., 2005) (Table 2).

Globally, these works showed complex transcriptome changes, with increased expression of several genes on the chromosome 21, and on other chromosomes. These observations confirm that transcript levels are elevated about 1.5-fold for the majority of trisomic genes (Table 2) in a few tissues from humans with trisomy 21 (FitzPatrick et al., 2002; Mao et al., 2003; 2005) and across a broad range of tissues in trisomic mouse models (Kahlem et al., 2004; Lyle et al., 2004). Other genes were overexpressed at different ratios and some genes show decreased expression (Table 2).

Interestingly, the level of the expression variation for a given gene can change in the different tissues, including the brain. In addition, not only trisomic genes show altered expression in tissues from individuals with Trisomy 21, and perturbation of gene expression levels has been demonstrated to extend beyond trisomic genes to those that are disomic, affecting expression levels of a substantial proportion of transcripts in trisomic tissues in mice (Saran et al., 2003; Dauphinot et al., 2005).

Variability of the used techniques, samples, and statistical methods does not allow yet understanding of transcriptional response to gene-dosage. Improvement of these techniques is in progress and they promise global understanding of gene-dosage response mechanisms.

c. Candidate Genes for Mental Retardation in Down Syndrome

Down syndrome may be regarded as a complex trait where the ultimate phenotypes could represent the epistatic and synergistic effects of overdosage of many genes, particularly those localized in the Down syndrome critical region DCR-1.

At this day, some genes have been studied as candidates for neurological Down syndrome phenotypes: DYRK1A (Smith et al., 1997; Altafaj et al., 2001), SIM2 (Chrast et al., 2000b; Vialard et al., 2000; Rachidi et al., 2005a), TPRD (Lopes et al., 1999; Rachidi et al., 2000), GIRK2 (Lesage et al., 1994; Gosset et al., 1997; Ohira et al., 1997; Rachidi et al., unpublished data) and DOPEY2 (Lopes et al., 2003; Rachidi et al., 2005b; 2006).

These genes were considered as good candidate genes for mental retardation in Down syndrome because of their strong expression in the brain regions that play crucial roles in cognitive functions and, in addition, are altered in Down syndrome patients. Consequently, studies of these candidate genes and of the effects of their overexpression may help understanding of the developmental brain alterations in Down syndrome.

GIRK2

KCNJ6 or GIRK2 (Lesage et al., 1994; Gosset et al., 1997; Ohira et al., 1997) encodes the G-protein coupled inward rectifying potassium channel subunit 2, a member of the ATP-sensitive potassium channels, also called K(ATP) channels, that are involved in increase in the intracellular ATP concentration of the cell, linking cellular metabolism to the electrical excitability of the plasma membrane.

GIRK2 mutation was responsible of the weaver phenotype in mouse (Lane, 1964; Patil et al., 1995), characterized by a cerebellum drastically reduced in size due to depletion of granular cell neurons. It is highly expressed in human fetal and adult mouse brain, particularly in the cerebellum, suggesting a role of Girk2 in normal and abnormal granule cell differentiation (Goldowitz and Smeyne, 1995; Rachidi et al., unpublished data).

In Ts65Dn, a Down syndrome mouse model, GIRK2 is overexpressed in the brain, particularly in the hippocampus (Lyle et al., 2004; Harashima et al., 2006) (Table 2), and determines an increase of GIRK channel density in Ts65Dn neurons and a 2 fold increase of GABAB-mediated GIRK current (Best et al., 2006). The GIRK2 overexpression seems to alter the GIRK1/GIRK2 ratio which likely affects the balance between excitatory and inhibitory neuronal transmission in Ts65Dn and thus to contribute to Down syndrome neurophysiological phenotypes (Best et al., 2006; Harashima et al., 2006).

TPRD

TPRD gene (Tsukahara et al., 1996; Ohira et al., 1996; Dahmane et al., 1998) contains three units of a 34-amino acid repeat similar to the tetratricopeptide (TPR) motif (Sikorski et al. 1990), involved in protein-protein interactions (Das et al. 1998; Groves and Barford, 1999).

Very early in the mouse and human development, and during all lifespan, *TPRD* was strongly expressed throughout the nervous system, with regional and cellular specificity in the brain regions (Lopes et al., 1999; Rachidi et al., 2000). In particular, the higher expression found in the differentiating area than in the proliferating ones suggested a role of *TPRD* in neuronal cell differentiation. Moreover, *TPRD* was characterized by differential expression in human fetal and mouse adult brain regions (Lopes et al., 1999; Rachidi et al., 2000), showing different intensity in specific neuronal cell types as estimated by a novel microscopy technology allowing gene transcription quantification (Rachidi et al., 2000).

Interestingly, the specific expression in the hippocampus and cerebellum corresponds to abnormal brain regions seen in DS (Golden and Hyman, 1994; Raz et al., 1995). In addition, the strong *TPRD* expression in the cortex and its evolution from 13 to 22 weeks gestation corresponds to crucial developmental stage when the size of the cortical mantle doubles in thickness and the cortical lamination begins. This expression pattern suggests a potential role of *TPRD* in neuronal cell differentiation and in cortical lamination.

TPRD, also called *TTC3*, has been found overexpressed at more than 1.5 fold in trisomic tissues (Saran et al., 2003; Amano et al., 2004; Lyle et al. 2004; Rachidi and Lopes, unpublished data) (Table 2). It could be hypothesized that overexpression of *TPRD* in the brain could be involved in neuroanatomical alterations observed in DS patients, and participate to mental retardation pathogenesis.

SIM2

The *Drosophila* sim ortholog, encoding a transcription factor (Crews, 1998), is a master gene of midline development in the central nervous system, functioning as transcriptional regulator in cell fate determination (Crews et al., 1988; Thomas et al., 1988; Nambu et al., 1991). *Sim* gene encodes a transcription factor, member of the protein family containing bHLH (basic helix-loop-helix) and PAS (*Per*, ARNT and *Sim*) association domains (Muralidhar et al., 1993; Frank and Crews, 1994; Crews, 1998).

The mammalian *Sim2* (Dahmane et al., 1995) is expressed in early central nervous system in delimited regions of the neuroepithelium of D1 and D2 neuromeric region and along the neural tube (Dahmane et al., 1995; Ema et al., 1996; Fan et al., 1996; Rachidi et al., 2005a). In later fetal stages and in adults, several discrete brain regions, including the cortical layers, the hippocampus, and the cerebellum, express *SIM2* (Rachidi et al., 2005a; unpublished data). Interestingly, *SIM2* differential expression was observed in human fetal brain regions, showing different intensities in specific neuronal cell types (Rachidi et al., 2005a). The *SIM2*-expressing regions in human fetal brain (cortex, hippocampus, dentate gyrus and cerebellum) correspond to key brain structures involved in learning and memory processes (Milner et al., 1998; Krasuski, 2002; Ito, 2002; Dalley et al., 2004; Miyashita, 2004) that, moreover, are altered in Down syndrome patients (Golden and Hyman, 1994; Raz et al., 1995).

Sim2 is overexpressed in Ts1Cje mouse fetuses, a segmental trisomy 16 mouse model of Down syndrome (Vialard et al., 2000) and in human trisomic tissues (Rachidi and Lopes, unpublished data) (Table 2). Transgenic mice overexpressing *Sim2* display reduced sensitivity to pain and mild impairment of two learning tasks, the fear conditioning and the spatial water maze test (Ema et al., 1999; Chrast et al., 2000b), depending on the function of hippocampus (Morris et al., 1982; Kim and Fanselow, 1992). These behavioral anomalies found in the *Sim2* transgenic mice remembered some phenotypes observed in mouse models for Down syndrome, Ts65Dn and Ts1Cje (Coussons-Read and Crnic, 1996; Sago et al., 1998; Martinez-Cue et al., 1999), and in Down syndrome patients.

DOPEY2

C21orf5 (Dahmane et al., 1998), recalled recently *DOPEY2* (Rachidi et al., 2005b), is a member of the Dopey family that contains leucine zipper-like domains, involved in multiple protein-protein interactions.

Human and mouse embryos showed a very high expression level in the whole developing nervous system during embryogenesis, with a relatively lower intensity in telencephalon (Lopes et al., 2003; Rachidi et al., 2006). Moreover, *DOPEY2* was more intensely expressed in brain zones containing differentiating cells than in proliferation zones, suggesting a role of *DOPEY2* in cell differentiation and developmental patterning. This potential role was also supported by the high homology of *DOPEY2* with the *C. elegans Pad-1*, required for embryonic patterning during gastrulation (Guipponi et al., 2000), the yeast *Dop1* (Dujon, 1996) and *DopA* (Pascon and Miller, 2000), required for normal growth patterning, cell differentiation and organogenesis (Pascon and Miller, 2000).

During fetal development and in adult brain, this gene becomes surprisingly selective to the cerebellum, the hippocampus, and the cortex, with regional and cellular specifity, particularly in the hippocampal formation (Lopes et al., 2003; Rachidi et al., 2006). In addition, *DOPEY2* transcription appeared differentially expressed in these three fetal brain structures, as demonstrated by an improved new optic technology, allowing estimation of relative transcription activity by comparison of cell density and expression intensity (Rachidi et al., 2006). Interestingly, the three brain regions that express *DOPEY2* play key roles in learning and memory and could present neuronal alterations in Down syndrome patients (Weis et al., 1991; Golden and Hyman, 1994; Raz et al., 1995).

DOPEY2 is overexpressed (Table 2) in Down syndrome human lymphoblasts 1.5-2 fold than in normal lymphoblasts (Lopes et al., 2003), suggesting that *DOPEY2* is a dosage-sensitive gene, although the hypothesis that other overexpressed genes may regulated it cannot be excluded.

Independent lines of transgenic mice containing human YAC 230E8 have been created (Smith et al., 1995), containing the entire *DOPEY2* gene (Lopes et al., 2003; Rachidi et al., 2005b), and overexpressing it at less than 2 fold (Lopes et al., 2003; Rachidi et al., 2005b). These transgenic mice showed increased cortical cells (Smith et al., 1997; Rachidi et al., 2005b) that overexpressed *DOPEY2* (Rachidi et al., 2005b). This phenotype well corresponds to the abnormal lamination pattern found in the cortex of Down syndrome patients (Golden and Hyman, 1994). Moreover, these transgenic mice showed also mild impairment in learning and memory (Smith et al., 1997) that could be caused by the cortical abnormalities.

In addition, the three *DOPEY2*-expressing fetal brain structures, the cortex, the cerebellum and the hippocampal formation, play central roles in learning and memory. The medial temporal-lobe system, highly and differentially expressing *DOPEY2*, includes hippocampal formation and perirhinal cortex, and works as control centres of the memory circuits and storage (Milner et al., 1998; Krasuski 2002). The cortex and the cerebellum also participate in elaboration of memory (Ito, 2002; Dalley et al., 2004; Miyashita, 2004). The patterned differential expression of *DOPEY2* restricted to these key brain regions altered in DS brains, suggested a potential role of this gene in the pathogenesis of neuroanatomical and neurological alterations that could contribute to mental retardation in Down syndrome patients (Lopes et al., 2003; Rachidi et al., 2005b; 2006).

DYRK1A

DYRK1A (Tejedor et al., 1995), the human homolog of the *Drosophila minibrain* gene, *MNB*, encodes a serine-threonine kinase (Kentrup et al., 1996).

Drosophila MNB is involved in neuroblast proliferation, causing reduction of the adult brain, particularly at the level of the optic lobe and central brain and learning deficits and hypoactivity (Tejedor et al, 1995).

DYRK1A gene is expressed in several regions of the central nervous system, from early embryonic stages to adulthood, especially in the cortex, the hippocampus and the cerebellum (Guimera et al., 1996; Rahmani et al., 1998; Guimera et al., 1999). Overexpression of *DYRK1A* has been found in Down syndrome fetal brain and its murine homolog *Dyrk1A* is also overexpressed in Ts65Dn mice (Guimera et al., 1999; Saran et al., 2003; Lyle et al., 2004) (Table 2), a murine model partial trisomic for mouse chromosome 16 (Reeves et al., 1995).

Two transgenic mouse models overexpressing *DYRK1A* have been generated. The first, carried a human YAC, 152F7, containing *DYRK1A* (Smith et al., 1995); the second, carried the full-length *DYRK1A* cDNA (Altafaj et al., 2001). In the Morris water maze the two models show a significant impairment in spatial learning and memory, indicating hippocampal and prefrontal cortex function alteration. Using the reversal learning paradigm, reference memory appeared more particularly concerned in dysfunction (Smith et al., 1997; Altafaj et al., 2001). Moreover, the transgenic mice overexpressing *DYRK1A* exhibit delayed craniocaudal maturation with functional consequences in neuromotor development, and show altered motor skill acquisition and hyperactivity (Altafaj et al., 2001). These alterations are comparable with those found in the partial trisomy chromosome 16 murine models of Down syndrome and suggest a causative role of *DYRK1A* in mental retardation and in motor anomalies of Down syndrome.

But these genes alone did not explain entirely the complex Down syndrome phenotype, suggesting that overdosage of other genes on the chromosome 21 may participate in Down syndrome pathogenesis. At the time, some genes on chromosome 21, not localized in DCR-1, and over-expressed in fetal trisomic brains, are also considered candidate genes for mental retardation in Down syndrome: *SOD1* (Epstein et al., 1987), *APP* (Lamb et al., 1993), *ETS2* (Sumarsono et al., 1996), *S100b* (Reeves et al., 1994) and *DSCR1* (Fuentes et al., 1995).

SOD1

SOD1 gene encodes the Cu-Zn superoxide dismutase, a key enzyme in the metabolism of oxygen-derived free radicals. *SOD1* products, mRNA and protein, have been found at increased level in human and mouse trisomic tissues (Table 2) (de Haan et al., 1997; Saran et al., 2003; Lyle et al., 2004; Kadota et al., 2004; Mao et al., 2005). The enzymatic activity also is increased in fetal Down syndrome brain (Ani et al., 2000) and could alter the normal steady state equilibrium of reactive oxygen species, leading to oxidative injury.

Transgenic mice have been used as a model for investigating the effects of the increased level of this enzyme in Down syndrome and showed increased activity of *Sod1* (Epstein et al., 1987). Overexpression of *Sod1* in transgenic mice led to an apparently specific defect in distal motor neuron terminals, indicating that this gene can selectively affect motor neurons (Gurney et al., 1994).

Premature ageing, one of the characteristics of Down syndrome, may involve oxidative stress and impairment of proteasome activity. Transgenic mice overexpressing the human *SOD1* gene show a reduction in proteasome activities in the cortex of *SOD1* transgenic mice and an associated increase in the content of oxidized SOD1 protein (Le Pecheur et al., 2005).

APP and ETS2

The *APP* gene encodes the beta-amyloid precursor protein, centrally involved in senile plaque formation in Down syndrome and Alzheimer disease. In Down syndrome, beta-APP was expressed at more than the expected 1.5-fold (Table 2) (Epstein, 2001; Lyle et al., 2004) suggesting that other genes on chromosome 21 directly or indirectly can further up-regulate *APP* gene.

The transcription factor ETS2 transactivates *APP* gene (Wolvetang et al., 2003a). Fibroblasts overexpressing *ETS2*, display molecular abnormalities also seen in Down syndrome, such as elevated expression of APP protein and an increase in beta-amyloid production (Wolvetang et al., 2003a), suggesting that *ETS2* overexpression in Down syndrome determines overexpression of *APP* and that may play a role in the pathogenesis of the brain abnormalities in Down syndrome and Alzheimer disease.

ETS2, a protooncogene and transcription factor expressed in neurons, is overexpressed in Down syndrome (Table 2) (Saran et al., 2003; Lyle et al., 2004; Dauphinot et al., 2005). Transgenic mice overexpressing *Ets2* developed neurocranial and cervical skeletal abnormalities (Sumarsono et al. 1996), similarly to trisomy-16 mice and humans with Down syndrome, in which the gene dosage of *ETS2* is increased (Table 2). Overexpression of *ETS2* also results in apoptosis of neuronal cells (Wolvetang et al. 2003b), suggesting that overexpression of *ETS2* may contribute to the increased rate of apoptosis of neurons in Down syndrome. *ETS2* may have important consequences into therapeutic interventions in Down syndrome.

S100b

S100b protein is a calcium-binding protein found within astroglial cells, synthesized and released by astrocytes in response to serotonin (5-HT)-mediated stimulation of 5-HT1A receptors and appears to be an important extracellular neurotrophic agent during normal fetal brain development, with effects on neuroblasts and glia, involving the neuronal cytoskeleton (Azmitia et al., 1992).

Both *S100b* RNA and protein are expressed at high levels in brain of Down syndrome and Alzheimer disease patients (Griffin et al., 1998; Epstein 2001). S100b is overexpressed along all life in Down syndrome brain (Griffin et al. 1998). Its mRNA is also increased in fetal Down syndrome brain (Epstein 2001) (Table 2).

Both astrocytosis and neurite proliferation occurred in transgenic mice expressing elevated levels of *S100b* (Reeves et al. 1994). Transgenic mice overexpressing human *S100b* show changes in cytoskeletal markers (Shapiro et al., 2004), suggesting involvement of *S100b* overexpression in glial-neuronal interactions, aging and neuronal growth pathology, in Down syndrome and Alzheimer disease. Early over-expression of S100b may therefore indicate a potential role of this protein in dendritic abnormalities and mental retardation. More importantly, it can provide an important clue to the link between 5-HT and Down syndrome (Whitaker-Azmitia 2001).

S100b is a glial-derived protein that is a well-established biomarker for severity of neurological injury and prognosis for recovery. Transgenic mice overexpressing human S100b were significantly more susceptible to perinatal hypoxic ischemia, showing increased neuropathologic injury, and increased ischemic brain volume loss, by accelerating neuroinflammatory processes (Wainwright et al., 2004). *S100b* transgenic mice also showed a marked increased in glial fibrillary acidic protein (GFAP) consistent with heightened glial activation and neuro-inflammation in response to injury (Wainwright et al., 2004).

DSCR1

DSCR1, also called myocyte-enriched calcineurin-interacting protein 1 (MCIP1) or calcipressin 1 (CSP1), is a developmentally regulated gene involved in neurogenesis, showing significant expression in brain and spinal cord. Within the brain, *DSCR1* was predominantly expressed in neurons of the cerebral cortex, hippocampus, substantia nigra, thalamus, and medulla oblongata (Ermak et al., 2001). Moreover, *DSCR1* expression in the cerebral cortex and hippocampus of Alzheimer disease patients is approximately double than normal indivudals (Ermak et al. 2001).

DSCR1 have increased expression in the brains of young rats compared with adults (Fuentes et al., 1995) suggesting a role during central nervous system development, and its overexpression may contribute to brain abnormalities through inhibition of calcineurin-dependent gene transcription (Fuentes et al. 2000).

DSCR1 products, RNA and protein, are overexpressed in the brain of Down syndrome fetuses (Table 2) and interact physically and functionally with calcineurin A, the catalytic subunit of the Ca(2+)/calmodulin-dependent protein phosphatase PP2B (Fuentes et al., 1995; 2000; Amano et al., 2004).

DSCR1 protein has dephosphorylation activity on nuclear factor of activated T-cells (NFAT) and overexpression of DSCR1 inhibits calcineurin-dependent gene transcription through the inhibition of NFAT translocation to the nucleus (Arron et al., 2006). This result constitutes the first proved interaction between two genes on chromosome 21 and explains a molecular pathway involved in Down syndrome phenotypes (Arron et al., 2006). The second gene involved in this mechanism is *DYRK1A* showing phosphorylation activity on NFAT. Overexpression of *DYRK1A* determines phosphorylation increase of NFAT and its cytoplasmic localization (Arron et al., 2006).

Consequently, in trisomy 21, the combined overexpression of *DSCR1* and *DYRK1A* can have cooperative and interactive effects on the homeostasis of the regulatory circuit leading to reduced NFAT activity (Arron et al., 2006), determining several phenotypes in Down syndrome, particularly in the brain, and could be a primary cause of the mental retardation.

III. Mouse Models of Down Syndrome

In human, magnetic resonance spectroscopy provides an indirect view of neurotransmission, as it cannot detect the transmitters themselves, but only their metabolites. Because of these limitations, mouse models remain the best way for investigating the fine neuronal and cellular mechanisms involved in Down syndrome and most genetic disorders, and will continue to do so for a long time yet. Mouse models are powerful tools because of the ability to genetically manipulate their genome, the accessibility at any tissues and the high degree of genomic conservation between the mouse and human genomes.

Models of Down syndrome, of which the most useful models so far have been mice, can be used both to elucidate molecular and cellular pathogenesis and to link these abnormalities to an increased dose of a specific gene(s) (Davisson and Costa, 1999; Antonarakis et al., 2001; Dierssen et al., 2001; Reeves et al., 2001; Epstein, 2002). Since understanding of the impact of increased gene expression throughout development is essential in Down syndrome research, animal models play a critical role especially for correlating the direct and cascading effects of trisomic gene expression on development and function. An animal model to study Down syndrome needs two characteristics. First, the phenotype of the animal model must possess features that are relevant to Down syndrome. Second, the animal model should be trisomic for a gene or genes that are present on human chromosome 21.

Two possible approaches are possible in mouse model studies for Down syndrome. First, mice carrying the largest extra part of human chromosome 21 or of the syntenic region of the mouse genome can be generated to reproduce equivalent Down syndrome features in mice. The limitation of this approach remains the genetic complexity and the impossibility to analyze single gene effect in Down syndrome pathogenesis. Second, transgenic mice overexpressing a candidate gene allow identification of a major effect of this gene in cognitive impairment. In these models, the limitation is the loss of the eventual gene interactions, the additive or also epistatic effects that the overexpressed genes should establish to mimic the trisomy 21 phenotypes, particularly the mental retardation. Consequently, to study Down syndrome candidate genes and their involvement in neurological phenotypes and mental retardation, it is necessary to use different mouse models to obtain complementary results giving the most complete and faithful representation of the Down syndrome molecular genetics.

Mouse models of Down syndrome can be used because of the syntenies existing between human gene on chromosome 21 and mouse genes on chromosome 16 (~26.5 Mb), chromosome 10 (~2.3 Mb) and chromosome 17 (~1.1 Mb) (Table 3). Several mouse models of Down syndrome, with full or segmental trisomy of mouse chromosome 16, have been produced (Figure 1).

Table 3. Known genes of Human q21 arm chromosome and indication of Synteny to mouse chromosomes

GENES	NAMES
Mouse Chromosome 16	
LIPI	Lipase, member I
RBM11	RNA binding motif protein 11
ABCC13	ATP-binding cassette protein C13 isoform b
STCH	Stress 70 protein chaperone
SAMSN1	SAM domain, SH3 domain and nuclear localisation signals, 1
NRIP1	Receptor interacting protein 140
C21irf116	*Hypothetical protein AF130090*
USP25	Ubiquitin specific protease 25
C21orf34	Hypothetical protein LOC388815 isoform a
CXADR	Coxsackie virus and adenovirus receptor
BTG3	B-cell translocation gene 3
AF338194	Hepatocellular carcinoma-associated antigen HCA25b
C21orf91	Hypothetical protein LOC54149 – EURL homolog
CHODL	Chondrolectin
PRSS7	Enterokinase
NCAM2	Neural cell adhesion molecule 2
AK124194	Hypothetical protein FLJ42200
MRPL39	Mitochondrial ribosomal protein L39
JAM2	Junctional adhesion molecule 2
ATP5J	ATP synthase H+ transporting mitochondrial F0
GABPA	GA binding protein transcription factor alpha
APP	Amyloid beta A4 protein

Table 3. (Continued)

GENES	NAMES
CYYR1	Cysteine and tyrosine-rich 1 protein
ADAMTS1	ADAM metallopeptidase with thrombospondin type 1
ADAMTS5	ADAM metallopeptidase with thrombospondin type 1
C21orf94	*Hypothetical protein LOC246705*
C21orf100	*Hypothetical protein LOC118421*
HEMK2	HemK methyltransferase family member 2
ZNF294	Zinc finger protein 294
C21orf6	*Hypothetical protein LOC10069*
USP16	Ubiquitin specific protease 16
CCT8	Chaperonin containing TCP1 subunit 8 (theta)
C21orf7	*Chromosome 21 open reading frame 7*
C21orf109	*Chromosome 21 open reading frame 109*
BACH1	BTB and CNC homology 1
GRIK1	Glutamate receptor ionotropic kainate 1
C21orf41	*Chromosome 21 open reading frame 41*
C21orf9	*Chromosome 21 open reading frame 9*
CLDN17	Claudin 17
CLDN8	Claudin 8
KRTAP (28 genes)	Keratin associated proteins
TIAM1	T-cell lymphoma invasion and metastasis 1
SOD1	Superoxide dismutase 1 soluble
SFRS15	Splicing factor arginini/serine-rich 15
HUNK	Hormonally upregulated Neu-associated kinase
C21orf45	Chromosome 21 open reading frame 45
AK125043	Hypothetical protein FLJ43053
MRAP	Melanocortin 2 receptor accessory protein
C21orf119	Chromosome 21 open reading frame 119
C21orf63	Chromosome 21 open reading frame 63
AK1001794	Hypothetical protein LOC55264
TCP10L	T-complex 10A-2
C21orf59	*Hypothetical protein* LOC56683
SYNJ1	Synaptojanin 1
C21orf66	GC-rich sequence DNA-binding factor candidate
C21orf62	*Hypothetical protein LOC56245*
OLIG2	Oligodendrocyte lineage transcription factor 2
OLIG1	Oligodendrocyte lineage transcription factor 1
IFNAR2	Interferon alpha/beta receptor 2
IL10RB	Interleukin 10 receptor beta
IFNAR1	Interferon-alpha receptor 1
IFNGR2	Interferon-gamma receptor beta chain
AK129657	Hypothetical protein FLJ26146
TMEM50B	Transmembrane protein 50B
C21orf55	*Hypothetical protein LOC54943*

Table 3. (Continued)

GENES	NAMES
GART	Phsphoribosylglycinamide formyltransferase
SON	SOM DNA-binding protein
DONSON	Downstream neighbor of SON
CRYZL1	Crystallin zeta-like 1
ITSN1	Intersectin 1
ATP5O	Mitochondrial ATP synthase O subunit
FLJ46020	Hypothetical protein LOC400863
MRPS6	Mitochondrial ribosomal protein S6
SLC5A3	Solute carrier family 5 (inositol transporters)
BC111996	Hypothetical protein C21orf82
KCNE2	Potassium voltage-gated channel Isk-related
C21orf51	*Hypothetical protein C21orf51*
KCNE1	Potassium voltage-gated channel Isk-related
DSCR1	Calcipressin 1
CLIC6	Chloride intracellular channel 6
RUNX1	Runt-related transcription factor 1
AK024509	Hypothetical protein C21orf96
SETD4/C21orf18	SET domain containing 4
DCR-1 Start	
CBR1	Carbonyl reductase 1
CR606022	Fragment
CBR3	Carbonyl reductase 3
DOPEY2	DOPEY2/C21orf5
MORC3	MORC family CW-type zinc finger 3
CHAF1B	Chromatin assembly factor 1 subunit B
CLDN14	Claudin 14
SIM2	single-minded 2
HLCS	Holocarboxylase synthetase
DSCR6	Down syndrome critical region protein 6
PIGP	Phosphatidylinositol glycan anchor biosynthesis/DSCR5
TTC3	Tetratricopeptide repeat domain 3 / TPRD
DSCR9	DSCR9
DSCR3	DSCR3
DYRK1A	Dual-specificity tyrosine-(Y)-phosphorylation
KCNJ6	Potassium inwardly-rectifying channel J6 / GIRK2
DSCR4	DSCR4
DSCR8	DSCR8
DSCR10	DSCR10
KCNJ15	Potassium inwardly-rectifying channel J15
ERG	v-ets erythroblastosis virus E26 oncogene like
DCR-1 End	
C21orf24	Hypothetical protein LOC400866
ETS2	v-ets erythroblastosis virus E26

Table 3. (Continued)

GENES	NAMES
FLJ45139	Hypothetical protein LOC400867
DSCR2	DSCR2
BRWD1	Bromodomain and WD repeat domain containing 1
C21orf87	Hypothetical protein LOC257357
HMGN1	High-mobility group nucleosome binding domain 1
WRB	Tryptopha, rich basic protein
C21orf13	C21orf13
SH3BGR	SH3-binding domain and glutamic acid-rich
AK129590	Hypothetical protein FLJ26079
C21orf88	Hypothetical protein LOC114041
B3GALT5	UDP-Gal:betaGlcNAc beta
PCP4	Purkinje cell protein 4
DSCAM	Down syndrome cell adhesion molecule
BACE2	Beta-site APP-cleaving enzyme 2
PLAC4	Placenta-specific 4
FAM3B	family with sequence similarity 3 member B
AK126107	Hypothetical protein FLJ44119
MX2	Myxovirus resistance protein 2
MX1	Myxovirus resistance protein 1
AK318374	Hypothetical protein pp9284
TMPRSS2	*transmembrane protease serine 2*
C21orf129	Hypothetical protein LOC150135
RIPK4	Ankyrin repeat domain 3
PRDM15	PR domain containing 15
C21orf25	C21orf25
ZNF295	Zinc finger protein 295
C21orf121	Hypothetical protein C21orf121
Mouse Chromosome 17	
UMODL1	*Uromodulin-like 1*
C21orf128	Hypothetical protein LOC150147
ABCG1	ATP-binding cassette sub-family G member 1
TFF3	Trefoil factor 3
TFF2	Trefoil factor 2
TFF1	Trefoil factor 1
TMPRSS3	transmembrane protease serine 3
UBASH3A	Ubiquitin associated and SH3 domain containing
TSGA2	Testis-specific gene A2
SLC37A1	Solute carrier family 37 member 1
AK127597	Hypothetical protein FLJ45693
PDE9A	Phosphodiesterase 9A
WDR4	WD repeat domain 4 protein
NDUFV3	NADH-ubiquinone oxidoreductase flavoprotein 3
PKNOX1	PBX/knotted 1 homeobox 1

Table 3. (Continued)

GENES	NAMES
CBS	cystathionine-beta-synthase
U2AF1	U2 small nuclear RNA auxillary factor 1
CRYAA	Crystallin alpha A
AK131425	Hypothetical protein FLJ16545
FLJ41733	Hypothetical protein LOC400870
SNF1LK	SNF1-like kinase
C21orf125	Hypothetical protein LOC284836
HSF2BP	Heat shock transcription factor 2 binding protein
KIAA0179	*Hypothetical protein LOC23076*
C21orf124	Hypothetical protein LOC85006
Mouse Chromosome 10	
PDXK	Pyridoxal kinase
CSTB	Cystatin B
D21S2056E	Nucleolar protein NOP52
LOC284837	Hypothetical protein LOC284837
AGPAT3	1-acylglycerol-3-phosphate O-acyltransferase 3
TMEM1	Transmembrane protein 1
PWP2H	PWP2 periodic tryptophan protein homolog
C21orf33	Es1 protein isoform I
ICOSLG	Inducible T-cell co-stimulator ligand
DNMT3L	Cytosine-5-methyltransferase 3-like protein
AIRE	Autoimmune regulator AIRE
PFKL	Liver phosphofructokinase
C21orf2	Hypothetical protein LOC755
TRPM2	Transient receptor potential cation channel
LRRC3	Leucine-rich repeat-containing 3
AL11578	Hypothetical protein C21orf30
C21orf29	Hypothetical protein C21orf29
KRTAP (16 genes)	Keratin associated proteins
UBE2G2	Ubiquitin-conjugating enzyme E2G 2
SUMO3	Small ubiquitin-like modifier protein 3
PTTG1IP	Pituitary tumor-transforming gene 1
AK097864	Hypothetical protein FLJ40545
ITGB2	Integrin beta 2
C21orf69	Hypothetical protein C21orf69
C21orf67	Hypothetical protein C21orf67
C21orf70	Hypothetical protein C21orf70
BC004343	Hypothetical protein C21orf122
ADARB1	RNA-specific adenosine deaminase B1
AF26268	Hypothetical protein C21orf89
POFUT2	Protein O-fucosyltransferase 2
C21orf86	Hypothetical protein LOC257103
C21orf93	Hypothetical protein LOC246704

Table 3. (Continued)

GENES	NAMES
COL18A1	alpha & type XVIII collagen
C21orf123	Hypothetical protein LOC378832
SLC19A1	Solute carrier family 19 member 1
AK127669	Hypothetical protein FLJ45767
AK123852	Hypothetical protein FLJ41858
PCBP3	Poly(rC) binding protein 3
COL6A1	Collagen type VI alpha 1
COL6A2	Collagen type VI alpha 2C2
AK128695	Hypothetical protein AK128695
FTCD	Formiminotransferase cyclodeaminase
C21orf56	Hypothetical protein LOC84221
LSS	Lanosterol synthase
AF426262	Hypothetical protein C21orf85
MCM3AP	Minichromosome maintenance protein 3 associated
C21orf57	*Hypothetical protein LOC54059*
C21orf58	Hypothetical protein LOC54058
PCNT	Pericentrin
DIP2A	DIP2-like protein
S100b	S100 calcium-binding protein beta
PRMT2	HMT1 hnRNP methyltransferase-like 1

a. Ts16 Mice

The Ts16 mice (Cox et al., 1984) have three full copies of chromosome 16, which contains not only the syntenic region to human chromosome 21 but also to human chromosomes 3, 8, 16 and 22. Ts16 mice are produced by mating heterozygote mice for two Robertsonian chromosomes containing chromosome 16 to wild type mice (Gearhart et al., 1986), and they are a potential animal model for human Down syndrome (Epstein 1986; Lacey-Casem and Oster-Granite 1994; Reeves et al. 1986).

Ts16 mice have many features that are reminiscent of Down syndrome and have been used profitably to study different aspects of Down syndrome. In fact, Ts16 fetuses have a number of phenotypic characteristics similar to those of Down syndrome individuals (Epstein et al., 1985; Gearhart et al., 1986). Overall features of Ts16 fetuses include small body and brain size, and cellular hypoplasia in several organ systems (Lacey-Casem and Oster-Granite, 1994). Ts16 embryos also show delayed development of the precursors of the sensory organs and skull ossification (Ludwig et al., 1997), abnormal neuronal migration and evidence of oxidative stress (Behar and Colton, 2003), abnormalities in calcium (Galdzicki et al., 1998), potassium and chloride channels (Peng et al., 2000) and cardiac defects (Webb et al., 1996).

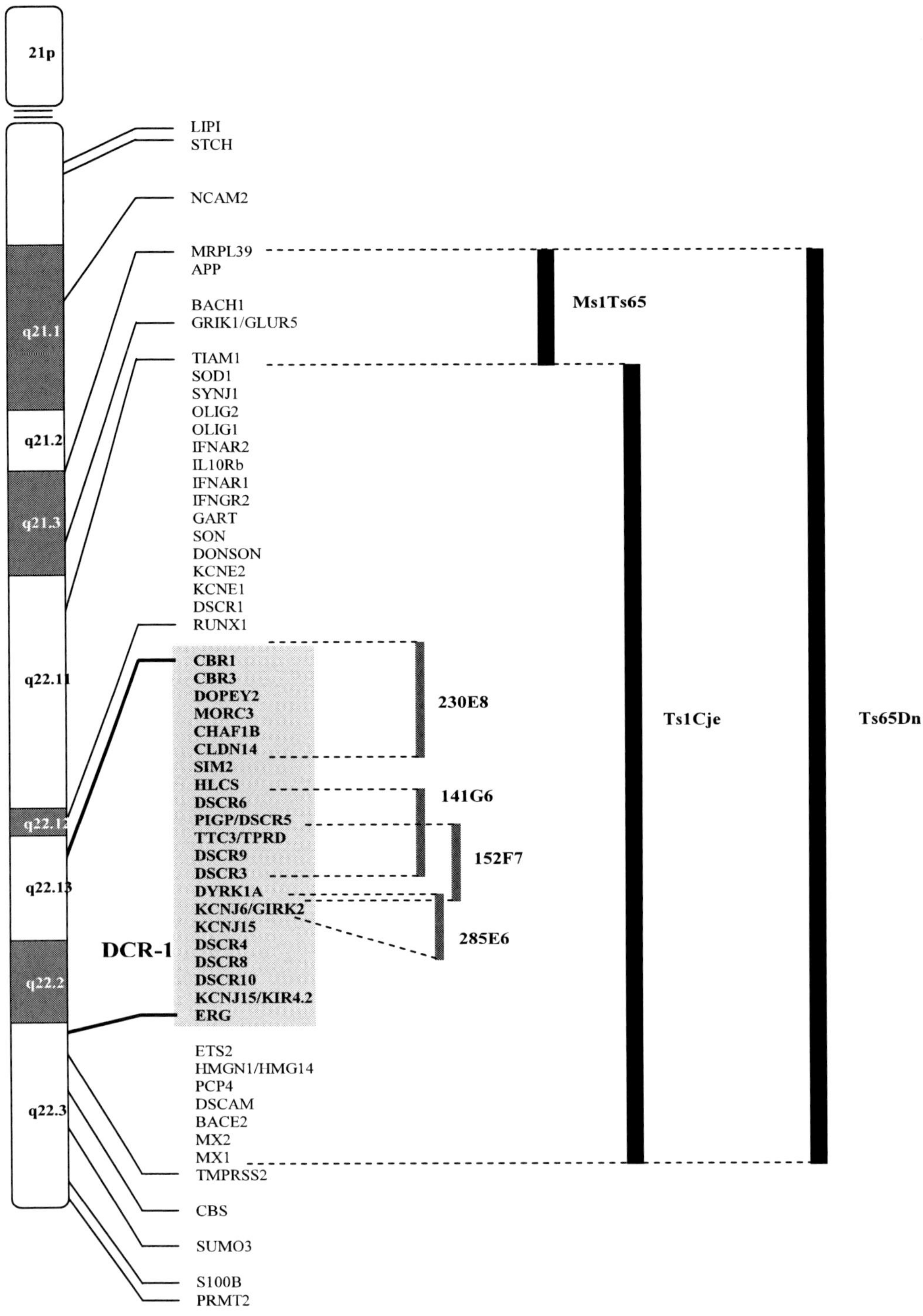

Figure 1. Syntenic regions to human chromosome 21 in segmental trisomic mice.

Although Ts16 mice show some of the characteristics of Down syndrome (Coyle et al., 1988), their value as a model for Down syndrome is limited because of the presence of triplicated genes on other than the human chromosome 21 syntenic region and also does not contain all the genes on human chromosome 21, and also because of its lethality in utero. So, their investigation has been limited to early developmental stages, cell culture systems and neuronal Ts16 tissue grafted into brain ventricles (Galdzicki et al. 2001; Lacey-Casem & Oster-Granite 1994; Rapoport and Galdzicki 1994).

Contrarily to Ts16 mice, other mouse models carrying triplication of a chromosomal 16 segment, survive to adulthood and enable post-natal studies including behavior, learning and memory.

b. Ts65Dn Mice

Genetics and Phenotypes

The Ts(1716)65Dn, named (Ts65Dn), produced by reciprocal translocation T(16C3-4; 17A2)65Dn, was the first segmental trisomy model created and is the best-characterized and most commonly used model (Davisson and Costa, 1999; Patterson and Costa, 2005). Ts65Dn mice are trisomic for most of the human chromosome 21 orthologs in the distal end of mouse chromosome 16, extending from the gene for mitochondrial ribosomal protein L39 (Mrpl39) (Kahlem et al., 2004) to the *Mx1* gene, at the distal telomere (Figure 1).

The Ts65Dn mouse has been used to model Down syndrome (Davisson and Costa, 1999) and Alzheimer disease (Granholm et al., 2000). Ts65Dn mice exhibit many physical, behavioural and neurological features that are reminiscent of those seen in people with Down syndrome, including craniofacial dysmorphogenesis, male sterility, developmental delay in neonatal life, reduced birth weight and slower body weight gain in Ts65Dn pups, as well as abnormal cognitive behaviors in both young and adult animals that may be analogous to mental retardation (Reeves et al., 1995; Holtzman et al., 1996; Coussons-Read and Crnic, 1996; Hyde et al., 2000; Richtsmeier et al., 2000; 2002; Cataldo et al., 2003; Hampton et al., 2004; Olson et al., 2004b; Stasko and Costa, 2004).

Neuropathology and Cognitive Behaviors

At the central nervous system level, they show related deficits, and notable learning and memory deficits, concerning motor dysfunction (Costa et al. 1999), and several adult-like reflexes (Holtzman et al., 1996). Ts65Dn mice have been reported to have several alterations in neurotransmitters (Dierssen et al., 1997; Megias et al., 1997), synaptic ultrastructure (Kurt et al., 2000), long-term potentiation (LTP) and long-term depression (LTD) in the CA1 region (Siarey et al., 1997; Kleschevnikov et al., 2004), and reduced noradrenergic function in the hippocampus (Dierssen et al., 1996; 1997), that globally demonstrated severe deficits in the limbic system. Cytological alterations in the hippocampal region of Ts65Dn mice include reduction in the number of neurons in the granule cell layer of the dentate gyrus, increased CA3 neurons, and reduced CA2 volume (Insausti et al., 1998; Kurt et al. 2000). Cerebellar volume is significantly reduced in Ts65Dn mice owing to reduced density of granular cells (to 80% of euploids) in Ts65Dn mice, such as in Down syndrome, while Purkinje cells are decreased about 10% (Baxter et al., 2000). The cerebellar deficit of Ts65Dn mice actually predicted a similar deficit that was subsequently confirmed in people with Down syndrome (Richtsmeier et al., 2000). (Table 4)

Table 4. Major Neurological phenotypes in mouse models of Down syndrome

Mouse models	Neurological phenotypes	References
Ts16	Decreased neuron time survival in primary hippocampal culture	Schuchmann et al., 1998
	Decreased brain size and cellular hypoplasia	Cox et al., 1984; Lacey-Casem and Oster-Granite, 1994
	Delayed development of the sensory organs	Ludwing et al., 1997
	Abnormal neuronal migration	Behar and Colton, 2003
Ts65Dn	Decreased LTP and increased LTD in CA1 and dentate gyrus	Siarey et al., 1997; Siarey et al., 1999; Kleschevnilov et al., 2004
	Increased β-amyloid level in hippocampus	Hunter et al., 2004
	Decreased cerebellum and granular cell layer	Baxter et al., 2000
	Decreased dentate gyrus	Kleschevnikov et al., 2004
	Decreased dentate gyrus and CA2, increased CA3	Insausti et al., 1998; Kurt et al., 2000
	BFCN age-related degeneration	Yates et al., 1983; Mann et al., 1984; Casanova et al., 1985
	Increased synapsis in CA1 and cortex	Kurt et al., 2000; Fiala et al., 2002; Belichenko et al., 2004
	Motor dysfunction	Costa et al., 1999
	Alterations of neurotransmitters	Dierssen et al., 1997; Megias et al., 1997
	Decreased noradrenergic function in hippocampus	Dierssen et al., 1996; Dierssen et al., 1997
	Altered NGF traffic	Cooper et al., 2001; Salehi et al., 2003
	Developmental delay	Holtzman et al., 1996
Ts1Cje	Decreased LTP and increased LTD	Siarey et al., 2005
	Decreased cerebellar volume	Sago et al., 2000; Olson et al., 2004b
YAC 152F7	Decreased LTP in hippocampus	Smith et al., 1997
	Increased brain weight and neuronal size	Branchi et al., 2004; Rachidi et al., unpublished
YAC 230E8	Increased neuronal cortical density	Smith et al., 1997; Rachidi et al., 2005b
SOD1	Decreased LTP in CA1	Harris-Cerruti et al., 2004
	Decreased cell number in several brain area	Zang et al., 2004
	Abnormal neuromuscular junction	Epstein et al., 1987
S100β	Increased CA1, CA3 and granular cell of dentate gyrus in old mice	Shapiro et al., 2004
	Abnormal dendrite development	Whitaker-Azmatia, et al., 1997
	Neurite degeneration and astrocytosis	Reeves et al., 1994
APP	Dystrophic neuritis with congophilic plaques	Sturchler-Pierrat et al., 1997

The medial septal nucleus of the basal forebrain cholinergic neurons (BFCNs), which project to the hippocampus and supply the major cholinergic input to the hippocampus and neocortex, shows age-related degeneration in Ts65Dn brains, beginning at 6 months of age (Holtzman et al., 1996; Granholm et al., 2000; 2002; Salehi et al., 2006). The age-related degeneration of BFCNs in Ts65Dn mice mimics the specific age-related decrease in cholinergic function seen in Down syndrome and Alzheimer disease (Yates et al., 1983, Mann et al., 1984; Casanova et al., 1985) and may contribute significantly to dementia (Coyle et al., 1988). The basal forebrain–hippocampus cholinergic system deficits appear to be related to abnormalities in nerve growth factor (NGF) trafficking (Cooper et al., 2001; Salehi et al. 2003) and dendritic spine abnormalities (Belichenko et al., 2004) (Table 4).

In the Ts65Dn brain, spine pathology can concern changes in spine density, shape, or distribution, and also changes in the structure of spines and includes increased spine size and alterations in spine content (Fiala et al., 2002). Both presynaptic and postsynaptic elements were enlarged in Ts65Dn, from postnatal day 21, in fascia dentata and motor cortex (Belichenko et al., 2004). Moreover, there was a significant decrease in the density of dendritic spines and in the pattern of innervation of dentate granule cell neurons (Belichenko et al., 2004). Also, there was reorganization of inhibitory inputs, with a relative decrease in inputs to dendrite shafts and an increase in inputs to the necks of spines (Belichenko et al., 2004). Similar findings have been also found in temporal cortex of Ts65Dn (Kurt et al., 2000). The findings are evident for marked and persistent changes in synaptic structure, the most prominent of which mimics the synaptic pathology described in Down syndrome.

Synaptic pathologies in Ts65Dn mice recapitulate some of those most frequently described in the changes seen in the Down syndrome brain. Marin-Padilla (1976) described very large spines on dendrites with decreased numbers of spines in pyramidal neurons of the motor cortex in a Down syndrome patient. Subsequent studies, examining hippocampus and cortex, documented similar findings, with consistent reports of reduced spine number in subjects beyond the early newborn period (Purpura, 1974; Suetsugu and Mehraein, 1980; Takashima et al., 1981, 1994; Ferrer and Gullotta, 1990; Fiala et al., 2002). Ferrer and Gullotta (1990) documented greater spine loss on pyramidal neurons in the CA1 and CA2–CA3 regions of hippocampus in Down syndrome patients with associated Alzheimer disease pathology. Taken together, these results are convincing that spines are abnormal in Down syndrome.

All these findings establish the Ts65Dn mouse as a model for abnormal synapse structure and function in Down syndrome, indicating the importance of studies to elucidate the mechanisms responsible for synapse enlargement.

The behavior of Ts65Dn animals was abnormal during the entire lifespan. The male Ts65Dn mouse appears abnormally aggressive in neutral areas (offensive), but less so in home areas (defensive) (Klein et al. 1996). Furthermore, the Ts65Dn mouse shows reduced responsiveness to painful stimuli (Martinez-Cue et al. 1999), potentially similar to abnormal nociception reported in Down syndrome individuals (Hennequin et al. 2000). Developmental delay and hyperactivity were noted during early development (Holtzman et al., 1996). These findings parallel what is observed in infants and children with Down syndrome (Epstein, 1986). Indeed, like Down syndrome children, Ts65Dn mice did achieve developmental sensorimotor milestones, albeit later than normal. Ts65Dn adults also exhibited spontaneous hyperactivity in open field testing. Moreover, adult subjects show deficiencies in some aspects of operant conditioning learning (Wenger et al., 2004), including impairment of hippocampal function as evidenced by impaired spatial memory (Reeves et al., 1995; Demas et al., 1996, 1998; Holtzman et al., 1996; Escorihuela et al., 1998; Sago et al., 2000) and context discrimination learning, that are dependent on the dorsal hippocampus in mice (Hyde et al., 2001). In the Morris water maze, Ts65Dn mice show learning impairment in the non-spatial test (visible platform) that ranges from mild to severe, depending on the report. They also show a severe impairment in spatial learning and reversal, but not visual discrimination learning and reversal (Reeves et al., 1995; Holtzman et al., 1996; Granholm et al. 2000; Hunter et al. 2003). Learning deficits in a hippocampal dependent task observed in Ts65Dn mice may be related to the loss of cholinergic input to the hippocampus (Hyde et al., 2001) (Tables 5).

c. Ts1Cje Mice

Genetics and Phenotypes

Another mouse model, Ts(16C-tel)1Cje (Ts1Cje), so-called Ts1Cje, has been developed as the result of a 12;16 translocation. Ts1Cje, a mouse model for Down syndrome, possesses a smaller extra segment of mouse chromosome 16 than that of the Ts65Dn mice (Sago et al. 1998). This mouse model, generated by a fortuitous translocation during the targeting of *Sod1* by homologous recombination, carries the translocation break-points proximal to *Sod1* and the very distal region of the mouse chromosome 12 (Huang et al., 1997). The heterozygous of these *Sod1* mutants, which are apparently balanced carriers for the translocation designated T(12;16)1Cje, have one each of normal mouse chromosome 12 and 16 and of 1216 and 1612 translocation chromosomes.

Partial trisomy of the distal region of mouse chromosome 16, Ts1Cje, is generated when a gamete carrying mouse chromosome translocation 1216 and mouse chromosome 16 combines with a normal gamete (Sago et al., 1998). Because the *Sod1* allele on mouse chromosome 12 is disrupted by the neomycin resistance sequence, the Ts1Cje animals have 100% rather than 150% of wild-type CuZn-SOD activity. Therefore, Ts1Cje is not functionally trisomic for *Sod1* (Sago et al., 1998). The Ts1Cje mouse is trisomic for about three-fourths of the genes that present in the Ts65Dn mouse. This segment spans superoxide dismutase 1 (Sod1) to Mx1 (Sago et al. 1998; 2000). This segment corresponds to human 21q22.1 to q22.3 (Figure 1).

Ts1Cje mice have fewer similarities to Down syndrome than Ts65Dn mice but are important to study the particular effects of trisomy for a subset of genes triplicated in Ts65Dn and not in Ts1Cje. Both male and female Ts1Cje mice are fertile and produce Ts1Cje progeny at the expected 50% segregation frequency when crossed to wild-type animals. Ts1Cje mice are viable and are indistinguishable from controls in gross appearance. There are no apparent limbic or facial malformations or other dysmorphic features (Sago et al., 1998). Craniofacial dysmorphology is also similar to Ts65Dn mice, but Ts1Cje mice lack the broadening of the cranium that confers brachycephaly in Ts65Dn mice (Richtsmeier et al., 2002).

Table 5. Major Behavioral phenotypes in mouse models of Down syndrome

Mouse models	Behavioral phenotypes	References
Ts65Dn	Decreased non spatial and spatial learning, and memory flexibility (Morris water test)	Holtzman et al., 1996; Smith et al., 1997; Sago et al., 2000; Stasko and Costa, 2004
	Decreased spatial learning (Radial-arm maze)	Demas et al., 1996; Demas et al., 1998
	Increased hyperactivity in open field test	Wenger et al., 2004
	Hyperactivity	Holtzman et al., 1996
	Decreased fear conditioning	Hyde et al., 2001
	Decreased spatial learning and memory flexibility (Water T-maze)	Granholm et al., 2000
	Decreased spatial learning and memory flexibility (Water radial-arm maze)	Bimonte-Nelson et al., 2003; Hunter et al., 2004
	Aggressive behavior	Klein et al., 1996
	Reduced responsiveness to painful stimuli	Martinez-Cue et al., 1999
Ts1Cje	Decreased spatial learning (Morris water test)	Sago et al., 1998; Sago et al., 2000
	Hypoactivity and decreased exploratory behavior	Sago et al., 1998
Ms1Ts65	Decreased spatial learning, and memory	Sago et al., 1998; Sago et al., 2000
HSA21 Chimera	Decreased fear conditioning	Shinohara et al., 2001
YAC 152F7	Decreased spatial learning and memory flexibility (Morris water test)	Smith et al., 1997
YAC 230E8	Decreased spatial learning (Morris water test)	Smith et al., 1997
SIM2	Decreased memory flexibility	Ema et al., 1999; Chrast et al., 2000b
	Increased fear conditioning	Ema et al., 1999
DYRK1A	Decreased spatial learning and memory flexibility (Morris water test)	Altafaj et al., 2001
	Motor dysfunction	Martinez de Lagrán et al., 2004
SOD1	Learning defects	Epstein et al., 1987
S100β	Decreased spatial learning and memory flexibility (Morris water test)	Gerlai and Roder, 1996; Whitaker-Azmitia et al., 1997
	Decreased spatial learning and memory flexibility (Radial arm maze; Y-maze test)	Roder et al., 1996; Winocur et al., 2001; Bell et al., 2003
APP	Learning defects	Lamb et al., 1993

Neuropathology and Cognitive Behaviors

In addition, the age-dependent degeneration of BFCN, which is observed in Ts65Dn mice and individuals with Down syndrome, is absent in Ts1Cje mice (Sago et al., 2000). Although these findings define a clear difference between Ts65Dn and Ts1Cje, they do not exclude the possibility that dysfunction of BFCN synapses in the Ts1Cje hippocampus contributes to the learning deficits (Tables 4).

Although the cerebellar volume is slightly reduced, the decrease in granule and Purkinje cell numbers is not significant (Sago et al., 2000; Olson et al., 2004b), in contrast to Ts65Dn.

As adults, Ts1Cje mice have a completely different spontaneous locomotor activity than the Ts65Dn and tend to be hypoactive, suggesting decreased exploratory behavior, whereas Ts65Dn tends to be hyperactive (Sago et al., 1998).

In the Ts1Cje DS mouse model, more subtle hippocampal behavioral deficits have been reported. The hippocampus from the Ts1Cje mouse had a smaller LTP and an increased LTD. The changes are less dramatic than had been reported previously for the Ts65Dn mouse (Siarey et al., 2005). These findings suggest that genes from Ts1Cje chromosome contribute to abnormal short- and long-term plasticity.

These mice also show behavioral deficits in the Morris water maze similar to the Ts65Dn but the reverse probe test indicates that impairments are less dramatic than the ones reported for the Ts65Dn mouse (Sago et al. 1998; Sago et al. 2000). Unlike Ts65Dn mice, they are able to perform as well as the controls in the cued or non-spatial (visible platform) part of the test and only show moderate to severe impairment in the hidden platform, probe and reverse learning parts of the test, that can be improved by previous training (Sago et al., 1998). Rats and mice with hippocampal lesions or in which the septohippocampal pathway is disrupted are impaired in the spatial version (invisible platform), but not in the cued version (visible platform) of the test (Morris et al., 1982). Hippocampal lesions also affect exploratory locomotion (Sandin et al., 1997). These findings suggest that the deficits exhibited by Ts1Cje mice are caused by abnormalities within the hippocampus determining abnormal hippocampal function (Tables 5).

d. Other Segmental Trisomic Mice

In addition to the above models, combinations of existing chromosome 16 aberrations can be used to further dissect the chromosome 16-conserved segment (Tables 4, 5). Mating Ts65Dn mice to mice carrying the reciprocal translocation T(12;16)1Cje, which gave rise to the Ts1Cje trisomic chromosome, produces offspring called Ms1Cje/Ts65Dn, or Ms1Ts65, that are trisomic for the genes present in Ts65Dn and missing from Ts1Cje, corresponding to the segment from *Mrpl39* to *Sod1* (Figure 1) (Sago et al., 2000). Spatial learning impairment is even less severe in Ms1Cje/Ts65Dn mice than in either Ts65Dn or Ts1Cje mice (Sago et al., 2000).

A duplication, Dp(16Cbr1-Mx1)1Rhr, or Ts1Rhr, and a deletion, Del1 Rhr, or Ms1Rhr, of the mouse chromosome 16 segment between *Cbr1* and *Mx1* have been created using Cre-loxP and embryonic stem (ES) cell technologies. These mice provide trisomy and monosomy, respectively, for a smaller segment of mouse chromosome 16 that is orthologous to the Down syndrome critical region of human chromosome 21 (Olson et al., 2004a). Ts1Rhr mice have even less severe craniofacial dysmorphology than either Ts1Cje or Ts65Dn. In particular, mating Ms1Rhr mice to Ts65Dn mice produces mice trisomic for the differential genes triplicated in Ts65Dn but not in Ts1Rhr (Olson et al., 2004a).

Like Ts1Cje, all of these other segmentally trisomic mice have fewer similarities to Down syndrome than do Ts65Dn mice, but they will be valuable models to further genetically dissect the effects of subsets of genes triplicated in Ts65Dn and to test therapies for phenotypes related to the genes in the specific triplicated segments.

e. Transgenic Mouse Models

Several transgenic mice that express from one or a few genes to entire segments of chromosome 21 have been produced. As expected, none of these recapitulate the entire phenotype of Down syndrome, but many have features that are reminiscent of aspects of the phenotype.

A panel of transgenic mice containing large fragments of human genome has been constructed (Figure 1) (Smith et al., 1995). This panel of transgenic mice constitutes an "in vivo library", in which human genome fragments are carried by mice and allow genotype/phenotype comparison studies (Smith et al., 1995; 1997). The human genome fragments used were 4 YAC (Yeast Artificial Chromosome) spanning the 2 Mb of the DCR-1 (Crété et al., 1993; Dufresne-Zacharia et al., 1994; Smith et al., 1995). The transgenic lines carrying the YAC 152F7 showed the most severe deficits on the Morris water maze, showing mildly impaired in probe test crossings, and severely impaired in the reverse versions of the tasks that assess learning flexibility, while milder deficits in learning flexibility were shown by the lines containing YAC 230E8 (Smith et al., 1997). Moreover, the YAC 230E8 lines also showed increased density of neurons in cerebral cortex (Smith et al., 1997; Rachidi et al., 2005b). This abnormal density of neurons may explain the learning and memory deficits of theses animals. Both learning deficits (Bauman, et al., 1995; Johnston et al., 1995) and cognitive abnormalities (Selemon et al., 1995) have been linked with increased neuronal density, by interfering with neuronal signalling (Tables 4, 5).

To localize the gene responsible for the learning and memory deficits of mice containing YAC 152F7, several lines have been generated carrying different fragments of the YAC. The line YAC152F7tel, carrying the telomeric fragment of YAC 152F7, showed the identical phenotype observed in the original lines. This YAC fragment contains only the *DYRK1A* gene indicating that the correct dosage of *DYRK1A* gene is crucial for normal development of the nervous system (Smith et al., 1997). Ts1Cje mice, in turn, are less severely impaired than Ts65Dn mouse model. This suggests that although the imbalance of *DYRK1A* has an impact on cognitive function, the learning and behavioral abnormalities of Ts1Cje cannot be attributed solely to the presence of an extra copy of this gene, but other genes in the region from *Sod1* to *Mx1* must contribute to the spatial learning deficits.

Single gene transgenic mice enable the functional analysis of specific genes that might play a role in Down syndrome. Such studies could have limited relevance to the Down syndrome phenotypes because of transgenic mice often carry multiple copies of a single inserted transgene in an otherwise euploid background and do not replicate the subtle interplay of the moderate elevation of protein products from many genes triplicated simultaneously.

Transgenic mice containing human *SOD1* were the first mice produced to contain a gene encoded on human chromosome 21 (Epstein et al., 1987). These mice have some features that are similar to those seen in people with Down syndrome (Avraham et al., 1991; Gahtan et al.,

1998) (Tables 4, 5). Many investigators have produced transgenic mice that express normal and mutant forms of *APP*, and have demonstrated learning and memory deficits in these mice, including performance decline with age (Tables 4, 5). In a recent experiment, compound transgenic mice that express human *SOD1* and *APP* were created (Harris-Cerruti et al., 2004). Other genes (see Tables 4, 5) that cause phenotypes that are relevant to Down syndrome when overexpressed in transgenic mice include *Pfkl* (Peled-Kamar et al., 1998), *Dyrk1a* (Martinez de Lagrán et al., 2004), *Sim2* (Chrast et al., 2000b), *S100* β (Bell et al., 2003) and *Ets2* (Wolvetang et al., 2003).

f. Human Chromosome 21 Chimeric Mice

Chimeric mice carrying an intact human chromosome 21 as a freely segregated extra chromosome have been generated via microcell-mediated chromosome transfer (MMCT) into TT2F mouse embryonic stem (ES) cells (Shinohara et al., 2001). These chimeric mice presented a wide variety of phenotypic traits of Down syndrome in humans, including impairment in learning and emotional behavior, and also hypoplastic thymus and cardiac defects (Shinohara et al., 2001) (Tables 4, 5). Increased susceptibility of the TT2F/hChr21 cell lines to apoptosis at the stage of neuronal stem cell differentiation in vitro was also issued (Kawasaki et al., 2000; Kadota et al., 2002).

IV. Discussion

Down syndrome, the more frequent genetic cause of mental retardation, is generally determined by the presence in all cells of three copies of chromosome 21. In human, the first great progress in the understanding of Down syndrome pathogenesis was allowed by genotype-phenotype studies in partial trisomic 21 patients, permitting the identification of DCR-1 critical region for mental retardation in Down syndrome.

In mouse, similar approaches were applied and two partial trisomic 16 mice were generated as Down syndrome models. The Ts65Dn mice, carrying three copies of about all the synthenic region corresponding to the human chromosome 21 (Davisson et al., 1990) and the Ts1Cje mice, carrying three copies of a smaller region containing about the syntenic sequence corresponding to the human DCR-1 (Sago et al., 1998). These major mouse models, such as other segmental trisomic mice, result indispensable to genetic dissection of neurological and behavioral phenotypes, and mental retardation in Down syndrome. This mouse model approach consists in a subtractive strategy, the goal of which is the identification of candidate genes contributing to mental retardation in Down syndrome.

The complete sequencing of the human chromosome 21 (Hattori et al., 2000), its transcriptional activity analysis (Kapranov et al., 2002) and the frequently update of the genomic sequence identified more than 300 genes at least 20 of which are localized in the critical region DCR-1. In particular, it is among these genes that etiological genes for mental retardation in Down syndrome will be identified.

Although the role of this region in Down syndrome pathogenesis remains controversial (Korenberg et al., 1994; Olson et al., 2004a), mouse models also evidenced that an extra-dose of DCR-1 may be important in the pathogenesis of mental retardation in Down syndrome patients (Reeves et al., 1995). Moreover, transgenic mice containing human YACs from DCR-1 (Smith et al., 1995) caused defects in learning and memory in the transgenic lines, demonstrating that DCR-1 region contribute to altered behaviour when present in an extra dose (Smith et al., 1997). In particular, it has been demonstrated that *DYRK1A,* a gene of the DCR-1, is involved in learning defects associated with DS (Smith et al., 1997).

To date, two groups of genes appear particularly attractive as candidate genes for neurological phenotypes and mental retardation in Down syndrome. The first group of candidate genes is localized in DCR-1, such as, *Girk2*, *TPRD*, *SIM2*, *DOPEY2* and *DYRK1A*. The second group is localized outside the DCR-1, such as *SOD1*, *APP*, *S100b* and *DSCR1*. All these candidate genes have been demonstrated to be overexpressed in the brain and seem involved in brain development or learning and memory process. In addition, the transgenic mice for these candidate genes have been established demonstrating their contribution in the pathogenesis of neuroanatomical and neurological alterations contributing to mental retardation in Down syndrome patients.

Studies to elucidate the pathological role of a given candidate gene in the mental retardation in Down syndrome are particularly difficult, considering that the genetic etiology of this pathology is a gene overdosage and not gene mutations. In this view, gene expression studies are a fundamental step to select and characterize candidate genes for mental retardation in Down syndrome. Several approaches have been used in these last years: on one hand, the genome-wide expression analyses, including different methods for transcriptome studies and, on the other hand, the single gene studies, generally using in situ expression (in situ hybridization or immunolocalization). These latter are high-resolution methods providing accurate descriptions of the spatiotemporal distribution of transcripts (Ballabio, 1993; Bulfone, et al., 1998; Lopes et al., 1999; Neidhardt, et al., 2000; Reymond, et al., 2001). In some cases, their application at large scale, analyzing the global transcribed sequences of chromosome 21, has been performed in "human chromosome 21 expression atlas" projects (Gitton et al., 2002; Reymond, et al., 2002).

These whole genome approaches results interesting for large gene screening and identification of candidate genes. But, the single gene approaches are necessary for precise expression study in the largest number of cell types during development and all lifespan. Most of the expression studies were performed on mouse tissues, because of their facility and availability, and generally, the expression pattern in human is extrapolated from mouse data with evident limitations due to the high but not complete conservation between the regulation mechanisms of the expression of ortholog genes in the two species. To avoid these extrapolations from mouse data, complete human embryogenesis and fetal brain development expression pattern could be investigated (Rachidi et al., 2000; 2005a; 2006). In addition, improvement of the in situ hybridization technique and the discovery of a novel technology to quantify the mRNA variations at cellular level during brain development (Rachidi et al., 2000; 2005a; 2006), allowed the in situ estimation of gene expression and overexpression, with the high advantage to identify expression variation in the different neuronal cell types.

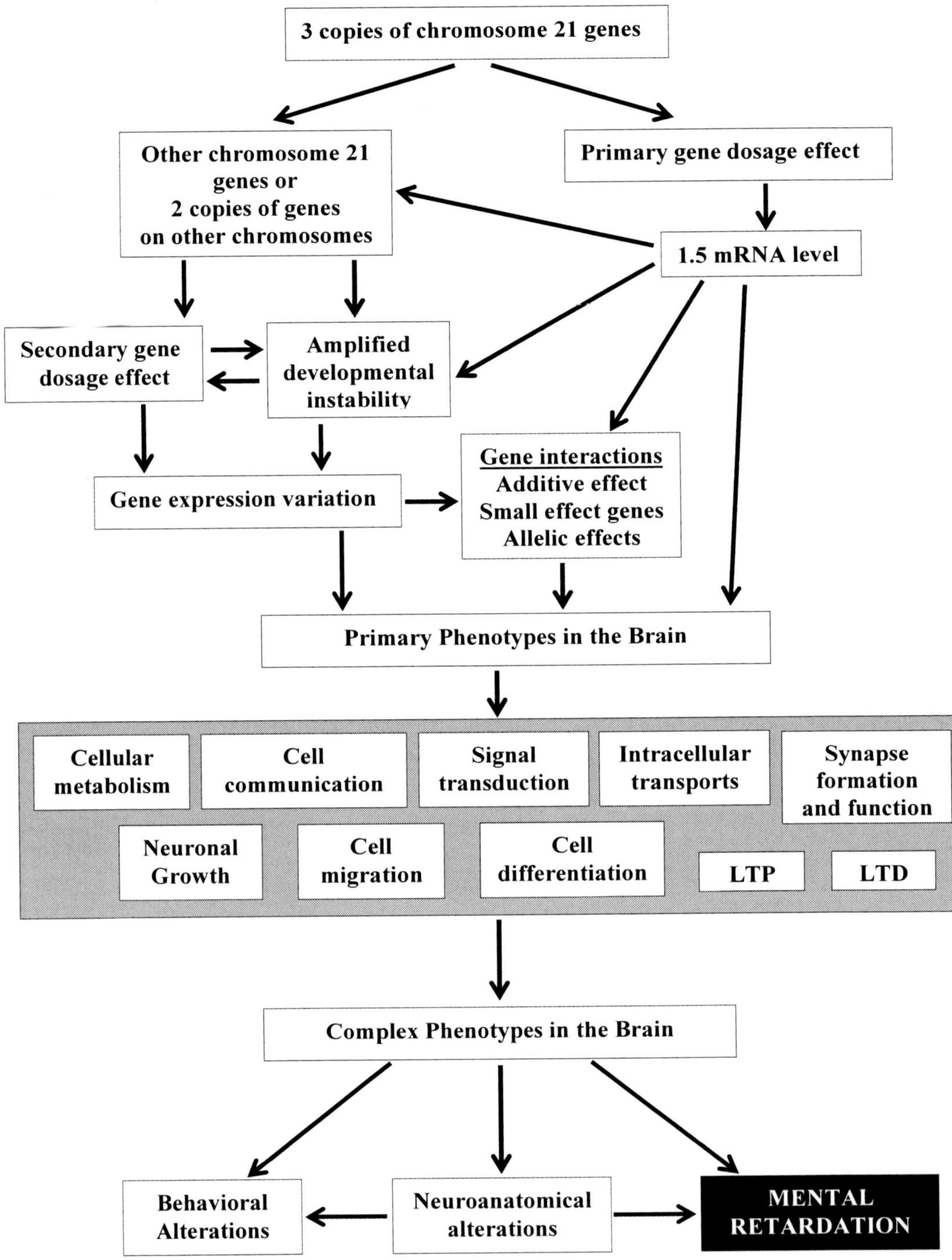

Figure 2. Possible global molecular mechanism of the mental retardation in Down syndrome.

As we have described above, several theoretical molecular mechanisms have been proposed to explain Down syndrome phenotype. At this time, any results of expression studies, both on single genes and transcriptome global analyses, seem unequivocally in agreement to one of these theories, and any of them alone seems explain the complex phenotype of Down syndrome.

In particular, mental retardation is the result of several developmental, structural, and biochemical primary alterations in different neuronal cell types (see Figure 2). These primary alterations in the brain are determined by the presence of three copies of the genes on chromosome 21, probably via several specific mechanisms for the different gene pathways (Figure 2).

We can hypothesize a global molecular mechanism leading to mental retardation (Figure 2). In this molecular model, some dosage-dependent genes are expressed 1.5 fold the normal level as a direct consequence of the 1.5 gene overdosage and could directly determine a primary phenotype in trisomic brain (Figure 2). In contrast, some of these dosage-dependent genes could modulate the expression of target genes that could be located on the chromosome 21 and also on the others. The modulation of the target gene expression could be different of 1.5 fold up-regulation and also could be down-regulated, depending of the nature of the dosage-dependent gene products, and thus determine a secondary gene dosage effect (Figure 2).

At the same time, all or some genes on chromosome 21, showing changes in their expression, could participate to the amplified developmental instability of the genome in trisomy 21, determining a general gene expression alteration and disequilibrium that could also be responsible of primary phenotypes in the brain and participate to pathogenesis of mental retardation. In addition, genes with altered expression can determine primary phenotypes in the brain by changes in gene interactions that, for the different cases, could be major or small additional effects, and interferences of the different allelic combinations (Figure 2).

Very recently, the first steps of a molecular pathway responsible of some Down syndrome phenotypes, in particular the mental retardation, have been elucidated (Arron et al., 2006). Two dosage-sensitive genes of chromosome 21 are involved, *DYRK1A* and *DSCR1*, that showed converging effects on the same pathways, which is responsible of NFAT-depending gene expression activation. Although, the products of these two chromosome 21 genes do not interact directly each others, they are involved in the control of the phosphorylation levels of NFAT and, consequently, of its activated nuclear localization (Arron et al., 2006; de la Luna and Estivill, 2006; Epstein, 2006).

One reason for the lack of drug treatments for mental retardation in Down syndrome is the limited understanding of the molecular and cellular mechanisms underlying this complex phenotype. At the time, we entry in a golden period for research to elucidate the molecular mechanisms of the mental retardation of Down syndrome, particularly with the development of powerful mouse models and molecular genetic technologies.

In this way, exemplary is the findings obtained using the Ts65Dn mouse model, in which estrogen treatment improved the learning performance and also reversed cholinergic impairment in old Ts65Dn females (Granholm et al., 2002). Previously, estrogen has been suggested to be neuroprotective, having beneficial effects on cognition (McEwen and Alves, 1999), and it modifies synapses in the hippocampal formation (Woolley et al., 1990; Woolley and McEwen, 1992).

Functional studies of candidate genes and of gene expression variations, and of their genomic controls are the two research priorities in the understanding of molecular mechanisms of mental retardation in Down syndrome. In addition, the development of new techniques in the regulation of gene expression by microRNAs or small interfering RNAs (He and Hannon, 2004) will provide potential powerful tools for correction of the aberrant gene expression in Down syndrome. So, actually, we could hope to rescue the basic molecular defects giving rise mental retardation in Down syndrome.

ACKNOWLEDGMENTS

We are grateful to our colleagues of the Jean-Pierre Changeux's Laboratory and Department of Molecular Biology-Jacques Monod at the Pasteur Institute (Paris) for their advices and support. We also thank J.M. Delabar (University Paris 7) for his continuous support.

REFERENCES

Aitken, D. A., McCaw, G., Crossley, J. A., Berry, E., Connor, J. M., Spencer, K. & Macri, J.N. (1993) First-trimester biochemical screening for fetal chromosome abnormalities and neural tube defects. *Prenat. Diagn., 13,* 681–689.

Altafaj, X., Dierssen, M., Baamonde, C., Marti, E., Visa, J., Guimera, J., Oset, M., Gonzalez, J. R., Florez, J., Fillat, C. & Estivill, X. (2001) Neurodevelopmental delay, motor abnormalities and cognitive deficits in transgenic mice overexpressing Dyrk1A (minibrain), a murine model of Down's syndrome. *Hum. Mol. Genet., 10,* 1915–1923.

Amano, K., Sago, H., Uchikawa, C., Suzuki, T., Kotliarova, S. E., Nukina, N., Epstein, C. J. & Yamakawa, K. (2004) Dosage-dependent over-expression of genes in the trisomic region of Ts1Cje mouse model for Down syndrome. *Hum. Mol. Genet., 13,* 1333-1340.

Ani, C., Grantham-McGregor, S. & Muller, D. (2000) Nutritional supplementation in Down syndrome: theoretical considerations and current status. *Dev. Med. Child. Neurol., 42*, 207-213.

Antonarakis, S. E. (1998) 10 years of genomics, chromosome 21, and Down syndrome, *Genomics 51,* 1–16.

Antonarakis, S. E. (2001) Chromosome 21: From sequence to applications. *Curr. Opin. Genet. Dev., 11,* 241–246.

Antonarakis, S. E., Lyle, R., Chrast, R. & Scott, H. S. (2001) Differential gene expression studies to explore the molecular pathophysiology of Down syndrome. *Brain Res. Brain Res. Rev., 36,* 265-274.

Antonarakis, S. E., Lyle, R., Dermitzakis, E. T., Reymond, A. & Deutsch, S. (2004) Chromosome 21 and Down syndrome: from genomics to pathophysiology. *Nat. Rev. Genet., 5,* 725-738.

Arai, Y., Ijuin, T., Takenawa, T., Becker, L. E. & Takashima, S. (2002) Excessive expression of synaptojanin in brains with Down syndrome. *Brain Dev., 24,* 67–72.

Arron, J. R., Winslow, M. M., Polleri, A., Chang, C. P., Wu, H., Gao, X., Neilson, J. R., Chen, L., Heit, J. J., Kim, S. K., Yamasaki, N., Miyakawa, T., Francke, U., Graef, I. A. & Crabtree, G. R. (2006) NFAT dysregulation by increased dosage of DSCR1 and DYRK1A on chromosome 21. *Nature, 441,* 595-600.

Avraham, K. B., Sugarman, H., Rotshenker, S. & Groner, Y. (1991) Down's syndrome: morphological remodelling and increased complexity in the neuromuscular junction of transgenic CuZn-superoxide dismutase mice. *J. Neurocytol., 20,* 208-215.

Aylward, E. H., Habbak, R., Warren, A. C., Pulsifer, M. B., Barta, P. E., Jerram, M. & Pearlson, G. D. (1997) Cerebellar volume in adults with Down syndrome. *Arch Neurol., 54,* 209-212.

Azmitia, E. C., Griffin, W. S. T., Marshak, D. R., Van Eldik, L. J. & Whitaker-Azmitia, P. M. (1992) S100b and serotonin: a possible astrocytic-neuronal link to neuropathology of Alzheimer's disease. *Prog. Brain Res., 92,* 459–473.

Bahn, S., Mimmack, M., Ryan, M., Caldwell, M. A., Jauniaux, E., Starkey, M., Svendsen, C. N. & Emson, P. (2002) Neuronal target genes of the neuron-restrictive silencer factor in neurospheres derived from fetuses with Down's syndrome: a gene expression study. *Lancet, 359,* 310–315.

Ballabio, A. (1993) The rise and fall of positional cloning? *Nature Genet., 3,* 277–279.

Bauman, M. L., Kemper, T. L. & Arin, D. M. (1995) Pervasive neuroanatomic abnormalities of the brain in three cases of Rett's syndrome. *Neurology, 45,* 1581-1586.

Baxter, L. L., Moran, T. H., Richtsmeier, J. T., Troncoso, J. & Reeves, R. H. (2000) Discovery and genetic localization of Down syndrome cerebellar phenotypes using the Ts65Dn mouse. *Hum. Mol. Genet., 9,* 195–202.

Becker, L. E., Armstrong, D. L. & Chan, F. (1986) Dendritic atrophy in children with Down's syndrome. *Ann. Neurol., 20,* 520–532.

Becker, L., Mito, T., Takashima, S. & Onodera, K. (1991) Growth and development of the brain in Down syndrome. In C. H. Epstein (Ed.), *The Morphogenesis of Down syndrome* (pp. 133–152). New York, Wiley-Liss.

Behar, T. N. & Colton, C. A. (2003) Redox regulation of neuronal migration in a Down syndrome model. *Free Radic. Biol. Med., 35,* 566-575.

Belichenko, P. V., Masliah, E., Kleschevnikov, A. M., Villar, A. J., Epstein, C. J., Salehi, A. & Mobley, W. C. (2004) Synaptic structural abnormalities in the Ts65Dn mouse model of Down syndrome. *J. Comp. Neurol., 480,* 281-298.

Bell, K., Shokrian, D., Potenzieri, C. & Whitaker-Azmitia, P. M. (2003) Harm avoidance, anxiety, and response to novelty in the adolescent S-100beta transgenic mouse: role of serotonin and relevance to Down syndrome. *Neuropsychopharmacology, 28,* 1810-1816.

Best, T. K., Siarey, R. J. & Galdzicki, Z. (2006) Ts65Dn, a mouse model of Down syndrome, exhibits increased GABAB induced potassium current. J. Neurophysiol. In press.

Bimonte-Nelson, H. A., Hunter, C. L., Nelson, M. E. & Granholm, A. C. (2003) Frontal cortex BDNF levels correlate with working memory in an animal model of Down syndrome. *Behav. Brain Res., 139,* 47-57.

Black, A. H., Nadel, L. & O'Keefe, J. (1977) Hippocampal function in avoidance learning and punishment. *Psychol. Bull., 84,* 1107-1129.

Branchi, I., Bichler, Z., Minghetti, L., Delabar, J. M., Malchiodi-Albedi, F., Gonzalez, M. C., Chettouh, Z., Nicolini, A., Chabert, C., Smith, D. J., Rubin, E. M., Migliore-Samour, D. & Alleva, E. (2004) Transgenic mouse in vivo library of human Down syndorme Critical

Region 1: association between *DYRK1A* overexpression, brain development abnormalities, and cell cycle protein alteration. *J. Neuropathol. Exp. Neurol., 63,* 429-440.

Brown, F. R., Greer, M. K., Aylward, E. H. & Hunt, H. H. (1990) Intellectual and adaptive functioning in individuals with Down syndrome in relation to age and environmental placement. *Pediatrics, 85,* 450–452.

Brown, J. H., Johnson, M. H., Patterson, S. J., Gilmore, R., Longhi, E. & Karmiloff-Smith, A. (2003) Spatial representation and attention in toddlers with Williams syndrome and Down syndrome. *Neuropsychologia, 41,* 1037-1046.

Bulfone, A., Gattuso, C., Marchitiello, A., Pardini, C., Boncinelli, E., Borsani, G., Banfi, S. & Ballabio, A. (1998) The embryonic expression pattern of 40 murine cDNAs homologous to Drosophila mutant genes (Dres): a comparativc and topographic approach to predict gene function. *Hum. Mol. Genet., 7,* 1997-2006.

Carlesimo, G. A., Marotta, L. & Vicari, S. (1997) Long-term memory in mental retardation: evidence for a specific impairment in subjects with Down's syndrome. *Neuropsychologia, 35,* 71-79.

Casanova, M. F., Walker, L. C., Whitehouse, P. J. & Price, D. L. (1985) Abnormalities of the nucleus basalis in Down's syndrome. *Ann Neurol., 18,* 310-313.

Cataldo, A. M., Petanceska, S., Peterhoff, C. M., Terio, N. B., Epstein, C. J., Villar, A., Carlson, E. J., Staufenbiel, M. & Nixon, R. A. (2003) App gene dosage modulates endosomal abnormalities of Alzheimer's disease in a segmental trisomy 16 mouse model of down syndrome. *J. Neurosci., 23,* 6788-6792.

Chapman, R. S. & Hesketh, L. J. (2000) Behavioral phenotype of individuals with Down syndrome. *Ment. Retard. Dev. Disabil. Res. Rev., 6,* 84-95.

Chapman, R. S., Seung, H-K., Schwartz, S. E. & Kay-Raining Bird, E. (1998) Language skills of children and adolescents with Down syndrome II: production deficits. *J. Speech Lang. Hear Res., 41*, 861–873.

Chen, H., Chrast, R., Rossier, V., Gos, A., Antonarakis, S. E., Kudoh, J., Yamaki, A., Shindoh, N., Maeda, H., Minoshima, S., et al. (1995) Single-minded and Down syndrome? *Nat. Genet., 10,* 9-10.

Chen, H., Chrast, R., Rossier, C., Morris, M. A., Lalioti, M. D. & Antonarakis, S. E. (1996) Cloning of 559 potential exons of genes of human chromosome 21 by exon trapping. *Genome Res., 6,* 747-760.

Chrast, R., Scott, H. S., Papasavvas, M. P., Rossier, C., Antonarakis, E. S., Barras, C., Davisson, M. T., Schmidt, C., Estivill, X., Dierssen, M., Pritchard, M. & Antonarakis, S. E. (2000a) The mouse brain transcriptome by SAGE: differences in gene expression between P30 brains of the partial trisomy 16 mouse model of Down syndrome (Ts65Dn) and normals. *Genome Res., 10,* 2006-2021.

Chrast, R., Scott, H. S., Madani, R., Huber, L., Wolfer, D. P., Prinz, M., Aguzzi, A., Lipp, H. P. & Antonarakis, S. E. (2000b) Mice trisomic for a bacterial artificial chromosome with the single-minded 2 gene (Sim2) show phenotypes similar to some of those present in the partial trisomy 16 mouse models of Down syndrome. *Hum. Mol. Genet., 9,* 1853-1864.

Clark, D. & Wilson, G. N. (2003) Behavioral assessment of children with Down syndrome using the Reiss psychopathology scale. *Am. J. Med. Genet., 118,* 210-216.

Cohen, W. I. (1999) Health care guidelines for individuals with Down syndrome: 1999 revision. *Down Syndrome Quarterly, 4,* 1-16.

Collacot, R. A., Cooper, S. A., Branford, D. & McGrother, C. (1998) Behaviour phenotype for Down's syndrome. *Br. J. Psychiatry, 172,* 85–89.

Connolly, B. H., Morgan, S. B., Russell, F. F. & Fulliton, W. L. (1993) A longitudinal study of children with Down syndrome who experienced early intervention programming. *Phys Ther., 73,* 170-9.

Connor, J. M., & Ferguson-Smith, M. A. (1997) *Essential medical genetics* (5th edn). Oxford, Blackwell Science.

Cooper, J. D., Salehi, A., Delcroix, J. D., Howe, C. L., Belichenko, P. V., Chua-Couzens, J., Kilbridge, J. F., Carlson, E. J., Epstein, C. J. & Mobley, W. C. (2001) Failed retrograde transport of NGF in a mouse model of Down's syndrome: reversal of cholinergic neurodegenerative phenotypes following NGF infusion. *Proc. Natl. Acad. Sci., 98,* 10439-10444.

Costa, A. C., Walsh, K. & Davisson, M. T. (1999) Motor dysfunction in a mouse model for Down syndrome. *Physiol. Behav., 68,* 211-220.

Coussons-Read, M. E. & Crnic, L. S. (1996) Behavioral assessment of the Ts65Dn mouse, a model for Down syndrome: altered behavior in the elevated plus maze and open field. *Behav. Genet., 26,* 7-13.

Cox, D. R., Smith, S. A., Epstein, L. B. & Epstein, C. J. (1984) Mouse trisomy 16 as an animal model of human trisomy 21 (Down syndrome): production of viable trisomy 16 diploid mouse chimeras. *Dev. Biol., 101,* 416-424.

Coyle, J. T., Oster-Granite, M. L. & Gearhart, J. D. (1986) The neurobiologic consequences of Down syndrome. *Brain Res. Bull., 16,* 773–787.

Coyle, J. T., Oster-Granite, M. L., Reeves, R. H. & Gearhart, J. D. (1988) Down syndrome, Alzheimer's disease and the trisomy 16 mouse. *Trends Neurosci., 11,* 390–394.

Crété, N., Gosset, P., Théophile, D., Duterque-Coquillaud, M., Blouin, J. L., Vayssettes, C., Sinet, P. M. & Creau-Goldberg, N. (1993) Mapping the Down syndrome chromosome region. Establishment of a YAC contig spanning 1.2 megabases. *Eur. J. Hum. Genet., 1,* 51-63.

Crews, S. T., Thomas, J. B. & Goodman, C. S. (1988) The Drosophila singleminded gene encodes a nuclear protein with sequence similarity to the per gene product, *Cell*, *52,* 143–151.

Crnic, L. S. & Pennington, B. F. (2000) Down syndrome: neuropsychology and animal models. *Prog. Infanc. Res., 1,* 69-111.

Dahmane, N., Charron, G., Lopes, C., Yaspo, M. L., Maunoury, C., Decorte, L., Sinet, P. M., Bloch, B. & Delabar, J. M. (1995) Down syndrome critical region contains a gene homologous to Drosophila sim expressed during rat and human central nervous system development, *Proc. Natl. Acad. Sci. USA*, *92,* 9191–9195.

Dahmane, N., Ait Ghezala, G. A., Gosset, P., Chamoun, Z., Dufresne-Zacharia, M. C., Lopes, C., Rabatel, N., Gassanova-Maugenre, S., Chettouh, Z., Abramowski, V., Fayet, E., Yaspo, M. L., Korn, B., Blouin, J. L., Lehrach, H., Poutska, A., Antonarakis, S. E., Sinet, P. M., Creau, N. & Delabar, J. M. (1998) Transcriptional map of the 2.5-Mb CBR–ERG region of chromosome 21 involved in Down syndrome. *Genomics, 48,* 12–23.

Dalley, J. W., Cardinal, R. N. & Robbins, T. W. (2004) Prefrontal executive and cognitive functions in rodents: neural and neurochemical substrates. *Neurosci. Biobehav. Rev., 28,* 771-784.

Dalton, A. J. & Crapper-McLachlan, D. R. (1986) Clinical expression of Alzheimer's disease in Down syndrome. *Psychiatr. Clin. North. Am., 9,* 959–70.

Das, A. K., Cohen, P. W. & Barford, D. (1998) The structure of the tetratricopeptide repeats of protein phosphatase 5: implications for TPR-mediated protein-protein interactions. *EMBO J., 17,* 1192-1199.

Dauphinot, L., Lyle, R., Rivals, I., Dang, M. T., Moldrich, R. X., Golfier, G., Ettwiller, L., Toyama, K., Rossier, J., Personnaz, L., et al. (2005) The cerebellar transcriptome during postnatal development of the Ts1Cje mouse, a segmental trisomy model for Down syndrome. *Hum. Mol. Genet., 14,* 373-384.

Davisson, M. & Costa, A. (1999). *Mouse Models in the Study of Genetic Neurological Disorders* (ed. Popko, K.). New York, Kluwer Academic_Plenum, pp. 297–327.

Delabar, J. M., Theophile, D., Rahmani, Z., Chettouh, Z., Blouin, J. L., Prieur, M., Noel, B. & Sinet, P. M. (1993) Molecular mapping of twenty-four features of Down syndrome on chromosome 21. *Eur. J. Hum. Genet., 1,* 114–124.

Demas, G. E., Nelson, R. J., Krueger, B. K. & Yarowsky, P. J. (1996) Spatial memory deficits in segmental trisomic Ts65Dn mice. *Behav. Brain Res., 82,* 85-92.

Demas, G. E., Nelson, R. J., Krueger, B. K. & Yarowsky, P. J. (1998) Impaired spatial working and reference memory in segmental trisomy (Ts65Dn) mice. *Behav. Brain Res., 90,* 199–201.

Devenny, D. A., Silverman, W. P., Hill, A. L., Jenkins, E., Sersen, E. A. & Wisniewski, K. E. (1996) Normal ageing in adults with Down's syndrome: a longitudinal study. *J. Intellect. Disabil. Res., 40,* 208-221.

Dierssen, M., Vallina, I. F., Baamonde, C., Lumbreras, M. A., Martinez-Cue, C., Calatayud, S. G. & Florez, J. (1996) Impaired cyclic AMP production in the hippocampus of a Down syndrome murine model. *Brain Res. Dev. Brain Res., 95,* 122-124.

Dierssen, M., Vallina, I. F., Baamonde, C., Garcia-Calatayud, S., Lumbreras, M. A. & Florez, J. (1997) Alterations of central noradrenergic transmission in Ts65Dn mouse, a model for Down syndrome. *Brain Res., 749,* 238-244.

Dierssen, M., Fillat, C., Crnic, L., Arbones, M., Florez, J. & Estivill, X. (2001) Murine models for Down syndrome. *Physiol. Behav., 73,* 859-871.

Down, J. L. H. (1866). Observations on an ethnic classification of idiots. *Lond. Hosp. Rep., 3,* 259–262.

Dufresne-Zacharia, M. C., Dahmane, N., Theophile, D., Orti, R., Chettouh, Z., Sinet, P. M. & Delabar, J. M. (1994) 3.6-Mb genomic and YAC physical map of the Down syndrome chromosome region on chromosome 21. *Genomics, 19,* 462-469.

Dujon, B. (1996) The yeast genome project: what did we learn? *Trends Genet., 12,* 263-270.

Ema, M., Suzuki, M., Morita, M., Hirose, K., Sogawa, K., Matsuda, Y., Gotoh, O., Saijoh, Y., Fujii, H., Hamada, H. & Fujii-Kuriyama, Y. (1996) cDNA cloning of a murine homologue of Drosophila single-minded, its mRNA expression in mouse development, and chromosome localization. *Biochem. Biophys. Res. Commun., 218,* 588-594.

Ema, M., Ikegami, S., Hosoya, T., Mimura, J., Ohtani, H., Nakao, K., Inokuchi, K., Katsuki, M. & Fujii-Kuriyama, Y. (1999) Mild impairment of learning and memory in mice overexpressing the mSim2 gene located on chromosome 16: an animal model of Down's syndrome, *Hum. Mol. Genet., 8,* 1409-1415.

Engidawork, E. & Lubec, G. (2003) Molecular changes in fetal Down syndrome brain. *J. Neurochem., 84,* 895–904.

Engidawork, E., Balic, N., Fountoulakis, M., Dierssen, M., Graber-Platzer, S. & Lubec, G. (2001) b-Amyloid precursor protein, ETS-2 and collagen alpha 1 (VI) chain precursor, encoded on chromosome 21, are not overexpressed in fetal Down syndrome: further evidence against gene dosage effect. *J. Neural Transm. Suppl., 61,* 335–346.

Epstein, C. J. (1986) *The Consequences of Chromosome Imbalance: Principles, Mechanisms, and Models,* New York, Cambridge University Press.

Epstein, C. J. (1988) Mechanisms of the effects of aneuploidy in mammals. *Annu. Rev. Genet., 22,* 51-75.

Epstein, C. J. (1995) Down syndrome (trisomy 21). In C. R. Scriver, A. L., Beaudet, W. S., Sly, & D. Valle (Eds.), *The Metabolic and Molecular Bases of Inherited Disease* (pp.749–794) New York, McGraw-Hill.

Epstein, J. (2001) Down syndrome. In C. R. Scriver, A. L. Beaudet, W. S. Sly., & D. Valle (Eds.), *The Metabolic and Molecular Bases of Inherited Disease* (7th edn., Vol. I, pp. 1223–1256) New York, McGraw-Hill, Inc.

Epstein, C. J. (2002). 2001 William Allan Award Address. From Down syndrome to the "human" in "human genetics". *Am. J. Hum. Genet., 70,* 300-313.

Epstein, C. J. (2006) Down's syndrome: critical genes in a critical region. *Nature, 441,* 582-583.

Epstein, C. J., Hofmeister, B. G., Yee, D., Smith, S. A., Philip, R., Cox, D. R. & Epstein, L. B. (1985) Stem cell deficiencies and thymic abnormalities in fetal mouse trisomy 16. *J. Exp. Med., 162,* 695–712.

Epstein, C. J., Avraham, K. B., Lovett, M., Smith, S., Elroy-Stein, O., Rotman, G., Bry, C. & Groner, Y. (1987) Transgenic mice with increased Cu/Zn-superoxide dismutase activity: animal model of dosage effects in Down syndrome. *Proc. Natl. Acad. Sci., 84,* 8044-8048.

Ermak, G., Morgan, T. E. & Davies, K. J. (2001) Chronic overexpression of the calcineurin inhibitory gene DSCR1 (Adapt78) is associated with Alzheimer's disease. *J. Biol. Chem., 276,* 38787-38794.

Escorihuela, R. M., Vallina, I. F., Martinez-Cue, C., Baamonde, C., Dierssen, M., Tobena, A., Florez, J. & Fernandez-Teruel, A. (1998) Impaired short- and long-term in Ts65Dn mice, a model for Down syndrome. *Neurosci. Lett., 247,* 171–174.

Esquirol, J. E. D. (1838) *Des maladies mentales considérées sous les rapports médical, hygiénique et médico-légal.* Paris: J.-B. Baillères.

Fan, C. M., Kuwana, E., Bulfone, A., Fletcher, C. F., Copeland, N. G., Jenkins, N. A., Crews, S., Martinez, S., Puelles, L., Rubenstein, J. L. & Tessier-Lavigne, M. (1996) Expression patterns of two murine homologs of Drosophila single-minded suggest possible roles in embryonic patterning and in the pathogenesis of Down syndrome. *Mol. Cell. Neurosci., 7,* 1-16.

Ferencz, C., Neill, C. A., Boughman, J. A., Rubin, J. D., Brenner, J. I. & Perry, L. W. (1989) Congenital cardiovascular malformations associated with chromosome abnormalities: An epidemiologic study. *J. Pediatr., 114,* 79-86.

Ferrando-Miguel, R., Cheon, M. S. & Lubec, G. (2004) Protein levels of genes encoded on chromosome 21 in fetal Down syndrome brain (Part V); overexpression of phosphatidyl-inositol-glycan class P protein (DSCR5). *Amino Acids., 26,* 255-261.

Ferrer, I. & Gullotta, F. (1990) Down's syndrome and Alzheimer's disease: dendritic spine counts in the hippocampus. *Acta Neuropathol. (Berl), 79,* 680-685.

Fiala, J. C. Spacek, J. & Harris, K. M. (2002) Dendritic spine pathology: cause or consequence of neurological disorders? *Brain Res. Brain Res. Rev., 39,* 29-54.

FitzPatrick, D. R. (2005) Transcriptional consequences of autosomal trisomy: primary gene dosage with complex downstream effects. *Trends Genet., 21,* 249-253.

FitzPatrick, D. R., Ramsay, J., McGill, N. I., Shade, M., Carothers, A.D. & Hastie, N. D. (2002) Transcriptome analysis of human autosomal trisomy. *Hum. Mol. Genet., 11,* 3249-3256.

Frank, R. G. & Crews, S. T. (1994) Transcriptional activation domains of the single-minded bHLH protein are required for CNS midline cell development. *Mech. Dev., 45,* 269-277.

Freeman, S. B., Taft, L. F., Dooley, K. J., Allran, K., Sherman, S. L., Hassold, T. J., Khoury, M. J. & Saker, D. M. (1998) Population-based study of congenital heart defects in Down syndrome. *Am. J. Med. Genet., 80,* 213-217.

Fuentes, J. J., Pritchard, M. A., Planas, A. M., Bosch, A., Ferrer, I. & Estivill, X. (1995) A new human gene from the Down syndrome critical region encodes a proline-rich protein highly expressed in fetal brain and heart. *Hum. Mol. Genet., 4,* 1935-1944.

Fuentes, J. J., Genesca, L., Kingsbury, T. J., Cunningham, K. W., Perez-Riba, M., Estivill, X. & de la Luna, S. (2000) DSCR1, overexpressed in Down syndrome, is an inhibitor of calcineurin-mediated signaling pathways. *Hum. Mol. Genet., 9,* 1681–1690.

Funahashi, S., Takeda, K. & Watanabe, Y. (2004) Neural mechanisms of spatial working memory: contributions of the dorsolateral pre-frontal cortex and the thalamic mediodorsal nucleus. Cogn. Affect. *Behav. Neurosci., 4,* 409-420.

Gahtan, E., Auerbach, J. M., Groner, Y. & Segal, M. (1998) Reversible impairment of long-term potentiation in transgenic Cu/Zn-SOD mice. *Eur. J. Neurosci., 10,* 538-544.

Galdzicki, Z., Coan, E. J., Rapoport, S. I. & Stoll, J. (1998) Increased expression of voltage-activated calcium channels in cultured hippocampal neurons from mouse trisomy 16, a model for Down syndrome. *Brain Res. Mol. Brain Res., 56,* 200-206.

Galdzicki, Z., Siarey, R., Pearce, R., Stoll, J. & Rapoport, S. I. (2001) On the cause of mental retardation in Down syndrome: extrapolation from full and segmental trisomy 16 mouse models. *Brain Res. Brain Res. Rev., 35,* 115-145.

Gardiner, K., Fortna, A., Bechtel, L. & Davisson, M. T. (2003) Mouse models of Down syndrome: how useful can they be? Comparison of the gene content of human chromosome 21 with orthologous mouse genomic regions. *Gene, 318,* 137–147.

Gardiner, K., Davisson, M. T. & Crnic, L. S. (2004) Building protein interaction maps for Down's syndrome. *Brief Funct. Genomic Proteomic., 3,* 142-56.

Gearhart, J. D., Davisson, M. T. & Oster-Granite, M. L. (1986) Autosomal aneuploidy in mice: generation and developmental consequences. *Brain Res. Bull., 16,* 789-801.

Gerlai, R. & Roder, J. (1998) Spatial and nonspatial learning in mice: effects of S100 beta overexpression and age. Neurobiol. *Learn. Mem., 66,* 143-154.

Gitton, Y., Dahmane, N., Baik, S., Ruiz, I., Altaba, A., Neidhardt, L., Scholze, M., Herrmann, B. G., Kahlem, P., Benkahla, A., Schrinner, S., Yildirimman, R., Herwig, R., Lehrach, H. & Yaspo, M. L. (2002) A gene expression map of human chromosome 21 orthologues in the mouse. *Nature, 420,* 586-590.

Golden, J. A. & Hyman, B. T. (1994) Development of the superior temporal neocortex is anomalous in trisomy 21. J. Neuropathol. *Exp. Neurol., 53,* 513–552.

Goldowitz, D. & Smeyne, R. J. (1995) Tune into the weaver channel. *Nat. Genet., 11,* 107-109.

Gosset, P., Ghezala, G. A., Korn, B., Yaspo, M. L., Poutska, A., Lehrach, H., Sinet, P. M. & Creau, N. (1997) A new inward rectifier potassium channel gene (KCNJ15) localized on chromosome 21 in the Down syndrome chromosome region 1 (DCR1). *Genomics, 44,* 237-241.

Granholm, A. C, Sanders, L. A. & Crnic, L. S. (2000) Loss of cholinergic phenotype in basal forebrain coincides with cognitive decline in a mouse model of Down's syndrome. *Exp. Neurol., 161,* 647-663.

Granholm, A. C., Ford, K. A., Hyde, L. A., Bimonte, H. A., Hunter, C. L., Nelson, M., Albeck, D., Sanders, L. A., Mufson, E. J. & Crnic, L. S. (2002) Estrogen restores cognition and cholinergic phenotype in an animal model of Down syndrome. *Physiol. Behav., 77,* 371-385.

Griffin, W. S. T., Sheng, J. G., McKenzie, L. E., Royston, M. C., Gentleman, S. M., Brumback, R. A., Cork, L. C., Del Bigio, M. R., Roberts, G. W. & Mrak, R. E. (1998) Life-long over-expression of S100b in Down's syndrome: implications for Alzheimer's pathogenesis. *Neurobiol. Aging, 19,* 401–405.

Groves, M. R. & Barford, D. (1999) Topological characteristics of helical repeat proteins. *Curr. Opin. Struct. Biol., 9,* 383-389.

Guimera, J., Casas, C., Pucharcos, C. Solans, A., Domenech, A., Planas, A. M., Ashley, J., Lovett, M., Estivill, X. & Pritchard, M. A. (1996) A human homologue of Drosophila minibrain (MNB) is expressed in the neuronal regions affected in Down syndrome and maps to the critical region. *Hum. Mol. Genet., 5,* 1305–1310.

Guimera, J., Casas, C., Estivill, X. & Pritchard, M. (1999) Human minibrain homologue (MNBH/DYRK1): characterization, alternative splicing, differential tissue expression, and overexpression in Down syndrome, Genomics, 57, 407–418.

Guipponi, M., Brunschwig, K., Chamoun, Z., Scott, H. S., Shibuya, K., Kudoh, J., Delezoide, A. L., El Samadi, S., Chettouh, Z., Rossier, C., Shimizu, N., Mueller, F., Delabar, J. M. & Antonarakis, S. E. (2000) *C21orf5*, a novel human chromosome 21 gene, has a *Caenorhabditis elegans* ortholog (*pad-1*) required for embryonic patterning. *Genomics, 68,* 30–40.

Gurney, M. E., Pu, H., Chiu, A. Y., Dal Canto, M. C., Polchow, C. Y., Alexander, D. D., Caliendo, J., Hentati, A., Kwon, Y. W., Deng, H. X. et al. (1994) Motor neuron degeneration in mice that express a human Cu,Zn superoxide dismutase mutation. *Science, 264,* 1772-1775.

de Haan, J. B., Wolvetang, E. J., Cristiano, F., Iannello, R., Bladier, C., Kelner, M. J. & Kola, I. (1997) Reactive oxygen species and their contribution to pathology in Down syndrome. *Adv. Pharmacol., 38,* 379–402.

Hampton, T. G., Stasko, M. R., Kale, A., Amende, I. & Costa, A. C. (2004) Gait dynamics in trisomic mice: quantitative neurological traits of Down syndrome. *Physiol Behav., 82,* 381-389.

Harashima, C., Jacobowitz, D. M., Witta, J., Borke, R. C., Best, T. K., Siarev, R. J. & Galdzicki, Z. (2006) Abnormal expression of the G-protein-activated inwardly rectifying potassium channel 2 (GIRK2) in hippocampus, frontal cortex, and substantia nigra of Ts65Dn mouse: a model of Down syndrome. *J. Comp. Neurol., 494,* 815-833.

Harris-Cerruti, C., Kamsler, A., Kaplan, B., Lamb, B., Segal, M., Groner, Y. (2004) Functional and morphological alterations in compound transgenic mice overexpressing

Cu/Zn superoxide dismutase and amyloid precursor protein. *Eur. J. Neurosci., 19,* 1174-90. (Erratum in: *Eur. J. Neurosci., 19,* 2913).

Hasle, H. (2001) Pattern of malignant disorders in individuals with Down's syndrome. *Lancet Oncol., 2,* 429-436.

Hassold, T. & Hunt, P. (2001) To err (meiotically) is human: The genesis of human aneuploidy. *Nat. Rev. Genet., 2,* 280-291.

Hattori, M., Fujiyama, A., Taylor, T. D., Watanabe, H., Yada, T., Park, H. S., Toyoda, A., Ishii, K., Totoki, Y., Choi, D. K., Groner, Y., Soeda, E., Ohki, M., Takagi, T., Sakaki, Y., Taudien, S., Blechschmidt, K., Polley, A., Menzel, U., Delabar, J., Kumpf, K., Lehmann, R., Patterson, D., Reichwald, K., Rump, A., Schillhabel, M., Schudy, A., Zimmermann, W., Rosenthal, A., Kudoh, J., Schibuya, K., Kawasaki, K., Asakawa, S., Shintani, A., Sasaki, T., Nagamine, K., Mitsuyama, S., Antonarakis, S. E., Minoshima, S., Shimizu, N., Nordsiek, G., Hornischer, K., Brant, P., Scharfe, M., Schon, O., Desario, A., Reichelt, J., Kauer, G., Blocker, H., Ramser, J., Beck, A., Klages, S., Hennig, S., Riesselmann, L., Dagand, E., Haaf, T., Wehrmeyer, S., Borzym, K., Gardiner, K., Nizetic, D., Francis, F., Lehrach, H., Reinhardt, R., Yaspo, M. L. Chromosome 21 mapping and sequencing consortium. (2000) The DNA sequence of human chromosome 21, *Nature, 405,* 311–319.

He, L. & Hannon, GH. (2004) MicroRNAs: small RNAs with a big role in gene regulation. *Nat. Rev. Genet., 5,* 522-531.

Hennequin, M., Morin, C. & Feine, J. S. (2000) Pain expression and stimulus localisation in individuals with Down's syndrome. *Lancet, 356,* 1882-1887. (Erratum in: *Lancet , 357,* 890.

Hodapp, R. M. & Zigler, E. (1990) Applying the developmental perspective to individuals with Down syndrome. In D. Cicchetti, & M. Beeghly (Eds.), *Children with Down syndrome: a developmental perspective* (pp. 1-28). New York: Cambridge University Press.

Hodapp, R. M., Ewans, D. E. & Gray, F. L. (1999) Intellectual development in children with Down syndrome. In J. A. Rondal, J. Perera, & L. Nadel (eds.) *Down syndrome: a review of current knowledge* (pp; 124-132) London, UK: Whurr publisher.

Holtzman, D. M., Santucci, D., Kilbridge, J., Chua-Couzens, J., Fontana, D. J., Daniels, S. E., Johnson, R. M., Chen, K., Sun, Y., Carlson, E., Alleva, E., Epstein, C. J. & Mobley, W. C. (1996) Developmental abnormalities and age-related neurodegeneration in a mouse model of Down syndrome. *Proc. Natl. Acad. Sci. USA, 93,* 13333–13338.

Huang, T. T., Yasunami, M., Carlson, E. J., Gillespie, A. M., Reaume, A. G., Hoffman, E. K., Chan, P. H., Scott, R. W. & Epstein, C. J. (1997) Superoxide-mediated cytotoxicity in superoxide dismutase-deficient fetal fibroblasts. *Arch. Biochem. Biophys., 344,* 424-432.

Hulme, C. & Mackenzie, S. (1992) *Working memory and severe learning difficulties.* Hove, UK: Erlbaum.

Hunter, C. L., Isacson, O., Nelson, M., Bimonte-Nelson, H., Seo, H., Lin, L., Ford, K., Kindy, M. S. & Granholm, A. C. (2003) Regional alterations in amyloid precursor protein and nerve growth factor across age in a mouse model of Down's syndrome. *Neurosci, Res., 45,* 437-445.

Hunter, C. L., Bimonte-Nelson, H. A., Nelson, M., Eckman, C. B. & Granholm, A. C. (2004) Behavioral and neurobiological markers of Alzheimer's disease in Ts65Dn mice: effects of estrogen. *Neurobiol. Aging, 25,* 873-884.

Hyde, L. A. & Crnic, L. S. (2001) Age-related deficits in context discrimination learning in Ts65Dn mice that model Down syndrome and Alzheimer's disease. *Behav. Neurosci., 115,* 1239–1246.

Hyde, L. A., Frisone, D. F. & Crnic, L. S. (2001) Ts65Dn mice, a model for Down syndrome, have deficits in context discrimination learning suggesting impaired hippocampal function. Behav. Brain Res., 118, 53–60.

Insausti, A. M., Megias, M., Crespo, D., Cruz-Orive, L. M., Dierssen, M., Vallina, I. F., Insausti, R., Florez, J. & Vallina, T. F. (1998) Hippocampal volume and neuronal number in Ts65Dn mice: a murine model of Down syndrome. *Neurosci. Lett., 253,* 175–178.

International Human Genome Sequencing Consortium (2004) Finishing the euchromatic sequence of the human genome. *Nature, 431,* 931-945.

Ito, M. (2002) The molecular organization of cerebellar long-term depression. *Nature Rev. Neurosci., 3,* 896-902.

Jernigan, T. L., Bellugi, U., Sowell, E., Doherty, S. & Hesselink, J. R. (1993) Cerebral morphologic distinctions between Williams and Down syndromes. *Arch. Neurol., 50,* 186–191.

Johnston, M. V., Hohmann, C. & Blue, M. E. (1995) Neurobiology of Rett syndrome. *Neuropediatrics, 26,* 119-122.

Kadota, M., Shirayoshi, Y. & Oshimura, M. (2002) Elevated apoptosis in pre-mature neurons differentiated from mouse ES cells containing a single human chromosome 21. *Biochem. Biophys. Res. Commun. 299,* 599–605.

Kadota, M., Nishigaki, R., Wang, C. C., Toda, T., Shirayoshi, Y., Inoue, Gojobori, T., Ikeo, K., Rogers, M. S. & Oshimura, M. (2004) Proteomic signatures and aberrations of mouse embryonic stem cells containing a single human chromosome 21 in neuronal differentiation: an *in vitro* model of Down syndrome. *Neuroscience, 129,* 325–335.

Kahlem, P., Sultan, M., Herwig, R., Steinfath, M., Balzereit, D., Eppens, B., Saran, N. G., Pletcher, M. T., South, S. T., Stetten, G. et al. (2004) Transcript level alterations reflect gene dosage effects across multiple tissues in a mouse model of downsyndrome. *Genome Res., 14,* 1258-1267.

Kampa, D., Cheng, J., Kapranov, P., Yamanaka, M., Brubaker, S., Cawley, S., Drenkow, J., Piccolboni, A., Bekiranov, S., Hclt, G., Tammana, H. & Gingeras, T. R. (2004) Novel RNAs identified from an in-depth analysis of the transcriptome of human chromosomes 21 and 22. *Genome Res., 14,* 331-342.

Kapranov, P., Cawley, S. E., Drenkow, J., Bekiranov, S, Strausberg, R. L., Fodor, S. P. & Gingeras, T. R. (2002) Large-scale transcriptional activity in chromosomes 21 and 22, *Science, 296,* 916–919.

Kawasaki, H., Mizuseki, K., Nishikawa, S. Kaneko, S., Kuwana, Y., Nakanishi, S., Nishikawa, S. I. & Sasai, Y. (2000) Induction of midbrain dopaminergic neurons from ES cells by stromal cell-derived inducing activity. *Neuron, 28,* 31–41.

Kentrup, H., Becker, W., Heukelbach, J., Wilmes, A., Schurmann, A., Huppertz, C., Kainulainen, H. & Joost, H. G. (1996) Dyrk, a dual specificity protein kinase with unique structural features whose activity is dependent on tyrosine residues between subdomains VII and VIII. *J. Biol. Chem., 271,* 3488-3495.

Kim, J. J. & Fanselow, M. S. (1992) Modality-specific retrograde amnesia of fear. *Science, 256,* 675-677.

Kish, S., Karlinsky, H., Becker, L., Gilbert, J., Rebbetoy, M., Chang, L. J., DiStefano, L. & Hornykiewicz, O. (1989) Down's syndrome individuals begin life with normal levels of brain cholinergic markers. *J. Neurochem., 52,* 1183-1187.

Klein, S. L., Kriegsfeld, L. J., Hairston, J. E., Rau, V., Nelson, R. J. & Yarowsky, P. J. (1996) Characterization of sensorimotor performance, reproductive and aggressive behaviors in segmental trisomic 16 (Ts65Dn) mice. *Physiol. Behav., 60,* 1159-1164.

Kleschevnikov, A. M., Belichenko, P. V., Villar, A. J., Epstein, C. J., Malenka, R. C. &, Mobley, W. C. (2004) Hippocampal long-term potentiation suppressed by increased inhibition in the Ts65Dn mouse, a genetic model of Down syndrome. *J. Neurosci., 24,* 8153-8160.

Korenberg, J. R., Kawashima, H., Pulst, S. M., Ikeuchi, T., Ogasawara, N., Yamamoto, K., Schonberg, S. A., West, R., Allen, L., Magenis, E. et al. (1990) Molecular definition of a region of chromosome 21 that causes features of the Down syndrome phenotype, *Am. J. Hum. Genet., 47,* 236–246.

Korenberg, J. R., Chen, X. N., Schipper, R., Sun, Z., Gonsky, R., Gerwehr, S., Carpenter, N., Daumer; C., Dignan, P., Disteche, C., Graham, Jr. J. M., Hugdins, L., McGillivray, B., Miyazaki, K., Ogasawara, N., Park, J. P., Pagon, R., Pueschel, S., Sack, G., Say, B., Schuffenhauer, S., Soukup, S. & Yamanaka, T. (1994) Down syndrome phenotypes: The consequences of chromosomal imbalance. *Proc. Natl. Acad. Sci. USA., 91,* 4997-5001.

Krasuski, J. S., Alexander, G. E., Horwitz, B., Rapoport, S. I. & Schapiro, M. B. (2002) Relation of medial temporal lobe volumes to age and memory function in nondemented adults with Down's syndrome: implications for the prodromal phase of Alzheimer's disease. *Am. J. Psychiatry, 159,* 74-81.

Krinsky-McHale, S. J., Devenny, D. A. & Silverman, W. P. (2002) Changes in explicit memory associated with early dementia in adults with Down's syndrome. *J. Intellect. Disabil. Res., 46,* 198-208.

Kurt, M. A., Davies, D. C., Kidd, M., Dierssen, M. & Florez, J. (2000) Synaptic deficit in the temporal cortex of partial trisomy 16 (Ts65Dn) mice. *Brain Res., 858,* 191–197.

Lacey-Casem, M. L. & Oster-Granite, M. L. (1994) The neuropathology of the trisomy 16 mouse. *Crit. Rev. Neurobiol., 8,* 293-322.

Lamb, B. T., Sisodia, S. S., Lawler, A. M., Slunt, H. H., Kitt, C. A., Kearns, W. G., Pearson, P. L., Price, D. L. & Gearhart, J. D. (1993) Introduction and expression of the 400 kilobase amyloid precursor protein gene in transgenic mice. *Nat. Genet., 5,* 22-30. (Erratum in: *Nat. Genet., 5,* 312.

Lane, P. W. (1964) New mutation: Weaver, wv. *Mouse News Lett., 30,* 32-33.

Lander, E. S., Linton, L. M., Birren, B., Nusbaum, C., Zody, M. C., Baldwin, J., Devon, K., Dewar, K., Doyle, M., FitzHugh, W., Funke, R., Gage, D., Harris, K., Heaford, A., Howland, J., Kann, L., Lehoczky, J., LeVine, R., McEwan, P., McKernan, K., Meldrim, J., Mesirov, J. P., Miranda, C., Morris, W., Naylor, J., Raymond, C., Rosetti, M., Santos, R., Sheridan, A., Sougnez, C., Stange-Thomann, N., Stojanovic, N., Subramanian, A., Wyman, D., Rogers, J., Sulston, J., Ainscough, R., Beck, S., Bentley, D., Burton, J., Clee, C., Carter, N., Coulson, A., Deadman, R., Deloukas, P., Dunham, A., Dunham, I., Durbin, R., French, L., Grafham, D., Gregory, S., Hubbard, T., Humphray, S., Hunt, A., Jones, M., Lloyd, C., McMurray, A., Matthews, L., Mercer, S., Milne, S., Mullikin, J. C., Mungall, A., Plumb, R., Ross, M., Shownkeen, R., Sims, S., Waterston, R. H., Wilson, R. K., Hillier, L. W., McPherson, J. D., Marra, M. A., Mardis, E. R., Fulton, L. A.,

Chinwalla, A. T., Pepin, K. H., Gish, W. R., Chissoe, S. L., Wendl, M. C., Delehaunty, K. D., Miner, T. L., Delehaunty, A., Kramer, J. B., Cook, L. L., Fulton, R. S., Johnson, D. L., Minx, P. J., Clifton, S. W., Hawkins, T., Branscomb, E., Predki, P., Richardson, P., Wenning, S., Slezak, T., Doggett, N., Cheng, J. F., Olsen, A., Lucas, S., Elkin, C., Uberbacher, E., Frazier, M., Gibbs, R. A., Muzny, D. M., Scherer, S. E., Bouck, J. B., Sodergren, E. J., Worley, K. C., Rives, C. M., Gorrell, J. H., Metzker, M. L., Naylor, S. L., Kucherlapati, R. S., Nelson, D. L., Weinstock, G. M., Sakaki, Y., Fujiyama, A., Hattori, M., Yada, T., Toyoda, A., Itoh, T., Kawagoe, C., Watanabe, H., Totoki, Y., Taylor, T., Weissenbach, J., Heilig, R., Saurin, W., Artiguenave, F., Brottier, P., Bruls, T., Pelletier, E., Robert, C., Wincker, P., Smith, D. R., Doucette-Stamm, L., Rubenfield, M., Weinstock, K., Lee, H. M., Dubois, J., Rosenthal, A., Platzer, M., Nyakatura, G., Taudien, S., Rump, A., Yang, H., Yu, J., Wang, J., Huang, G., Gu, J., Hood, L., Rowen, L., Madan, A., Qin, S., Davis, R. W., Federspiel, N. A., Abola, A. P., Proctor, M. J., Myers, R. M., Schmutz, J., Dickson, M., Grimwood, J., Cox, D. R., Olson, M. V., Kaul, R., Raymond, C., Shimizu, N., Kawasaki, K., Minoshima, S., Evans, G. A., Athanasiou, M., Schultz, R., Roe, B. A., Chen, F., Pan, H., Ramser, J., Lehrach, H., Reinhardt, R., McCombie, W. R., de la Bastide, M., Dedhia, N., Blocker, H., Hornischer, K., Nordsiek, G., Agarwala, R., Aravind, L., Bailey, J. A., Bateman, A., Batzoglou, S., Birney, E., Bork, P., Brown, D. G., Burge, C. B., Cerutti, L., Chen, H. C., Church, D., Clamp, M., Copley, R. R., Doerks, T., Eddy, S. R., Eichler, E. E., Furey, T. S., Galagan, J., Gilbert, J. G., Harmon, C., Hayashizaki, Y., Haussler, D., Hermjakob, H., Hokamp, K., Jang, W., Johnson, L. S., Jones, T. A., Kasif, S., Kaspryzk, A., Kennedy, S., Kent, W. J., Kitts, P., Koonin, E. V., Korf, I., Kulp, D., Lancet, D., Lowe, T. M., McLysaght, A., Mikkelsen, T., Moran, J. V., Mulder, N., Pollara, V. J., Ponting, C. P., Schuler, G., Schultz, J., Slater, G., Smit, A. F., Stupka, E., Szustakowski, J., Thierry-Mieg, D., Thierry-Mieg, J., Wagner, L., Wallis, J., Wheeler, R., Williams, A., Wolf, Y. I., Wolfe, K. H., Yang, S. P., Yeh, R. F., Collins, F., Guyer, M. S., Peterson, J., Felsenfeld, A., Wetterstrand, K. A., Patrinos, A., Morgan, M. J., de Jong, P., Catanese, J. J., Osoegawa, K., Shizuya, H., Choi, S. & Chen, Y. J. International Human Genome Sequencing Consortium. (2001) Initial sequencing and analysis of the human genome. *Nature, 409,* 860-921.

Laws, G. (2002) Working memory in children and adolescents with Down syndrome: evidence from a colour memory experiment. *J. Child Psychol. Psychiatry, 43,* 353-364.

Lejeune, J., Gautier, M., & Turpin, R. (1959) Etude des chromosomes somatiques de neufs enfants Mongoliens, *C. R. Acad. Sci. Paris*, *248,* 1721-1722.

Lejeune, J., Turpin, R. & Gautier, M. (1958) Le mongolisme. Premier exemple d'aberration autosomique humaine. *Ann. Génét. Paris, 1,* 41-49.

Lejeune, J. (1990) Pathogenesis of mental deficiency in trisomy 21. *Am. J. Med. Genet. Suppl., 7,* 20-30.

Le Pecheur, M., Bourdon, E., Paly, E., Farout, L., Friguet, B., London, J. (2005) Oxidized SOD1 alters proteasome activities in vitro and in the cortex of SOD1 overexpressing mice. *FEBS Lett., 579,* 3613-3618.

Lesage, F., Duprat, F., Fink, M., Guillemare, E., Coppola, T., Lazdunski, M. & Hugnot, J. P. (1994) Cloning provides evidence for a family of inward rectifier and G-protein coupled K+ channels in the brain. *FEBS Lett., 353,* 37-42.

Lopes, C., Chettouh, Z., Delabar, J. M., & Rachidi, M. (2003) The differentially expressed *C21orf5* gene in the medial temporal-lobe system could play a role in mental retardation in Down syndrome and transgenic mice, *Biochem. Biophys. Res. Commun., 305,* 915-924.

Lopes, C., Rachidi, M., Gassanova, S., Sinet, P. M. & Delabar, J. M. (1999) Developmentally regulated expression of mtprd, the murine ortholog of tprd, a gene from the Down syndrome chromosomal region 1. *Mech. Dev., 84,* 189-193.

Lott, I. T. & Head, E. (2005) Alzheimer disease and Down syndrome: factors in pathogenesis. *Neurobiol. Aging, 26,* 383-389.

Lucente, D., Chen, H. M., Shea, D., Samec, S. N., Rutter, M., Chrast, R., Rossier, C., Buckler, A., Antonarakis, S. E. & McCormick, M. K. (1995) Localization of 102 exons to a 2.5 Mb region involved in Down syndrome. *Hum. Mol. Genet., 4,* 1305-1311.

Ludwig, M., Busch, L. C. & Winking, H. (1997) The embryonic development of sensory organs and the skull in the trisomy 16 mouse, an animal model for Down's syndrome. *Ann. Anat., 179,* 525-33.

de la Luna, S. & Estivill, X. (2006) Cooperation to amplify gene-dosage-imbalance effects. *Trends Mol. Med., 12,* 451-454.

Lyle, R., Gehrig, C., Neergaard-Henrichsen, C., Deutsch, S. & Antonarakis, S. E. (2004) Gene expression from the aneuploid chromosome in a trisomy mouse model of down syndrome. *Genome Res., 14,* 1268-1274.

Mann, D. M., Yates, P. O. & Marcyniuk, B. (1984) Alzheimer's presenile dementia, senile dementia of Alzheimer type and Down's syndrome in middle age form an age related continuum of pathological changes. *Neuropathol. Appl. Neurobiol., 10,* 185-207.

Mao, R., Zielke, C. L., Zielke, H. R. & Pevsner, J. (2003) Global up-regulation of chromosome 21 gene expression in the developing Down syndrome brain. *Genomics, 81,* 457-467.

Mao, R., Wang, X., Spitznagel Jr, E. L., Frelin, L. P., Ting, J. C., Ding, H., Kim, J-W., Ruczinski, I., Downey T. J. & Pevsner, J. (2005) Primary and secondary transcriptional effects in the developing human Down syndrome brain and heart. *Genome Biology, 6,* R107.

Marin-Padilla, M. (1976) Pyramidal cell abnormalities in the motor cortex of a child with Down's syndrome. *J. Comp. Neurol., 167,* 63–75.

Martinez de Lagran, M., Altafaj, X., Gallego, X., Marti, E., Estivill, X., Sahun, I., Fillat, C. & Dierssen, M. (2004) Motor phenotypic alterations in TgDyrk1a transgenic mice implicate DYRK1A in Down syndrome motor dysfunction. *Neurobiol. Dis., 15,* 132-142.

Martinez-Cue, C., Baamonde, C., Lumbreras, M. A., Vallina, I. F., Dierssen, M. & Florez, J. (1999) A murine model for Down syndrome shows reduced responsiveness to pain. *Neuroreport, 10,* 1119–1122.

McEwen, B. S. & Alves, S. E. (1999) Estrogen actions in the central nervous system. *Endocr. Rev., 20,* 279-307.

Megias, M., Verduga, R., Dierssen, M., Florez, J., Insausti, R. & Crespo, D. (1997) Cholinergic, serotonergic and catecholaminergic neurons are not affected in Ts65Dn mice. *Neuroreport., 8,* 3475-3478.

Miguel, R. F., Pollak, A. & Lubec, G. (2005) Metalloproteinase ADAMTS-1 but not ADAMTS-5 is manifold overexpressed in neurodegenerative disorders as Down syndrome, Alzheimer's and Pick's disease. *Brain Res. Mol. Brain Res., 133,* 1-5.

Milner, B., Squire, L. R. & Kandel, E. R. (1998) Cognitive neuroscience and the study of memory, *Neuron, 20,* 445–468.

Miyashita, Y. (2004) Cognitive memory: cellular and network machineries and their top-down control. *Science, 306,* 435-440.

Morris, R. G., Garrud, P., Rawlins, J. N. & O'Keefe, J. (1982) Place navigation impaired in rats with hippocampal lesions. *Nature, 297,* 681-683.

Morris, J. K., Wald, N. J. & Watt, H. C. (1999) Fetal loss in Down syndrome pregnancies. *Prenat. Diagn., 19,* 142-145.

Muralidhar, M. G., Callahan, C. A. & Thomas, J. B. (1993) Single-minded regulation of genes in the embryonic midline of the Drosophila central nervous system. *Mech. Dev., 41,* 129-138.

Murdoch, J. C., Rodger, J. C., Rao, S. S., Fletcher, C. D. & Dunnigan, M.G. (1977) Down's syndrome: An atheroma-free model. *Br. Med. J., 2,* 226-228.

Nadel, L. (2003) Down's syndrome: a genetic disorder in biobehavioral perspective. *Genes Brain Behav., 2,* 156-166.

Nadel, L. & Willner, J. (1980) Context and conditioning: a place for space. *Physiol. Psychol., 8,* 218-228.

Nambu, J. R., Lewis, J. O., Wharton, K. A. & Crews, S. T. (1991) The Drosophila single-minded gene encodes a helix-loop-helix protein that acts as a master regulator of CNS midline development. *Cell, 67,* 1157-1167.

Neidhardt, L., Gasca S., Wertz, K., Obermayr, F., Worpenberg, S., Lehrach, H. & Herrmann, B. G. (2000) Large-scale screen for genes controlling mammalian embryogenesis, using highthroughput gene expression analysis in mouse embryos. *Mech. Dev., 98,* 77–94.

Newby, D., Aitken, D. A., Crossley, J. A., Howatson, A. G., Macri, J. N. & Connor, J. M. (1997) Biochemical markers of trisomy 21 and the pathophysiology of Down's syndrome pregnancies. *Prenat. Diagn., 17,* 941–951.

Nicolaidis, P. & Petersen, M. B. (1998) Origin and mechanisms of nondisjunction in human autosomal trisomies. *Hum. Reprod., 13,* 313–319.

Ohira, M., Ootsuyama, A., Suzuki, E., Ichikawa, H., Seki, N., Nagase, T., Nomura, N. & Ohki, M. (1996) Identification of a novel human gene containing the tetratricopeptide repeat domain from the Down syndrome region of chromosome 21. *DNA Res., 3,* 9-16.

Ohira, M., Seki, N., Nagase, T., Suzuki, E., Nomura, N., Ohara, O., Hattori, M., Sakaki, Y., Eki, T., Murakami, Y., Saito, T., Ichikawa, H. & Ohki, M. (1997) Gene identification in 1.6-Mb region of the Down syndrome region on chromosome 21. *Genome Res., 7,* 47-58.

Ohr, P.S. & Fagen, J.W. (1994) Contingency learning in 9-month-old infants with Down syndrome. *Am. J. Mental Retard., 99,* 74-84.

Olson, L. E., Richtsmeier, J. T., Leszl, J. & Reeves, R. H. (2004a) A chromosome 21 critical region does not cause specific Down syndrome phenotypes. *Science, 306,* 687-690.

Olson, L. E., Roper, R. J., Baxter, L.L., Carlson, E. J., Epstein, C. J. & Reeves, R.H. (2004b) Down syndrome mouse models Ts65Dn, Ts1Cje, and Ms1Cje/Ts65Dn exhibit variable severity of cerebellar phenotypes. *Dev. Dyn., 230,* 581-589.

Pascon, R. C. & Miller, B. L. (2000) Morphogenesis in Aspergillus nidulans requires Dopey (DopA), a member of a novel family of leucine zipper-like proteins conserved from yeast to humans. *Mol. Microbiol., 36,* 1250-1264.

Patil, N., Cox, D. R., Bhat, D., Faham, M., Myers, R. M. & Peterson, A. S. (1995) A potassium channel mutation in weaver mice implicates membrane excitability in granule cell differentiation. *Nat. Genet., 11,* 126-129.

Patterson, D. & Costa, A. C. (2005) Down syndrome and genetics - a case of linked histories. *Nat. Rev. Genet., 6,* 137-147.

Peled-Kamar, M., Degani, H., Bendel, P., Margalit, R. & Groner, Y. (1998) Altered brain glucose metabolism in transgenic-PFKL mice with elevated L-phosphofructokinase: in vivo NMR studies. *Brain Res., 810,* 138-145.

Peng, S., Rapoport, S. I., Pearce, R. J. & Galdzicki, Z. (2000) Abnormal chloride and potassium conductances in cultured embryonic tongue muscle from trisomy 16 mouse. *Brain Res. Dev. Brain Res., 122,* 193-197.

Pennington, P. F., Moon, J., Edgin, J., Stedron, J. & Nadel, L. (2003) The neuropsychology of Down syndrome: evidence for hippocampal dysfunction. *Child Dev., 74,* 75-93.

Potier, M. C., Rivals, I., Mercier, G., Ettwiller, L., Moldrich, R. X., Laffaire, J., Personnaz, L., Rossier, J. & Dauphinot, L. (2006) Transcriptional disruptions in Down syndrome: a case study in the Ts1Cje mouse cerebellum during post-natal development. *J. Neurochem., 97 Suppl. 1,* 104-109.

Pritchard, M. A. & Kola, I. (1999) The "gene dosage effect" hypothesis versus the "amplified development instability" hypothesis in Down syndrome. *J. Neural. Transm Suppl., 57,* 293-303.

Pucharcos, C., Fuentes, J.-J., Casas, C., de la Luna, S., Alcàntara, S., Arbonés, M. L., Soriano, E., Estivill, X. & Pritchard, M. (1999) Alu-splice cloning of the human intersectin (ITSN), a putative multivalent binding protein expressed in proliferating and differentiating neurons and over-expressed in Down syndrome. *Eur. J. Hum. Genet., 7,* 704–712.

Puffenberger, E. G., Kauffman, E. R., Bolk, S., Matise, T. C., Washington, S. S., Angrist, M., Weissenbach, J., Garver, K. L., Mascari, M. & Ladda, R. (1994) Identity-by-descent and association mapping of a recessive gene for Hirschsprung disease on human chromosome 13q22, *Hum. Mol. Genet., 3,* 1217–1225.

Pulsifer, M B. (1996) The neuropsychology of mental retardation. *J. Int. Neuropsychol. Soc., 2,* 159-176.

Purpura, D. P. (1974) Dendritic spine dysgenesis and mental retardation. *Science, 186,* 1126-1128.

Rachidi, M., Lopes, C., Delezoide, A. L. & Delabar, J. M. (2006) C21orf5, a human candidate gene for brain abnormalities and mental retardation in Down syndrome. *Cytogenet. Genome Res., 112,* 16-22. (Erratum in: *Cytogenet. Genome Res., 112,* 226.)

Rachidi, M., Lopes, C., Charron, G., Delezoide, A. L., Paly, E., Bloch, B. & Delabar, J. M. (2005a) Spatial and temporal localization during embryonic and fetal human development of the transcription factor SIM2 in brain regions altered in Down syndrome. *Int. J. Dev. Neurosci., 23,* 475-484.

Rachidi, M., Lopes, C., Costantine, M. & Delabar, J. M. (2005b) C21orf5, a new member of dopey family involved in morphogenesis, could participate in neurological alterations and mental retardation in down syndrome. *DNA Res., 12,* 203-210.

Rachidi, M., Lopes, C., Gassanova, S., Sinet, P. M., Vekemans, M., Attie, T., Delezoide, A. L. & Delabar, J. M. (2000) Regional and cellular specificity of the expression of TPRD, the tetratricopeptide Down syndrome gene, during human embryonic development. *Mech. Dev., 93,* 189–193.

Rahmani, Z., Blouin, J. L., Creau-Goldberg, N., Watkins, P. C., Mattei, J. F., Poissonnier, M., Prieur, M., Chettouh, Z., Nicole, A., Aurias, A., Sinet, P. M. & Delabar, J. M. (1989)

Critical role of the D21S55 region on chromosome 21 in the pathogenesis of Down syndrome. *Proc. Natl. Acad. Sci. USA, 86,* 5958–5962.

Rahmani, Z., Lopes, C., Rachidi, M. & Delabar, J. M. (1998) Expression of the mnb (dyrk) protein in adult and embryonic mouse tissues. *Biochem. Biophys. Res. Commun., 253,* 514–518.

Rapoport, S. I. & Galdzicki, Z. (1994) Electrical studies of cultured fetal human trisomy 16 and mouse neurons identify functional deficits that may lead to mental retardation in Down syndrome. *Dev. Brain Dysfunct., 7,* 265-288.

Raz, N., Torres, I. J., Briggs, S. D., Spencer, W. D., Thornton, A. E., Loken, W. J., Gunning, F. M., McQuain, J. D., Driesen, N. R. & Acker, J.D. (1995) Selective neuroanatomic abnormalities in Down_s syndrome and their cognitive correlates: evidence from MRI morphometry. *Neurology, 45,* 356–366.

Reeves, R. H., Gearhart, J. D. & Littlefield, J. W. (1986) Genetic basis for a mouse model of Down syndrome. *Brain Res. Bull., 16,* 803-814.

Reeves, R. H., Yao, J., Crowley, M. R., Buck, S., Zhang, X., Yarowsky, P., Gearhart, J. D. & Hilt, D. C. (1994) Astrocytosis and axonal proliferation in the hippocampus of S100b transgenic mice. *Proc. Natl. Acad. Sci. USA., 91,* 5359-5363.

Reeves, R. H., Irving, N. G., Moran, T. H., Wohn, A., Kitt, C., Sisodia, S. S., Schmidt, C., Bronson, R. T. & Davisson, M. T. (1995) A mouse model for Down syndrome exhibits learning and behaviour deficits. *Nat. Genet., 11,* 177-184.

Reeves, R. H., Baxter, L. L. & Richtsmeier, J. T. (2001) Too much of a good thing: mechanisms of gene action in Down syndrome. *Trends Genet., 17,* 83-88.

Reymond, A., Meroni, G., Fantozzi, A., Merla, G., Cairo, S., Luzi, L., Riganelli, D., Zanaria, E., Messali, S., Cainarca, S., Guffanti, A., Minucci, S., Pelicci, P. G. & Ballabio, A. (2001) The tripartite motif family identifies cell compartments. *EMBO J., 20,* 2140–2151.

Reymond, A., Marigo, V., Yaylaoglu, M.B., Leoni, A., Ucla, C., Scamuffa, N., Caccioppoli, C., Dermitzakis, E. T., Lyle, R., Banfi, S., Eichele, G., Antonarakis, S.E. & Ballabio, A. (2002) Human chromosome 21 gene expression atlas in the mouse. *Nature, 420,* 582-586.

Richtsmeier, J. T., Baxter, L. L. & Reeves, R. H. (2000) Parallels of craniofacial maldevelopment in Down syndrome and Ts65Dn mice. *Dev. Dyn., 217,* 137–145.

Richtsmeier, J. T., Zumwalt, A., Carlson, E. J., Epstein, C. J. & Reeves, R. H. (2002) Craniofacial phenotypes in segmentally trisomic mouse models for Down syndrome. *Am. J. Med. Genet., 107,* 317–324.

Risser, D., Lubec, G., Cairns, N. & Herrera-Marschitz, M. (1997) Excitatory amino acids and monoamines in parahippocampal gyrus and frontal cortical pole of adults with Down syndrome. *Life Sci., 60,* 1231–1237.

Roder, J. K., Roder, J. C. & Gerlai, R. (1996) Conspecific exploration in the T-maze: abnormalities in S100 beta transgenic mice. *Physiol. Behav., 60,* 31-36.

Roper, R. J. & Reeves, R.H. (2006) Understanding the basis for Down syndrome phenotypes. *PloS Genet., 2,* e50.

Sago, H., Carlson, E. J., Smith, D. J., Kilbridge, J., Rubin, E. M., Mobley, W. C., Epstein, C. J. & Huang, T. T. (1998) Ts1Cje, a partial trisomy 16 mouse model for Down syndrome, exhibits learning and behavioural abnormalities. *Proc. Natl. Acad. Sci. USA., 95,* 6256-6261.

Sago, H., Carlson, E. J., Smith, D. J., Rubin, E. M., Crnic, L. S., Huang, T.-T. & Epstein, C. J. (2000) Genetic dissection of region associated with behavioral abnormalities in mouse models for Down syndrome. *Pediatr. Res., 48,* 606–613.

Salehi, A., Delcroix, J. D. & Mobley, W. C. (2003) Traffic at the intersection of neurotrophic factor signaling and neurodegeneration. *Trends Neurosci., 26,* 73-80.

Salehi, A., Delcroix, J. D., Belichenko, P. V., Zhan, K., Wu, C., Valletta, J. S., Takimoto-Kimura, R., Kleschevnikov, A. M., Sambamurti, K., Chung, P. P., Xia, W., Villar, A., Campbell, W. A., Kulnane, L. S., Nixon, R. A., Lamb, B. T., Epstein, C. J., Stokin, G. B., Goldstein, L. S. & Mobley, W. C. (2006) Increased App expression in a mouse model of Down's syndrome disrupts NGF transport and causes cholinergic neuron degeneration. *Neuron, 51,* 29-42.

Sandin, J., Georgieva, J., Schott, P. A., Ogren, S. O. & Terenius, L. (1997) Nociceptin/orphanin FQ microinjected into hippocampus impairs spatial learning in rats. *Eur. J. Neurosci., 9,* 194-197.

Saran, N. G., Pletcher, M. T., Natale, J. E., Cheng, Y. & Reeves, R. H. (2003) Global disruption of the cerebellar transcriptome in a Down syndrome mouse model. *Hum. Mol. Genet., 12,* 2013-2019.

Schimmel, M. S., Hammerman C., Bromiker, R. & Berger, I. (2006) Third ventricle enlargement among newborn infants with trisomy 21. *Pediatrics, 117,* e928-e931.

Schmidt-Sidor, B., Wisniewski, K. E., Shepard, T. H. & Sersen, E. A. (1990) Brain growth in Down syndrome subjects 1–22 weeks of gestation age and birth to 60 months. *Clin. Neuropathol., 4,* 181–190.

Schneider, C., Risser, D., Kirchner, L., Kitzmuller, E., Cairns, N., Prast, H., Singewald, N. & Lubec, G. (1997) Similar deficits of central histaminergic system in patients with Down syndrome and Alzheimer disease, *Neurosci. Lett., 222,* 183–186.

Schuchmann, S., Muller, W. & Heinemann, U. (1998). Altered Ca2+ signaling and mitochondrial deficiencies in hippocampal neurons of trisomy 16 mice: a model of Down's syndrome. *J. Neurosci., 18,* 7216–7231.

Selemon, L. D., Rajkowska, G. & Goldman-Rakic, P. S. (1995) Abnormally high neuronal density in the schizophrenic cortex. A morphometric analysis of prefrontal area 9 and occipital area 17. *Arch. Gen. Psychiatry, 52,* 805-820.

Séguin, E. (1846). *Traitement moral, hygiène et éducation des idiots et autres enfants arriérés ou retardés dans leurs mouvements, agités de mouvements volontaires.* Paris: J.-B. Ballières.

Shapiro, B. (1983) Down syndrome – A disruption of homeostasis. *Amer. J. Medical Genet., 14,* 241-269.

Shapiro, B. L. & Whither, (1997) Down syndrome critical regions? *Hum. Genet., 99,* 421-423.

Shapiro, L. A. & Whitaker-Azmitia, P. M. (2004) Expression levels of cytoskeletal proteins indicate pathological aging of S100B transgenic mice: an immunohistochemical study of MAP-2, drebrin and GAP-43. *Brain Res., 1019,* 39-46.

Shinohara, T., Tomizuka, K., Miyabara, S., Takehara, S., Kazuki, Y., Inoue, J., Katoh, M., Nakane, H., Iino, A., Ohguma, A., Ikegami, S., Inokuchi, K., Ishida, I., Reeves, R. H. & Oshimura, M. (2001) Mice containing a human chromosome 21 model behavioral impairment and cardiac anomalies of Down's syndrome. *Hum. Mol. Genet., 10,* 1163–1175.

Shumway-Cook, A. & Woollacott, MH. (1985) Dynamics of postural control in the child with Down syndrome. *Psys. Ther., 65,* 1315-1322.

Siarey, R. J., Carlson, E. J., Epstein, C. J., Balbo, A., Rapoport, S. I. & Galdzicki, Z. (1999). Increased synaptic depression in the Ts65Dn mouse, a model for mental retardation in Down syndrome. *Neuropharmacology, 38,* 1917–1920.

Siarey, R. J., Stoll, J., Rapoport, S. I. & Galdzicki, Z. (1997). Altered long-term potentiation in the young and old Ts65Dn mouse, a model for Down Syndrome. *Neuropharmacology, 36,* 1549–1554.

Siarey, R. J., Villar, A. J., Epstein, C. J. & Galdzicki, Z. (2005) Abnormal synaptic plasticity in the Ts1Cje segmental trisomy 16 mouse model of Down syndrome. *Neuropharmacology, 49,* 122-128.

Sikorski, R. S., Boguski, M. S., Goebl, M. & Hieter, P. (1990) A repeating amino acid motif in CDC23 defines a family of proteins and a new relationship among genes required for mitosis and RNA synthesis. *Cell, 60,* 307-317.

Smith, D. J., Zhu, Y., Zhang, J., Cheng, J. F. & Rubin, E. M. (1995) Construction of a panel of transgenic mice containing a contiguous 2-Mb set of YAC/P1 clones from human chromosome 21q22.2. *Genomics, 27,* 425-434.

Smith, D. J., Stevens, M. E., Sudanagunta, S. P., Bronson, R. T., Makhinson, M., Watabe, A. M., O'Dell, T. J., Fung, J., Weier, H. U., Cheng, J. F. & Rubin, E. M. (1997) Functional screening of 2Mb of human chromosome 21q22.2 in transgenic mice implicates minibrain in learning defects associated with Down syndrome. *Nature Genet., 16,* 28–36.

Spencer, K. (2001) What is the true fetal loss rate in pregnancies affected by trisomy 21 and how does this influence whether first trimester detection rates are superior to those in the second trimester? *Prenat. Diagn., 21,* 788-789.

Stasko, M. R. & Costa, A. C. (2004). Experimental parameters affecting the Morris water maze performance of a mouse model of Down syndrome. *Behav. Brain Res., 154,* 1–17.

Stoll, C., Alembik Y., Dott, B. & Roth, M. P. (1990) Epidemiology of Don syndrome in 118,265 consecutive births. *Am. J. Med. Genet., 7(Suppl.),* 79-83.

Sturchler-Pierrat, C., Abramowski, D., Duke, M., Wiederhold, K. H., Mistl, C., Rothacher, S., Ledermann, B., Burki, K., Frey, P., Paganetti, P. A., Waridel, C., Calhoun, M. E., Jucker, M., Probst, A., Staufenbiel, M. & Sommer, B. (1997) Two amyloid precursor protein transgenic mouse models with Alzheimer disease-like pathology. *Proc. Natl. Acad. Sci. USA., 94,* 13287-13292.

Suetsugu, M. & Mehraein, P. (1980) Spine distribution along the apical dendrites of the pyramidal neurons in Down's syndrome. A quantitative Golgi study. *Acta Neuropathol. (Berl.), 50,* 207-210.

Sumarsono, S. H., Wilson, T. J., Tymms, M. J., Venter, D. J., Corrick, C. M., Kola, R., Lahoud, M. H., Papas, T. S., Seth, A. & Kola, I. (1996) Down's syndrome-like skeletal abnormalities in Ets2 transgenic mice. *Nature, 379,* 534-537.

Takashima, S., Becker, L. E., Armstrong, D. L. & Chan, F. (1981) Abnormal neuronal development in the visual cortex of the human fetus and infant with Down's syndrome. A quantitative and qualitative Golgi study. *Brain Res., 225,* 1–21.

Takashima, S., Iida, K., Mito, T. & Arima, M. (1994) Dendritic and histochemical development and aging in patients with Down's syndrome. *J. Intellect. Disabil. Res., 38(Pt3),* 265–273.

Teipel, S. J. & Hampel, H. (2006) Neuroanaotmy of Down syndrome in vivo: a moldel of preclinical Alzheier's disease. *Behav. Genet., 36,* 405-415.

Teipel, S. J., Schapiro, M. B., Alexander, G. E., Krasuski, J. S., Horwitz, B., Hoehne, C., Moller, H. J., Rapoport, S. I. & Hampel, H. (2003) Relation of corpus callosum and hippocampal size to age in non-demented adults with Down's syndrome. *Am. J. Psychiatry, 160,* 1870-1878.

Tejedor, F., Zhu, X. M., Kaltenbach, E., Ackermann, A. Baumann, A., Canal, I., Heisenberg, M., Fischbach, K. F. & Pongs, O. (1995) Minibrain: a new protein kinase family involved in postembryonic neurogenesis in Drosophila. *Neuron, 14,* 287–301.

Thomas, J. B., Crews, S. T. & Goodman, C. S. (1988) Molecular genetics of the single-minded locus: a gene involved in the devclopment of the Drosophila nervous system. *Cell, 52,* 133-141.

Thomas, K. G., Hsu, M., Laurance, H. E., Nadel, L. & Jacobs, W. J. (2001) Place learning in virtual space. III: Investigation of spatial navigation training procedures and their application to fMRI and clinical neuropsychology. *Behav. Res. Methods Instrum. Comput., 33,* 21-37.

Tsukahara, F., Hattori, M., Muraki, T. & Sakaki, Y. (1996) Identification and cloning of a novel cDNA belonging to tetratricopeptide repeat gene fa mily from Down syndrome-critical region 21q22.2. *J. Biochem., 120,* 820-827.

Turrigiano, G. G. & Nelson, S. B. (2004) Homeostatic plasticity in the developing nervous system. *Nat. Rev. Neurosci., 5,* 97-107.

Vialard, F., Toyama, K., Vernoux, S., Carlson, E. J., Epstein, C. J., Sinet, P. M. & Rahmani, Z. (2000) Over-expression of mSim2 gene in the zona limitans of the diencephalon of segmental trisomy 16 Ts1Cje fetuses, a mouse model for trisomy 21: a novel whole-mount RNA hybridization assay. *Dev. Brain Res., 121,* 73–78.

Venter, J. C., Adams, M. D., Myers, E. W., Li, P. W., Mural, R. J., Sutton, G. G., Smith, H. O., Yandell, M., Evans, C. A., Holt, R. A., Gocayne, J. D., Amanatides, P., Ballew, R. M., Huson, D. H., Wortman, J. R., Zhang, Q., Kodira, C. D., Zheng, X. H., Chen, L., Skupski, M., Subramanian, G., Thomas, P. D., Zhang, J., Gabor Miklos, G. L., Nelson, C., Broder, S., Clark, A. G., Nadeau, J., McKusick, V. A., Zinder, N., Levine, A. J., Roberts, R. J., Simon, M., Slayman, C., Hunkapiller, M., Bolanos, R., Delcher, A., Dew, I., Fasulo, D., Flanigan, M., Florea, L., Halpern, A., Hannenhalli, S., Kravitz, S., Levy, S., Mobarry, C., Reinert, K., Remington, K., Abu-Threideh, J., Beasley, E., Biddick, K., Bonazzi, V., Brandon, R., Cargill, M., Chandramouliswaran, I., Charlab, R., Chaturvedi, K., Deng, Z., Di Francesco, V., Dunn, P., Eilbeck, K., Evangelista, C., Gabrielian, A. E., Gan, W., Ge, W., Gong, F., Gu, Z., Guan, P., Heiman, T. J., Higgins, M. E., Ji, R. R., Ke, Z., Ketchum, K. A., Lai, Z., Lei, Y., Li, Z., Li, J., Liang, Y., Lin, X., Lu, F., Merkulov, G. V., Milshina, N., Moore, H. M., Naik, A. K., Narayan, V. A., Neelam, B., Nusskern, D., Rusch, D. B., Salzberg, S., Shao, W., Shue, B., Sun, J., Wang, Z., Wang, A., Wang, X., Wang, J., Wei, M., Wides, R., Xiao, C., Yan, C., Yao, A., Ye, J., Zhan, M., Zhang, W., Zhang, H., Zhao, Q., Zheng, L., Zhong, F., Zhong, W., Zhu, S., Zhao, S., Gilbert, D., Baumhueter, S., Spier, G., Carter, C., Cravchik, A., Woodage, T., Ali, F., An, H., Awe, A., Baldwin, D., Baden, H., Barnstead, M., Barrow, I., Beeson, K., Busam, D., Carver, A., Center, A., Cheng, M. L., Curry, L., Danaher, S., Davenport, L., Desilets, R., Dietz, S., Dodson, K., Doup, L., Ferriera, S., Garg, N., Gluecksmann, A., Hart, B., Haynes, J., Haynes, C., Heiner, C., Hladun, S., Hostin, D., Houck, J., Howland, T., Ibegwam, C.,

Johnson, J., Kalush, F., Kline, L., Koduru, S., Love, A., Mann, F., May, D., McCawley, S., McIntosh, T., McMullen, I., Moy, M., Moy, L., Murphy, B., Nelson, K., Pfannkoch, C., Pratts, E., Puri, V., Qureshi, H., Reardon, M., Rodriguez, R., Rogers, Y. H., Romblad, D., Ruhfel, B., Scott, R., Sitter, C., Smallwood, M., Stewart, E., Strong, R., Suh, E., Thomas, R., Tint, N. N., Tse, S., Vech, C., Wang, G., Wetter, J., Williams, S., Williams, M., Windsor, S., Winn-Deen, E., Wolfe, K., Zaveri, J., Zaveri, K., Abril, J. F., Guigo, R., Campbell, M. J., Sjolander, K. V., Karlak, B., Kejariwal, A., Mi, H., Lazareva, B., Hatton, T., Narechania, A., Diemer, K., Muruganujan, A., Guo, N., Sato, S., Bafna, V., Istrail, S., Lippert, R., Schwartz, R., Walenz, B., Yooseph, S., Allen, D., Basu, A., Baxendale, J., Blick, L., Caminha, M., Carnes-Stine, J., Caulk, P., Chiang, Y. H., Coyne, M., Dahlke, C., Mays, A., Dombroski, M., Donnelly, M., Ely, D., Esparham, S., Fosler, C., Gire, H., Glanowski, S., Glasser, K., Glodek, A., Gorokhov, M., Graham, K., Gropman, B., Harris, M., Heil, J., Henderson, S., Hoover, J., Jennings, D., Jordan, C., Jordan, J., Kasha, J., Kagan, L., Kraft, C., Levitsky, A., Lewis, M., Liu, X., Lopez, J., Ma, D., Majoros, W., McDaniel, J., Murphy, S., Newman, M., Nguyen, T., Nguyen, N., Nodell, M., Pan, S., Peck, J., Peterson, M., Rowe, W., Sanders, R., Scott, J., Simpson, M., Smith, T., Sprague, A., Stockwell, T., Turner, R., Venter, E., Wang, M., Wen, M., Wu, D., Wu, M., Xia, A., Zandieh, A. & Zhu, X. (2001) The sequence of the human genome. *Science, 291,* 1304-1351. (Erratum in: *Science, 292,* 1838.)

Vicari, S. (2004) Memory devlopment and intellecutal disabilities. *Acta Paediatr., Suppl. 93,* 60-63.

Vicari, S. (2006) Motor development and neuropsychological patterns in persons with trisomy 21. *Behav. Genet., 36,* 355-364.

Wainwright, M. S., Craft, J. M., Griffin, W. S., Marks, A., Pineda, J., Padgett, K. R. & Van Eldik, L. J. (2004) Increased susceptibility of S100B transgenic mice to perinatal hypoxia-ischemia. *Ann Neurol., 56,* 61-67.

Wang, P. P, Doherty, S., Hesselink, J. R. & Bellugi, U. (1992) Callosal morphology concurs with neurobehavioral and neuropathological findings in two neurodevelopmental disorders. *Arch. Neurol., 49,* 407–411.

Wang, C. C., Kadota, M., Nishigaki, R., Kazuki, Y., Shirayoshi, Y., Rogers, M. S., Gojobori, T., Ikeo, K. & Oshimura, M. (2004) Molecular hierarchy in neurons differentiated from mouse ES cells containing a single human chromosome 21. *Biochem. Biophys. Res. Commun., 314,* 335–350.

Webb, S., Anderson, R. H. & Brown, N. A. (1996) Endocardial cushion development and heart loop architecture in the trisomy 16 mouse. *Dev. Dyn., 206,* 301-309.

Weis, S., Weber, G., Neuhold, A. & Rett, A. (1991) Down syndrome: MR quantification of brain structures and comparison with normal control subjects. *Am. J. Neuroradiol., 12,* 1207–1211.

Weitzdoerfer, R., Fountoulakis, M., Dierssen, M. & Lubec, G. (2001) Aberrant expression of dihydropyrimidinase-related proteins-2-3, and -4 in fetal Down syndrome brain. *J. Neural. Transm., Suppl. 61,* 95–107.

Wenger, G. R., Schmidt, C. & Davisson, M. T. (2004). Operant conditioning in the Ts65Dn mouse: learning. *Behav. Genet., 34,* 105–119.

Whitaker-Azmitia, P. M. (2001) Serotonin and brain development: role in human developmental diseases. *Brain Res. Bull., 56,* 479–485.

Whitaker-Azmitia, P. M., Wingate, M., Borella, A., Gerlai, R., Roder, J. & Azmitia, E. C. (1997) Transgenic mice overexpressing the neurotrophic factor S-100 beta show neuronal cytoskeletal and behavioral signs of altered aging processes: implications for Alzheimer's disease and Down's syndrome. *Brain Res., 776,* 51–60.

Wierzba-Bobrowicz, T., Lewandowska, E., Schmidt-Sidor, B. & Gwiazda E. (1999) The comparison of microglia maturation in CNS of normal human fetuses and fetuses with Down's syndrome. *Folia Neuropathol., 37,* 227–234.

Winocur, G., Roder, J. & Lobaugh, N. (2001). Learning and memory in S100-beta transgenic mice: an analysis of impaired and preserved function. *Neurobiol. Learn. Mem., 75*, 230–243.

Wishart, J. G. (1995) Cognitive abilities in children with Down syndrome: developmental instability and motivational deficits. In C. J. Epstein, T. Hassold, I. T. Lott, et al. (Eds.) *Etiology and pathogenesis of Down syndrome* (pp. 57-91) New York: Wiley-Liss.

Wisniewski, K. E. (1990) Down syndrome children often have brain with maturation delay, retardation of growth, and cortical dysgenesis. *Am. J. Med. Genet. 7,* 274–281.

Wisniewski, K. E. & Bobinski, M. (1991) Hypothalamic abnormalities in Down syndrome, *Prog. Clin. Biol. Res., 373,* 153–167.

Wisniewski, K. E. & Schmidt-Sidor, B. (1989) Postnatal delay of myelin formation in brains from Down syndrome infants and children. *Clin. Neuropathol., 8*, 55–62.

Woolley, C. S., Gould, E., Frankfurt, M. & McEwen, B. S. (1990) Naturally occurring fluctuation in dendritic spine density on adult hippocampal pyramidal neurons. *J. Neurosci., 10,* 4035-4039.

Woolley, C. S. & McEwen, B. S. (1992) Estradiol mediates fluctuation in hippocampal synapse density during the estrous cycle in the adult rat. *J. Neurosci., 12,* 2549-2554.

Wolvetang, E. W., Bradfield, O. M., Tymms, M., Zavarsek, S., Hatzistavrou, T., Kola, I. & Hertzog, P.J. (2003a) The chromosome 21 transcription factor ETS2 transactivates the beta-APP promoter: implications for Down syndrome. *Biochim Biophys Acta., 1628,* 105-110.

Wolvetang, E. J., Bradfield, O. M., Hatzistavrou, T., Crack, P. J., Busciglio, J., Kola, I. & Hertzog, P.J. (2003b) Overexpression of the chromosome 21 transcription factor Ets2 induces neuronal apoptosis. *Neurobiol. Dis., 14,* 349-356.

Yang, Q., Rasmussen, S. A. & Friedman, J. M. (2002) Mortality associated with Down's syndrome in the USA from 1983 to 1997: A population-bases study. *Lancet, 359,* 1019-1025.

Yaspo, M. L., Gellen, L., Mott, R., Korn, B., Nizetic, D., Poustka, A. M. & Lehrach, H. (1995) Model for a transcript map of human chromosome 21: isolation of new coding sequences from exon and enriched cDNA libraries. *Hum. Mol. Genet., 4,* 1291-1304.

Yates, C. M., Simpson, J., Gordon, A., Maloney, A. F., Allison, Y., Ritchie, I. M. & Urquhart, A. (1983) Catecholamines and cholinergic enzymes in pre-senile and senile Alzheimer-type dementia and Down's syndrome. *Brain Res., 280,* 119-126.

Yla-Herttuala, S., Luoma, J., Nikkari, T. & Kivimaki, T. (1989) Down's syndrome and atherosclerosis. *Atherosclerosis, 76,* 269-272.

Zang da, W., Yang, Q., Wang, H. X., Egan, G., Lopes, E. C. & Cheema, S. S. (2004). Magnetic resonance imaging reveals neuronal degeneration in the brainstem of the superoxide dismutase 1 transgenic mouse model of amyotrophic lateral sclerosis. *Eur. J. Neurosci., 20,* 1745–1751.

In: Focus on Mental Retardation Research
Editor: Marina I. Carson, pp. 135-151
ISBN: 978-1-60021-647-3

Chapter 5

DOWN SYNDROME AND IMMUNITY

Diego Franciotta, Annapia Verri and Luigi Nespoli

(DF) Laboratory of Neuroimmunology and (AV) Department of Clinical Neurology, IRCCS, Foundation "Neurological Institute C. Mondino", University of Pavia, I-27100 Pavia, Italy

(LN) Department of Pediatrics, University of the Insubria, I-21100 Varese, Italy

ABSTRACT

Down's syndrome (DS) is the most frequent genetic disorder associated with mental retardation. The syndrome is the phenotypic result of a triplicated chromosome 21, or from a triplication of its restricted regions. Despite entire DNA sequence of human chromosome 21 is now complete, little is known about the mechanisms by which the increased gene copy number leads to the characteristic DS phenotype. The phenotype can be variable in severity, on the basis of allelic composition of chromosome 21 genes and of the interaction with environment and with expression of genes that are not located on chromosome 21. Dysregulation of the immune system is one characteristic pathological feature of the syndrome and likely contributes to increased susceptibility to viral and bacterial infections, autoimmune diseases, and haematologic malignancies. Chromosome 21 contains the interferon cytokine receptors cluster of genes that are structurally and functionally related. Interferon has pleiotropic effects that manifest mainly on immune system but even in the brain, as shown in DS and in its animal model, the trisomy 16 mouse. Interferon-γ plays a pivotal role in the polarization of immunity towards Th1-mediated responses, which are mainly involved in protection from virus infection and in autoimmunity. It could also cause neurodegeneration and β-amyloid production in DS, thus accounting for cognitive impairment. Notwithstanding these recent discoveries, most of the studies on immunological aspects in DS are old. Investigation with upgraded technologies is needed to improve knowledge in this field. In particular, studies on the expression of proteins, whose genes are encoded on chromosome 21 and that are directly or indirectly involved in immunity, may provide a better understanding of genotype-phenotype correlation in DS and, possibly, a rationale for therapeutic strategies aimed at contrasting the immune derangement and neurodegeneration that are typical of this syndrome.

Introduction

Down syndrome (DS) was firstly described by J. Down (London) in XIX century [1], and only in 1959 associated with a supernumerary chromosome 21 (trisomy 21) by J. Lejeune in France [2] and P. Jacobs in Scotland [3]. Complete DNA sequence of chromosome 21, which is the smallest human autosome, was published in 2000 [4]. Chromosome 21 consists of about 50 Mb of DNA, with a very small short arm and a concentration of transcriptional units in two regions of the long arm. Many genes that are linked with more or less frequent genetic or familial diseases in humans map to this chromosome. These diseases include DS, about 5% of familial amyotrophic lateral sclerosis, a small percentage of familial Alzheimer disease, Ewings sarcoma, and acute myeloid leukaemia. The study of chromosome 21 is therefore very interesting, as it means approaching the cause of major public health issues of the whole population, such as Alzheimer disease-related, or even age-related, neurodegeneration, increased risk of leukemia, and protection from cancer of solid tissues.

DS offers a unique opportunity to explore biological and phenotypic effects of the overdose of otherwise perfectly normal genes located on this chromosome and possibly related to the above-mentioned pathology-driving or from-pathology-protecting mechanisms. The degree of overexpression of these unbalanced gene is about 50%, which raises the issue of how correlating a so relatively small increase in the expression of normal genes with the profound biological consequences on DS phenotypes. Functional non-protein-coding DNA sequences could also contribute to the abnormal phenotypes.

Good news from chromosome 21 DNA sequencing was that the number of genes there located is only about a few hundreds [4], though the knowledge about their functions is limited. Moreover, studies on animal models suggest that only a few genes with major phenotipic effect could likely contribute to the determination of DS phenotypes. Effectively, elucidating the contribution of single genes to DS syndrome, and thus shedding light on the function of such genes, is very difficult. The syndrome indeed seems to adhere to the model of a “contiguous gene syndrome”, in which some groups of genes have prevalent roles over others, with concerted dose effects on few cell pathways.

Trisomy 21 is detected in about 1 out of 43 spontaneous abortions [5] and in about 1 out of 750 live births [6], resulting in the most common chromosome disease. Underlying mechanisms recalls meiotic maternal nondisjunction that is related to the age of the mother. DS incidence increases with increasing maternal age, being about 1 in 1400 at maternal age 25, and 1 in 30 at maternal age 45. The origin of nondisjunction is likely linked to errors in recombination and to age-dependent loss of meiotic chromosome cohesion [7]. The risk of recurrence (not allowing for maternal age) is low. About 2% of DS results from an unbalanced translocation (material from one chromosome breaking off and "sticking to" another). This often involves chromosomes 21 and 14, and is usually a "one-off" event. In some cases a parent also has a possibly balanced translocation without overall disruption of genetic material, and the risk of recurrence is high. 21 to 21 translocations also occur. Mosaicism is a term used to describe the presence of two, or more, cell lines within the body.

In DS this means that one cell line with trisomy 21 coexists with another unaffected cell line. About 3% of DS probably results from mosaicism, and therefore many cases may not be diagnosed. The proportion of affected and unaffected cell lines varies, as the intellectual impairment does.

DS manifests with more than 30 phenotypic features, which can be present with varying frequencies in affected individuals. Cognitive impairment is common in all DS subjects [8], as well as muscle hypotonia and, in subjects over 35 years of age, neuropathological abnormalities. These abnormalities, which comprise neurofibrillary tangles and the deposition of amyloid plaques in the brain, are identical to those observed in the brains of patients with Alzheimer disease [9]. Variable phenotypic features include congenital heart defects (mainly atrioventricular septal defect) that occur in about 40% of the cases, anomalies of the gastrointestinal tract, typical craniofacial and skeletal features, atlanto-axial instability, abnormal audiovestibular and visual functions, congenital cataracts, and seizures. Duodenal stenosis/atresia, Hirschsprung disease and acute megakaryocytic leukemia occur in subjects with DS, respectively, 250-, 30- and 300-times more frequently than in the general population. Most adults with DS are of short stature (70%), with a characteristic facial appearance. The eyes seem to slope upwards and outwards as a result of alterations in the structure of the surrounding tissues. Iris Brushfield spots are present in 55% of the subjects. The nose has a wide bridge, and the head an unusual shape ("brachycephaly"). Protruding tongue is present in 45% of the cases. Limb abnormalities include a single transverse crease on the palm, a large cleft between the first and second toes, and relatively short upper arms. People with DS are prone to abnormalities of the thyroid gland (15% develop hypothyroidism during childhood or adolescence). Ninety percent of all DS individuals have a significant hearing loss, usually of the conductive type.

Moreover, DS is characterized by a 50-70 fold higher incidence of childhood leukaemias, variable degree of compromission of immune system with immunodeficiency and predisposition to respiratory infections and autoimmunity. Conversely, the risk of developing solid tumors and some autoimmune diseases, such as multiple sclerosis [10], is lower than that expected in the general population.

Life expectancy has improved markedly over the past 50 years, largely as a result of antibiotic treatment of respiratory tract infections. Survival into the 8th decade is unusual but not extraordinary. The presence of an atrioventricular septal defect often leads to heart and lung failure early in adult life.

DS individuals manifest fewer behaviour problems in comparison to controls with cognitive disability, but more frequently than in sibling or in controls with normal intelligence quotient. About 18% of individuals with DS under 20 years of age have a psychiatric disorder, most frequently a disruptive behaviour disorder such as attention deficit hyperactivity disorder (~ 6%), conduct/oppositional disorder (~ 5%), or aggressive behaviour (~ 6%). In the adult age, about 26% of DS subjects likewise manifest a psychiatric disorder, most frequently, in these cases, a major depressive disorder (~ 6%), or aggressive behaviour (~ 6%).

The dual diagnoses of DS and autism has recently gained much attention. Although the association has invariably been appreciated, recent reports suggest a frequency as high as 7%, and great delays in diagnosis. The stereotype of people with DS as happy, placid individuals with a gift for mimicry has not borne out by recent behavioural research. "Stubbornness" and obsessional features seem to be over-represented, and many people with DS react adversely in situations involving conflicts.

Cognitive disability is a typical feature of DS. Most children and adults with DS fall into the range of mild-to-moderate intellectual disability. About 10% of them have a low average-borderline degree of intellectual disability, namely a cognitive impairment that is not so severe to be classifiable as a learning disability, whereas only a minority of them suffer from a severe or profound cognitive impairment .

Almost all children with DS have a relatively specific impairment in the expressive language. Expressive language deficit in syntax is greater than that in the lexicon. Comprehension of words is typically more advanced than nonverbal cognition. Cognition deficits in verbal working-memory and delayed recall has been described.

Cognitive abilities tend to be less severely affected in people in whom DS is caused by mosaicism for trisomy 21.

In adults with DS, neuropathological changes typical of Alzheimer disease usually develop by the fifth decade of life. Although almost all adults with DS over the age of 35 show these neuropathological abnormalities on post-mortem examination, only about 45% of those over 45 years of age have clinically apparent dementia that is cumulatively present in 75% of DS individuals. Over 60 years of age, they frequently manifest seizures (58%), change in personality (46%), focal neurological signs (46%), apathy (36%), and loss of conversational skills (36%).

Animal Models

Human chromosome 21 shares significant homology with mouse chromosome 16. Therefore, trisomy 16 mice have been generated and investigated as a mouse model for DS [11]. These mice have similarities in some characteristics to human individuals with DS, and these characteristics have been morphologically, biochemically and immunologically investigated. Trisomy 16 mice show overexpression of many more genes than those overexpressed in human trisomy 21, and lack of trisomy of the genes that are not syntenic with the homologue human chromosome. Mouse chromosome 16 has also homology to human chromosome 3, and genes from the more terminal part of human chromosome 21 are located on other mouse chromosomes such as 10 and 17 [12]. As a result, the mouse model does not completely resemble DS. Moreover, trisomy 16 mice are not usually viable, given that, as in the case of human trisomy 21 conceptions [13], trisomy 16 fetuses rarely survive until birth. Therefore, partially trisomy 16 mice, which have homology to human chromosome 21 from 21q21 to 21q22.3 regions, have been developed [14]. These mice show some characteristic that are reminiscent of DS, but the phenotype is not so severe like that found in DS and trisomy 16 mice. Notwithstanding these limitations, partially trisomy 16 mice represent a useful model to study the histopathological abnormalities that occur in DS in later life and, more extensively, in Alzheimer disease. Shukkur and Colleagues studied a segmental trisomy 16 mouse model for DS, namely Ts1Cje, which has a subset of triplicated human chromosome 21 gene orthologs that exclude amyloid-β precursor protein (APP) and Cu/Zn superoxide dismutase (SOD1) [15]. The overexpression of APP and SOD1 genes, which are located on chormosome 21, is considered to be responsible for increased oxidative stress and neurodegeneration commonly described in DS. Although APP and SOD1 were thus normally expressed in Ts1Cje mice, analysis of their brains showed a decrease in mitochondrial membrane potential and ATP production, an increase in reactive oxygen species, hyperphosphorylation of tau without neurofibrillary tangles formation, and an increase in GSK3β and JNK/SAPK activities, with the expected unaffected APP metabolism [15]. Therefore, genes on the trisomic Ts1Cje segment other than APP and SOD1 can cause profound metabolic and structural alterations that may play critical roles in the pathogenesis of mental retardation in DS. These findings also confirm that DS phenotypes likely result from a very complex interplay between many, and possibly related, genes.

The opportunity of approaching the study of both DS and the animal model has been recently exploited the use of transgenic mice that overexpress single genes. The availability of evaluating the direct phenotype-genotype relationship of genes from human chromosome 21, partially compensates for the production of mice that are not complete models for DS, in which many genes are contemporarily involved. For example, transgenic mice for the S100β protein, thus expressing elevated levels of the protein, showed abnormalities in astrocyte morphology and axonal sprouting, especially in the dentate gyrus, with astrocytosis and axonal proliferation [16]. This study provides unique insight into the role of S100β in glial-neuronal interactions that are applicable both to normal development and to DS or Alzheimer disease.

By manipulating mouse embryonic stem cells, O'Doherty and Colleagues have recently generated a trans-species aneuploid mouse line that stably transmits a freely segregating, almost complete human chromosome 21 (Hsa21). This "transchromosomic" mouse line, Tc1, is a model of trisomy 21, which manifests as DS in humans, given that shows phenotypic alterations in behavior, synaptic plasticity, cerebellar neuronal number, heart development, and mandible size [17]. This is a unique tool for studying DS and even other human aneuploidies, and has already generated immunological data that are shown in the appropriate section.

TRISOMY 21 AND CANCER

The relationship between human chromosome 21 and cancer is quite puzzling, as epidemiological data clearly indicate that people with DS are at 20-fold increased risk of childhood leukemia [18], whereas they seem to be protected from development of solid tumors. Defects in immunosurveillance can act as co-factors. Trisomy 21 is also one of the most frequent non-random changes in malignant cells in a variety of hematological malignancies of euploid children and adults [19]. Transient myeloproliferative disorder and megakaryoblastic leukemia of DS are also associated with mutations in the GATA1 gene in conjunction with trisomy 21. On the contrary, neuroblastomas and nephroblastomas in DS children and, gynecologic, digestive and breast cancers in DS adults have been only occasionally reported, and occur with a frequency significantly lower than that found in age-matched euploid controls: these strong epidemiological data suggest that chromosome 21 could contain genes with suppressive roles in the development of solid tumors [20]. Many genes can be involved in the complex pathways that possibly influence the largely unknown tumorigenesis. These genes include 10 kinases, 5 cell adhesion molecules, a lot of transcription factors, and 7 ion channel proteins, in addition to particularly interesting genes that code for proteins that regulate the rate of cell division, cell cycle arrest, apoptosis, and the response to DNA damage [21]. The genes that play prominent roles in cell cycle and cell growth are HSP70-like chaperone STCH (stress 70 protein chaperone, microsome-associated, 60 kD human homolog), B-cell translocation gene 3 (BTG3) of tumor suppressor gene family, T-lymphoma invasion and metastasis gene (TIAM)-1 protein, ets-2 proto-oncogene, BACH-1 gene, SOD-1, and 5 genes of the ubiquitin-proteasome pathway: 2 proteases, one conjugating enzyme, one ligase, and the small ubiquitin-like modifier (SUMO). From a purely speculative point of view, it is possible to hypothesize that a convergence of an increased dose of a group of genes that arrest cell cycle, are pro-apoptotic, and tumor suppressing could produce the low number of neurons in the brain, reduced brain size, hypocellularity in cervical spine vertebrae and in atrioventricular septa in the heart, defects in ability to mount proliferative responses in the field of immunity, and, finally, tumor suppression for solid tissue tumors.

Down Syndrome and Immunity

Dysregulation of the immune system is one characteristic pathological feature of DS, and accounts for increased susceptibility to viral and bacterial infections and, possibly, to childhood leukemia [18]. Understanding the causes of this relative immunodeficiency remains a challenge. Similarly to other aspects, such as Alzheimer-like brain lesions and neurodegeneration, a precocious senescence of the immune system has been hypothesized as a co-factor at least [22, 23]. The immunodeficiency also affects the lower response rate to vaccination in DS children and adults, in comparison with age-matched subjects [24]. It has been shown that both thymus dependent and independent functions were impaired in DS with a characteristic age sequence. In DS subjects, lymphocyte phytohemagglutinin responsiveness was in the normal range during the first decade, but it decreased thereafter progressively [25]. Another characteristic of the immunodeficiency seems to be the trend of starting early, during the initial phases of the development of the immune system, and of worsening progressively with ageing [26].

Lymphocyte function associated antigen-1 (LFA-1), which belongs to the family of integrins, is a fundamental adhesion molecule located at the lymphocyte surface that plays a crucial role in cell activation and trafficking. Abnormalities that affect the function of LFA-1 usually compromise the steps that lead to lymphocyte maturation and, above all, activation [27]. Mice with a null mutation in the gene that code for LFA-1 showed defects in immune function [28]. These mice displayed impairment in the cytotoxic activity towards allogenic spleen cells as well as cell line targets. Interestingly, LFA-1 seems to be important in tumor rejection, since mice that are deficient for LFA-1 gene are susceptible to metastasis of B16 melanoma cells, even though their in vitro NK cell activity appears normal [28]. The β-chain (CD18) of LFA-1 is encoded on chromosome 21, and LFA-1 gene expression resulted to be upregulated in lymphocytes of DS patients [29]. The overexpression, in turn, could be responsible for the increased adhesiveness of DS lymphocytes that would result in abnormalities in their development and function [30]. Moreover, the increased expression of intercellular adhesion molecule (ICAM)-1, which is the counter-receptor of LFA-1, on thymic epithelium might be fit with the theory that the immunodeficiency in DS individuals is likely due to excessive thymic deletion caused by overexpression of adhesion molecules [30]. The theory that lymphocyte hyperadhesiveness could be one of the factor that contribute to immunodeficiency in DS has not been supported by Lin and Colleagues, who failed in confirming an age-associated LFA-1 up-regulation and impaired ICAM-1 binding in lymphocytes from DS individuals [31]. They also found that DS children less than 2 years of age expressed a higher level of LFA-1 when compared with age-matched controls, but the difference in LFA-1 expression was much less significant in older DS individuals, when compared with age-matched children [31]. The Authors concluded that a generalized pathological process, such as early senescence of the immune system and ineffectiveness in activating lymphocytes, rather than pure lymphocyte hyperadhesiveness, might underlie the immune function defects in older DS individuals [31].

More recently, a gene named AIRE (autoimmune regulator) has been identified on chromosome 21q22.3 by positional cloning [32]. This gene codes for a protein that contains DNA-binding domains and is located in both the nucleus and cytoplasm [32]. Nonsense or missense mutations of AIRE gene has been identified as the cause of a familial immunodeficiency and autoimmune endocrinopathy [33]. The role for this gene, which is likely to be up-regulated in DS individuals, could be detrimental, especially in a condition characterized by the impaired LFA-1 upregulation and activation of integrin-mediated adhesion.

Significant differences in the lymphocyte subpopulations in DS children and adults, when compared with age-matched normal subjects, have also been reported [34]. The number of CD8+ T cells was increased in DS individuals, whereas that of CD4+ T cells was decreased; this decrease in the CD4+ subset subpopulation was due to the low proportion of CD4+ CD45RA+ naive lymphocytes [34]. These data suggest that abnormalities in the development of the lymphocytes can occur in DS. Corsi and Colleagues analogously found that peripheral CD4+ T cells were decreased in children with DS, but in their series mean values of cytotoxic CD8+ T cells were comparable with those in healthy children [35]. They also reported other immune abnormalities in DS such as an increase in circulating activated (CD3/HLA-DR positive) T cells, and in purified T cells that were positive for APO-I/Fas (CD95) antigen [35]. A particularly notable idiopathic CD4+ T lymphocytopenia in a child with DS has also been reported [36]. However, these data on CD4+ T cell decrease in DS have not been confirmed in an independent study [31], whereas proportions of memory lymphocytes expressing the CD45RO isoform were found to be higher in both younger and older DS individuals, when compared with age-matched control groups [31].

By using a novel animal model of DS (Tc1 mouse), O'Doherty and Colleagues studied the T cell receptor (TCR)–induced activation of T lymphocytes [17], which has been reported to be defective in DS [37]. The Authors consistently found that both CD4+ and CD8+ T cells from both spleen and lymph nodes of Tc1 mice upregulated CD25 (a marker of regulatory T cells) and CD69 (a marker of T cell activation) to a lesser extent than wild-type cells, in response to stimulation either through the TCR alone with antibodies to CD3ε, or in combination with antibodies to the costimulatory receptor CD28 [17]. Scotese and Colleagues also reported that a T cell activation defect seems to particularly depend on a partial impairment of signal transduction after TCR/CD3 complex engagement [37]. This defect did not prevent phorbol ester and ionomycin from inducing proliferative responses of DS lymphocytes. Cumulatively, these data suggest that regulatory circuitries, which involve specific T cell subsets, and defects in T cell activation could contribute to the generation of abnormal immune responses in DS.

Consistent data indicate that DS individuals have also abnormalities in the humoral immunity [38]. Before 6 years of age, serum immunoglobulin concentration did not differ between DS children and age-matched healthy controls, whereas, after that age, considerable hyper-IgG and hyper-IgA were found [38]. DS was also characterized by high concentrations of IgG1 and IgG3 subclasses, which are involved in IgM switch and are related to IFN-γ stimulation and Th1 activation, and a progressive age-dependent decline of IgG2 and IgG4 subclasses, which are mostly related to Th2 activation and allergy [38]. Response to vaccination was shown to be impaired, as the percentage of DS children vaccinated for hepatitis B virus showing a protective antibody titer was 17%, in comparison with 75% detected in healthy controls [38]. In contrast, the frequency of certain autoantibodies, such as anti-gliadin, anti-transglutaminase, and anti-thyroid in serum of DS individuals is higher than that found in the general population [38]. Recently, Chaushu and Colleagues reported that the concentration of parotid salivary immunoglobulins was decreased (IgG by 83%, and IgA by 75%) in DS individuals in comparison with age- and sex-matched healthy controls [39]. These data would be in line with the observed high prevalence of infections in the mucosae of gastrointestinal and respiratory system, and link these clinical manifestations with a specific immunodeficiency in the humoral mucosal immune response.

Analogously with other systems or organs, the chromosomal anomaly in DS involves many genes that encode molecules that are potentially important for the immune responses and lymphocyte development, but the complex interaction between these genes and, possibly, between these genes and other non up-regulated genes, might lead to immunological phenotypes that are not expected by simply assuming the overexpression of a single molecule.

Down Syndrome and Associated Autoimmune Disorders

Table 1 shows how DS preferably associates with some autoimmune diseases or with serum autoantibodies, whereas some other autoimmune diseases are only occasionally reported as co-occurring in DS individuals. The incidence and prevalence rates of autoimmune disorders, such as celiac disease [40], insulin-dependent diabetes mellitus [41], autoimmune thyroiditis [42, 43], and alopecia areata [44] are unequivocally increased in DS. On the contrary, there are only case reports on other autoimmune diseases, such as Crohn disease and ulcerative colitis [45], or systemic lupus erythematosus [46]. Particularly interesting is the extraordinary low rate of association with multiple sclerosis, the most frequent autoimmune, inflammatory demyelinating disease that affects young adults. One case of coincidence has been reported in the literature [47]. Multiple sclerosis is a complex disease, for which well-known associations with the major histocompatibility complex as well as with at least two important loci within this region have been repeatedly confirmed [48]. Links with other diseases are few for multiple sclerosis, but the association with diabetes in the Sardinian population and, perhaps, a putative protective effect of DS can now be added. The discovery of the genetic basis of this protective effect is a real challenge for researchers. However, the possibility of underdiagnosis of multiple sclerosis in DS cannot be excluded, as well as the possibility of underreporting in the retrospective literature. The diagnosis of multiple sclerosis is a complex task, and may take many years after onset of possibly mild and remitting clinical symptoms. Moreover, clinical symptoms, such as bladder disturbances or paresthesias, may not be detected in mentally retarded DS individuals. Notwithstanding these considerations, today a large part of DS individuals can communicate sufficiently with their caregivers, and have full access to health care [10]. Likewise, magnetic resonance imaging instruments, which help neurologists in diagnosing multiple sclerosis, are largely available in most countries.

The explanation for the co-occurrence, or the lack of the expected co-occurrence, between DS and various autoimmune diseases or autoimmune phenomena is difficult to find. The overexpression of genes such as SOD1 accounts for the increase in concentration of biomarkers of oxidative stress [15], which, in turn, are considered to be responsible for oxidative DNA damage and lipid peroxidation. These processes could contribute to the exposure of sequestrated self-antigens, while the more o less pronounced abnormalities [22-38] in the humoral and cellular immune responses might play a prominent role in the induction of autoimmunity. This scenario is particularly likely in the autoimmune disorders that are associated with thymus-dependent T cell functions [22]. On the contrary, the protective effect of DS against the development of autoimmune diseases, such as systemic lupus erythematosus or multiple sclerosis, is less easy to explain. Generically, such effect might depend on a gain of function due to a triplication of various genes (gene dosage effect), on a loss of function, or on the very complex interactions that regulate protein expression, which include the recently discovered and fascinating mechanisms of RNA interference [49]. Gain of function may apply to the well-known interferon (IFN) hypersensitivity [50], to which the next session is dedicated. Type 1 IFNs are a class of immunoregulatory molecules that are particularly interesting in multiple sclerosis, as IFN-β1b has been the first drug used, and that is currently used, to modify the course of the disease [51], whereas IFN-γ, administered as an anti-viral agent when multiple sclerosis was considered to be a putative viral-induced disease, was able to induce severe worsening and relapses [52]. Moreover, S100β protein, which is present on chromosome 21 and has been shown to produce astrocytosis in a transgenic mouse [16], is a potential autoantigen for multiple sclerosis. If these considerations on multiple sclerosis suggest that the multifaceted immunological abnormalities in DS can be organ-specific, on the other hand this theory is difficult to reconcile with the evidence that DS has protective effect on other non-neurological autoimmune diseases. From a genetic point of view, multiple sclerosis affects some ethnic groups (e.g., Caucasians) more frequently than others (e.g., Black Africans) [53], and these differences, together with those deriving from the study of chromosome 21, could help define a set of genes particularly important for understanding both protective and pathogenic factors in multiple sclerosis.

Table 1. Prevalence data, expressed per 100,000 people, for autoimmune diseases or serum autoantibodies in the general population and in individual with Down syndrome; the correlated risk ration has been also reported [modified from ref. # 10]

	Celiac disease	Juvenile rheumatoid arthritis	Anti-thyroid antibodies	Insulin-dependent diabetes mellitus	Alopecia areata	CIDP	Crohn disease	Ulcerative colitis	SLE
Prevalence in general population	100-200	0.2-1.0	1000-3000	220-260	100	3-5	20-40	70-150	15-50
Prevalence in Down syndrome	$7\text{-}17 \times 10^3$	1200	$23\text{-}85 \times 10^3$	$1.4\text{-}10.6 \times 10^3$	$6\text{-}9 \times 10^3$	occasional report	occasional report	occasional report	occasional report
Risk ratio in Down syndrome	35-169	12-59	8-39	5-41	60-88	n.a.	n.a.	n.a.	n.a.

CIDP, chronic inflammatory demyelinating polyneuropathy; SLE, systemic lupus erythematosus; n.a., not applicable.

THE INTERFERON SYSTEM IN DOWN SYNDROME

Data in the literature suggest that molecules and receptors usually operating in adaptive immunity may also be implicated in neurodevelopmental abnormalities and neurodegeneration in DS and trisomy 16 mouse [54-57]. In addition to the brain abnormalities that are detectable both in DS and Alzheimer dementia [9], other neuropathological features shared by DS and trisomy 16 mouse include decreased brain weight and decreased neuron number and density [58-59]. In vitro experiments on cultured fetal neurons from trisomy 21 human [60] and trisomy 16 mouse [61, 62] brains demonstrated that the decrease in neuronal viability was due to an increase in cell apoptosis frequency. IFN-γ regulates many genes involved in apoptosis [63], and contributes to many pathways that induce appreciable effects on neurons, such as: a) alterations in cell differentiation [64]; b) expression of major histocompatibility complex class I genes [65], which are, in turn, correlated to brain inflammation; and c) glia-mediated neurotoxicity [66]. However, IFN-γ can also exert protective roles in the brain after traumatic injury, since, for example, it enables microglia to remove glutamate that, in turn, contributes substantially to neuronal degeneration [67]. These findings would support a novel concept, namely that autoreactive T cells protect neurons against glutamate toxicity and, more in general, that autoimmunity can be beneficial.

In the field of the immune response to viruses, IFN-producing cells were identified in the 1980s as a small subset of leukocytes specialized in the secretion of high levels of type I IFNs (i.e., IFN-α, IFN-β, and IFN-ω) [68]. These cells have brought the attention of immunologists for their peculiar role in innate immunity and in shaping T cell responses [69]. The cells act in the T cell area of lymph nodes and express markers such as CD31, CD36, CD68, and the IL-3 receptor α chain, which is typical of myeloid cells. Given, in addition, the ability of stimulating T helper cell proliferation and differentiation, these cells were thus classified as a subset of dendritic cells [70].

The above-mentioned considerations indicate that IFN-γ is a molecule that links together innate and adaptive immunity, with a fundamental role in the immune response to viral infections. The chromosome 21 complete DNA sequencing shows that several structurally and functionally related genes form clusters, for examples the keratin-associated proteins, the trefoil peptides, and, interestingly, the interferon cytokine receptors [4]. Table 2 shows the genes that are located on chromosome 21 and are involved in immunity. The two genes IFNAR1 and IFNAR2 code for IFN-α, -β. and -ω receptor 1 and receptor 2, the IFNGR2 codes for IFN-γ receptor 2. Knock out mice that lack IFNAR1 demonstrated a compromised ability to withstand viral infections since they died significantly earlier after exposure to viruses such as Semliki Forest virus and encephalomyocarditis virus in comparison with control mice [71]. These data, together with other experimental data obtained in vitro by the same Authors [71], prove that the type I interferon system functions as an antiviral, antiproliferative, differentiation-modulating and natural killer cell-stimulating agents, thus protecting cells against viral infections. Other genes on chromosome 21 that are linked to the IFN system are MX1 and MX2 that code for IFN inducible proteins involved in responses to virus infections (Table 2). Mutant mice that did not produce Mx proteins showed increased susceptibility to influenza virus infection [72]. An additional gene on chromosome 21, namely CRFB4, is a member of the class II cytokine receptor family, which includes the IFN receptors [73]. Therefore, many genes that function in the IFN signalling pathways, or that are structurally related to IFN receptors, localize to human chromosome 21. However, knock out studies on some of these genes have to be carried out to more precisely define their exact biological functions.

Table 2. Genes mapped to human chromosome 21 that are specifically involved in immunity

Gene	Protein	Gene location	GDB accession #
CRFB4	CRF2-4 cytokine receptor family II, member 4	21q22.1- 21q22.2	138168
IFNAR1	IFRC IFNAR interferon (α, β and ω) receptor 1	21q22.1- 21q22.1	120078
IFNAR2	IFNABR interferon (α, β and ω) receptor 2	21q22.1- 21q22.1	568494
IFNGR2	IFNGT1 interferon γ receptor 2 (interferon γ transducer 1)	21pter- 21qter	142306
ITGB2	MF17 CD18 LFA-1 integrin, β2 [macrophage antigen 1 (mac-1) β subunit; antigen CD18 (p95), lymphocyte function-associated antigen 1]	21q22.3- 21q22.3	120574
MX1	IFI-78K MxA myxovirus (influenza) resistance 1	21q22.3- 21q22.3	120206
MX2	myxovirus (influenza) resistance 2	21q22.3- 21q22.3	120207

Additional effects of IFN-γ on immunity in DS include abnormalities in thymus anatomy, which would depend on both IFN-γ and tumour necrosis factor-α overexpression [74], and increased neopterin/biopterin urinary ratio [75].

All these lines of evidence on a genetic-dependent dysregulation of the IFN system in DS led us to investigate the percentages of IFN-γ- and IL-4-producing T cells in the peripheral blood of patients with DS, individuals with mental retardation, and healthy controls [76]. It is well-established that IL-12/IFN-γ polarize Th0 cells towards the Th1 phenotype, whereas IL-4 towards the Th2 phenotype, and that IFN-γ-producing T cells can be CD4+ (Th1), or CD8+ (Tc1), and IL-4-producing T cells CD4+ (Th2) and CD8+ (Tc2) [77]. The aim of our study was to ascertain whether the unbalanced IFN system in DS could be mirrored by abnormal proportions of peripheral blood Th1, Tc1, Th2, and Tc2 subsets. Intracellular cytokine staining, which was performed with a slightly-modified standard technique [78], was used for T cell typing. We found that the percentages of IFN-γ-producing $CD4^+$ and $CD8^+$ T cells, namely Th1 and Tc1 cells, and the Th1/Th2 ratio in DS were significantly higher than in individuals with mental retardation and in healthy controls [76]. Interestingly, nearly all the DS subjects with high Th1 or Tc1 cell percentages were also seropositive for anti-transglutaminase IgA, a biomarker of celiac disease. No correlation between high Th1 or Tc1 cell percentages and sex, age, APOE genotypes, coexisting autoimmune diseases, susceptibility to infections, or cognitive impairment was found. Therefore, it is likely that the substantial up-modulation of IFN-γ-producing $CD4^+$ and $CD8^+$ T cells that we found in our DS series could be among the many factors involved in DS-correlated immune dysregulation, although this abnormality had no clinical correlate in the areas of autoimmunity, infections, and cognition. The role of IFN-γ in immunity is not one-way oriented, given that it can promote both inflammation and countermechanisms that lead to the clearance of T cells by apoptosis [79]. Our data thus suggest that the hypothesized direct link between hyperactivity of IFN-γ-regulated circuitries and Th1-mediated autoimmune diseases and of acute/chronic infections [80] could not be invariably applied. A possible explanation of the phenomenon might refer to changes in the T cell repertoire that is under the pressure of recurrent infections in DS, so yielding the accumulation of effector T cells which have a strong IFN-γ production. Experimental and immunopathological data indicate that IFN-γ may play a role in DS neurodegeneration [54-62]. We found that high percentages of Th1 or Tc1 cell did not correlate either with the level of cognitive impairment, or with the ApoE ε4 allele in DS patients [76]. This allele marked severe cognitive impairment in a few DS patients, in accordance with previous reports [81].

CONCLUSION

DS is a condition that is very difficult to study, even after complete DNA sequencing of chromosome 21 [4]. These difficulties are mainly related to the complex gene interactions, the multiplicity of systems involved, and the high degree of variability of the phenotype. From the immunological point of view, many abnormalities have been described in both innate and adaptive immunity, although they have not been directly associated to a particular, infection-prone DS phenotype. A general point is that most of the studies on immunological function in DS are not recent and, therefore, investigations with upgraded technologies is warranted. Moreover, recent developments, especially in genetics, proteomics, genomics, developmental biology and neuroscience promise significant advancements in DS knowledge, with a rapid translation of the research products into benefits for DS individuals.

REFERENCES

[1] Down JL. Observation on an ethnic classification of idiots. *London Hospital Reports* 1866;3:259-62.

[2] Lejeune J, Gautier M, Turpin R. Etudes des chromosomes somatique de neuf enfants mongoliens. *Comptes Rendus Academie des Sciences Paris* 1959;248:1721-2.

[3] Jacobs P, Baikie W, Court-Brown W, Strong J. The somatic chromosomes in mongolism. *Lancet* 1959;i:710-1.

[4] Hattori M, Fujiyama A, Taylor TD, Watanabe H, Yada T, Park HS, et al. The DNA sequence of human chromosome 21. *Nature* 2000;405:311-9.

[5] Hsu L Y, in Genetic Disorders and the Fetus, Milunsky A Ed. (Johns Hopkins Univ. Press, Baltimore, MD, 1998), pp. 179–248.

[6] Antonarakis SE, Lyle R, Dermitzakis ET, Reymond A, Deutsch S. *Nat Rev Genet* 2004;5:725-38.

[7] Hassold T, Hunt P. To err (meiotically) is human: the genesis of human aneuploidy. *Nat Rev Genet* 2001;2:280-91.

[8] Jackson JF, North ER 3rd, Thomas JG. Clinical diagnosis of Down syndrome. *Clin Genet* 1976;9:483-7.

[9] Wisniewski KE, Wisniewski HM, Wen GY. Occurrence of neuropathological changes and dementia of Alzheimer's disease in Down's syndrome. *Ann Neurol* 1985;17:278-82.

[10] Weilbach FX, Toyka KV. Does Down's syndrome protect against multiple sclerosis? *Eur Neurol* 2002;47:52-5.

[11] Epstein CJ, Cox DR, Epstein L. Mouse trisomy 16: An animal model of human trisomy 21 (Down Syndrome). *Ann N Y Acad Sci* 1985;450:157–68.

[12] Davisson MT, Lalley PA, Peters J, et al. Report of the comparative subcommittee for human and mouse homologies. *Cytogen Cell Gene* 1990;55:434–56.

[13] Hassold TJ, Jacobs PA. Trisomy in man. *Annu Rev Genet* 1984;18:69-97.

[14] Reeves RH, Irving NG, Moran TH, et al. A mouse model for Down syndrome exhibits learning and behaviour deficits. *Nature Genet* 1995;11:77–84.

[15] Shukkur EA, Shimohata A, Akagi T, et al. Mitochondrial dysfunction and tau hyperphosphorylation in Ts1Cje, a mouse model for Down syndrome. *Hum Mol Genet* 2006;15:2752-62.

[16] Reeves RH, Yao J, Crowley MR, et al. Astrocytosis and axonal proliferation in the hippocampus of S100b transgenic mice. *Proc Natl Acad Sci USA* 1994;91:5359-63.

[17] O'Doherty A, Ruf S, Mulligan C, et al. An aneuploid mouse strain carrying human chromosome 21 with Down syndrome phenotypes. *Science* 2005;309:2033-7.

[18] Fong CT, Brodeur GM. Down syndrome and leukemia: epidemiology, genetics, cytogenetics and mechanisms of leukemogenesis. *Cancer Genet Cytogenet* 1987;28:55-76.

[19] Berger R. Acute lymphoblastic leukemia and chromosome 21. *Cancer Genet Cytogenet* 1997;94:8-12.

[20] Yang QH, Rasmussen SA, Friedman JM. Down syndrome associated mortality in the U.S. from 1983 to 1997: improved survival and paucity of cancer. *Am J Hum Genet* 2000;67(Suppl 2):26.

[21] Groet J, Ives JH, Jones TA, et al. Narrowing of the region of allelic loss in 21q11-21 in squamous non-small cell lung carcinoma and cloning of a novel ubiquitin-specific protease gene from the deleted segment. *Genes Chromosomes Cancer* 2000;27:153-61.

[22] Cuadrado E, Barrena MJ. Immune dysfunction in Down's syndrome: primary immune deficiency or early senescence of the immune system? *Clin Immunol Immunopathol* 1996; 78:209-4.

[23] Novo E, Garcia MI, Lavergne J. Non-specific immunity in Down syndrome. *Am J Med Genet* 1993; 46:384-91.

[24] Ahman L, Back E, Bensch K, Olcen P. Non-efficiency of low-dose intradermal vaccination against hepatitis B in Down's syndrome. *Scand J Infect Dis* 1993; 25:16-23.

[25] Burgio GR, Ugazio AG, Nespoli L, Marcioni AF, Bottelli AM, Pasquali F. Derangements of immunoglobulin levels, phytohemagglutinin responsiveness and T and B celll markers in Down's syndrome at different ages. *Eur J Immunol* 1975;5:600-3.

[26] Lockitch G, Singh VK, Puterman ML, Godolphin WJ. Age related changes in humoral and cell-mediated immunity in Down syndrome children living at home. *Pediatr Res* 1987;22:536-40.

[27] Larson RS, Springer TA. Structure and function of leukocyte integrins. *Immunol Rev* 1990;114:181-217.

[28] Shier P, Otulakowski G, Ngo K, et al. Impaired immune responses toward alloantigens and tumor cells but normal thymic selection in mice deficient in the beta2 integrin leukocyte function-associated antigen-1. *J Immunol* 1996;157:5375–86.

[29] Taylor GM, Haigh H, Williams A, et al. Down's syndrome lymphoid cell lines exhibit increased adhesion due to the over-expression of lymphocyte function-associated antigen (LFA-1). *Immunology* 1988; 64:451-6.

[30] Murphy M, Insoft RM, Pike-Nobile L, Derbin KS, Epstein LB. Overexpression of LFA-1 and ICAM-1 in Down syndrome thymus. *J Immunol* 1993; 150:5696-703.

[31] Lin S-J, Wang J-Y, Klickstein LB. Lack of age-associated LFA-1 up-regulation and impaired ICAM-1 binding in lymphocytes from patients with Down syndrome. *Clin Exp Immunol* 2001;126:54-63.

[32] Aaltonen J, Bjorses P. Cloning of the APECED gene provides new insight into human autoimmunity. *Ann Med* 1999;31:111-6.

[33] Bjorses P, Halonen M, Palvimo JJ, et al. Mutations in the AIRE gene: effects on subcellular location and transactivation function of the autoimmune polyendocrinopathy-candidiasis-ectodermal dystrophy protein. *Am J Hum Genet* 2000;66:378-92.

[34] Barrena MJ, Echaniz P, Garcia-Serrano C, Cuadrado E. Imbalance of the CD41 subpopulations expressing CD45RA and CD29 antigens in the peripheral blood of adults and children with Down syndrome. *Scand J Immunol* 1993; 38:323-6.

[35] Corsi MM, Ponti W, Venditti A, et al. Proapoptotic activated T-cells in the blood of children with Down's syndrome: relationship with dietary antigens and intestinal alterations. *Int J Tissue React* 2003;25:117-25.

[36] Tanaka S, Teraguchi M, Hasui M, et al. Idiopathic CD4+ T-lymphocytopenia in a boy with Down syndrome. Report of a patient and a review of the literature. *Eur J Pediatr* 2004;163:122-3.

[37] Scotese I, Gaetaniello L, Matarese G, et al. T cell activation deficiency associated with an aberrant pattern of protein tyrosine phosphorylation after CD3 perturbation in Down's syndrome. *Pediatr Res* 1998;44:252-8.

[38] Nespoli L, Burgio GR, Ugazio AG, Maccario R. Immunological features of Down's syndrome: a review. *J Intellect Disabil Res* 1993;37:543-51.

[39] Chaushu S, Yefenof E, Becker A, et al. Severe impairment of secretory Ig production in parotid saliva of Down syndrome individuals. *J Dent Res* 2002;81:308-12.

[40] Jansson U, Johansson C. Down syndrome and celiac disease. *J Pediatr Gastroenterol Nutr* 1995;21:443-5.

[41] Van Goor JC, Massa GG, Hirasing R. Increased incidence and prevalence of diabetes mellitus in Down's syndrome. *Arch Dis Child* 1997;77:186.

[42] May P, Kawanishi H. Chronic hepatitis B infection and autoimmune thyroiditis in Down syndrome. *J Clin Gastroenterol* 1996;23:181-4.

[43] Burgio GR, Severi F, Rossoni R, Vaccaro R. Mongolism and thyroid autoimmunity. Lancet 1965;i:166-7.

[44] Carter DM, Jegasothy BV. Alopecia areata and Down's syndrome. *Arch Dermatol* 1976;112:1397-9.

[45] Vajro P, Cucchiara S, Vegnente A, et al. Primary sclerosis cholangitis preceding Crohn's disease in a child with Down's syndrome. *Dig Dis Sci* 1998;43:166-9.

[46] Bakkaloglu A, Ozen S, Besbas N, et al. Down syndrome associated with systemic lupus erythematosus: a mere coincidence or a significant association? *Clin Genet* 1994;46:322-3.

[47] Solaro C, Uccelli MM, Mancardi GL. A patient with multiple sclerosis and Down's syndrome with a rare paroxysmal symptom at onset. *Eur J Neurol* 1999;6:505-7.

[48] Herrera BM, Ebers GC. Progress in deciphering the genetics of multiple sclerosis. *Curr Opin Neurol* 2003;16:253-8.

[49] Fire A, Xu S, Montgomery MK, et al. Potent and specific genetic interference by double-stranded RNA in Caenorhabditis elegans. *Nature* 1998;391:806-11.

[50] Maroun LE. Interferon action and chromosome 21 trisomy (Down syndrome): 15 years later. *J Theor Biol* 1996;181:41-6.

[51] Ann Marrie R, Rudick RA. Drug Insight: interferon treatment in multiple sclerosis. *Nat Clin Pract Neurol* 2006;2:34-44.

[52] Panitch HS, Hirsch RL, Haley AS, Johnson KP. Exacerbations of multiple sclerosis in patients treated with gamma interferon. *Lancet* 1987;1:893-5.

[53] Compston A. 'The marvellous harmony of the nervous parts': the origins of multiple sclerosis. *Clin Med* 2004;4:346-54.

[54] Tan YH. Chromosome 21 and the cell growth inhibitory effect of human interferon preparations. *Nature* 1976;260:141-3.

[55] Tan YH. Schneider BL, Tischfield J, et al. Human chromosome 21 dosage: effect on the expression of the interferon induced antiviral state. *Science* 1974;186: 61-3.

[56] Lin PF, Slate DL, Lawyer FC, Ruddle FH. Assignment of the murine interferon sensitivity and cytoplasmic superoxide dismutase genes to chromosome 16. *Science* 1980;209:285-7.

[57] Epstein CJ, Epstein LB. Genetic control of the response to interferon in man and mouse. *Lymphokines* 1983;8:277.

[58] Coyle JT, Oster-Granite ML, Gearhart JD. The neurobiologic consequences of Down syndrome. *Brain Res Bull* 1986;16:773-87.

[59] Lacey-Casem ML, Oster-Granite ML. The neuropathology of the trisomy 16 mouse. *Crit Rev Neurobiol* 1994;8:293–322.

[60] Busciglio J, Yankner BA. Apoptosis and increased generation of reactive oxygen species in Down's syndrome neurons in vitro. *Nature* 1995;378:776-9.

[61] Hallam DM, Maroun LE. Anti-gamma interferon can prevent the premature death of trisomy 16 mouse cortical neurons in culture. *Neurosci Lett* 1998;252:17-20.

[62] Bambrick LL, Krueger BK. Neuronal apoptosis in mouse trisomy 16: mediation by caspases. *J Neurochem* 1999;72:1769-72.

[63] Regis G, Conti L, Boselli D, Novelli F. IFNgammaR2 trafficking tunes IFNgamma-STAT1 signaling in T lymphocytes. *Trends Immunol* 2006;27:96-101.

[64] Barish ME, Mansdorf NB, Raissdana SS. Gamma-interferon promotes differentiation of cultured cortical and hippocampal neurons. *Dev Biol* 1991;144:412-23.

[65] Neumann H, Cavalie A, Jenne DE, Wekerle H. Induction of MHC class I genes in neurons. *Science* 1995;269:549-52.

[66] Jeohn GH, Kong LY, Wilson B, et al. Synergistic neurotoxic effects of combined treatments with cytokines in murine primary mixed neuron/glia cultures. *J Neuroimmunol* 1998;85;1-10.

[67] Shaked I, Tchoresh D, Gersner R, et al. Protective autoimmunity: interferon-gamma enables microglia to remove glutamate without evoking inflammatory mediators. *J Neurochem* 2005;92:997-1009.

[68] Fitzgerald-Bocarsly P. Human interferon-alpha producing cells. *Pharmacol Ther* 1993;60:39-62.

[69] Colonna M, krug A, Cella M. Interfeon-producing cells: on the front line in immune responses against pathogens. *Curr Opin Immunol* 2002;14:373-9.

[70] Cella M, Facchetti F, Lanzavecchia A, Colonna M. Plasmacytoid dendritic cells activated by influenza virus and CD40L drive a potent TH1 polarization. *Nat Immunol* 2000;1:305-10.

[71] Hwang SY, Hertzog PJ, Holland KA, et al. A null mutation in the gene encoding a type I interferon receptor component eliminates antiproliferative and antiviral responses to interferons α and β and alters macrophage responses. *Proc Natl Acad Sci USA* 1995;92:11284–8.

[72] Staeheli P, Grob R, Meier E, et al. Influenza virus-susceptible mice carry Mx genes with a large deletion or a nonsense mutation. *Mol Cell Biol* 1988;8: 4518-23.

[73] Lutfalla G, McInnis MG, Antonarakis SE, Uze G. Structure of the human CRFB4 gene: comparison with its IFNAR neighbour. *J Mol Evol* 1995;41:338-44.

[74] Murphy M, Friend DS, Pike-Nobile L, Epstein LB. Tumor necrosis factor-alpha and IFN-gamma expression in human thymus. Localization and overexpression in Down syndrome (trisomy 21). *J Immunol* 1992;149:2506-12.

[75] Cattel RJ, Hamon CG, Corbett JA, et al. Neopterin:biopterin ratios in Down's syndrome. *J Neurol Neurosurg Psychiatry* 1989;52:1015-6.

[76] Franciotta D, Verri A, Zardini E, et al. Interferon-gamma- and interleukin-4-producing T cells in Down's syndrome. *Neurosci Lett* 2006;395:67-70.

[77] Sad S, Marcotte R, Mosmann T. Cytokine-induced differentiation of precursor mouse $CD8^+$ T cells secreting Th1 and Th2 cytokines. *Immunity* 1995;2:271-9.

[78] Franciotta D, Zardini E, Bergamaschi R, et al. Interferon γ and interleukin 4 producing cells in peripheral blood of multiple sclerosis patients undergoing immunomodulatory treatment. *J Neurol Neurosurg Psychiatry* 2003;74:123-6.

[79] Refaeli Y, Van Parijs L, Alexander SI, Abbas AK. Interferon gamma is required for activation-induced death of T lymphocytes. *J Exp Med* 2002;196;999-1005.

[80] Sad S, Marcotte R, Mosmann T. Cytokine-induced differentiation of precursor mouse $CD8^+$ T cells secreting Th1 and Th2 cytokines. *Immunity* 1995;2:271-9.

[81] Del Bo R, Comi GP, Bresolin N, et al. The apolipoprotein E ε4 allele causes a faster decline of cognitive performances in Down's syndrome subjects. *J Neurol Sci* 1997;145:87-91.

In: Focus on Mental Retardation Research
Editor: Marina I. Carson, pp. 153-184

ISBN: 978-1-60021-647-3

Chapter 6

New Insights into X-Linked Mental Retardation: From Clinical to Molecular Approaches

C. B. Santos-Rebouças** and M. M. G. Pimentel
Department of Cell Biology and Genetics, State University of Rio de Janeiro, Rio de Janeiro, Brazil

Abstract

Mental retardation (MR) has long been known to be a common and etiologically heterogeneous disorder, affecting 2-3% of the general population. Over 10% of MR cases with a Mendelian pattern of inheritance have been assigned to the X chromosome, even though it carries less than 4% of all human genes, leading to a recognized excess of hemizygous males with intellectual disability than females. Clinically, X-Linked Mental Retardation (XLMR) appears as syndromic (MRXS) and non-syndromic (MRX) forms, according to the presence or absence of somatic, neurological, behavioral, or metabolic findings in addition to the MR. Therefore, at molecular level this usual classification is questionable as mutations in some genes have been found in both syndromic and nonsyndromic XLMR. Genetic and epigenetic mutations that give rise to XLMR are not evenly distributed along the X-chromosome and seem to cluster in regions Xp11, Xp22 and Xq26-q28. Recent breakthroughs have shown that genes located at these specific regions encode for proteins involved in signaling pathways, responsible for regulate cytoskeleton organization and synaptic efficacy, besides acting in other essential functions, like chromatin remodeling and microRNAs-mediated modulation. In this chapter, we provide an up-to-date review of the remarkable progress in the XLMR field, its promise for understanding neural function, memory and learning, and the implications of this research area for developing new diagnostic tools and pharmacological approaches for therapeutic intervention.

* Corresponding author: Professor C.B. Santos-Rebouças, Universidade do Estado do Rio de Janeiro, Instituto de Biologia Roberto Alcântara Gomes, Departamento de Biologia Celular e Genética, Serviço de Genética Humana, Rua São Francisco Xavier, 524, PHLC – sala 500, Maracanã, 20550-013. Rio de Janeiro, RJ, Brazil. Tel:+55 -21 2587-7107; FAX: +55 -21 2568-5891; E-mail: cbs@uerj.br

INTRODUCTION

Mental retardation (MR), a failure to develop cognitive abilities appropriately, affects ~2-3% of the general population and is the most frequent reason for referral to genetic services, although its underlying etiology is established in less than half of all cases (Chelly, 1999). This cognitive impairment condition is associated with an intelligence quotient (IQ) of less than 70 and can be divided by the World Health Organization into the following categories: borderline (70<IQ<85), mild (50<IQ<70), moderate (35<IQ<49), severe (20<IQ<34) and profound MR (IQ<20) (WHO, 1980).

MR is a high etiologically heterogeneous disorder and could result from genetic causes, environmental factors, as mother malnutrition, perinatal accidents, and *in utero* exposure to teratogenic agents, or the combination of both. However, a substantial genetic component is present in 60% of the unknown aetiology MR cases (Thapar *et al.*, 1994). The significant involvement of genetic causes in XLMR could be explained by the complex cytoarchiteture and cellular signaling mechanisms of the nervous system reflected at the molecular level with more genes being expressed in this tissue than in any other (Mattson, 2003).

It is vastly recognized that the number of mental impaired males overcomes in approximately 30% the number of females (Stevenson, 2000), pointing to a great importance of X-linked genes in MR. Between the 221 known human genetic defects that can cause mental impairment, some 10% reside on the X chromosome even though it carries less than 4% of known human genes (Zechner *et al*, 2001).

The aim of this chapter is to review the recent genetic and epigenetic progress in the field of XLMR, its promise for understanding neural function, memory and learning, and the role of this increasing and fascinating puzzle for developing new therapeutic tools.

CHROMOSOME X AND ITS ORIGIN

The finished sequence of X chromosome has almost been completed in 2005 and approximately 1100 genes have been annotated on it, of which at least 800 are protein-coding (Ross *et al*, 2005; Harsha *et al*, 2005). Based on large cohorts, more than 60 genes have been described with MR and X-linked inheritance (XLMR Genes Update WebSite, 2006).

The molecular evolution of the X-chromosome from an autosomal pair ~300 million years ago was accompanied by a disproportional enrichment of genes involved with brain development and function, either by recruitment of new genes to the X or by acquisition of a new function by ancient X-borne genes. Many XLMR genes (e.g. *FMR1* and *ATRX*) are probably ancient, since their orthologues lie on chicken chromosome 4 (Graves *et al*, 2006). From all the protein-coding genes located at X chromosome listed in Ensembl, roughly 40% are currently known to be expressed in the brain (Ropers, 2006).

The higher accumulation of cognitive genes on the X chromosome rather than on autosomes might be a result of a rapid fixation of recessive alleles that conferred advantage to hemizygous males, which could explain the huge enlargement of the hominid brain over the past million years. Such evidence of a higher frequency of X-linked genes involved in intellectual functioning compared to autosomes has lead some authors to speculate that natural selection may have driven the accumulation of intelligence modulators genes on the X chromosome and suggests that both MR and exceptional intelligence may be more frequent in males (Lubs, 1999; Zechner *et al*, 2001; Mandel and Chelly, 2004). The existence of intelligence X-linked genes may be sustained mainly by the observation that a human brain has more X-linked genes highly expressed than in a mouse brain (Nguyen and Disteche, 2006). Curiously, a study involving females with 45,X karyotype proposed that a paternally X inheritance chromosome was associated with enhanced social-cognitive abilities (Skuse *et al*, 1997). Concerning the effects of X-linked imprinting in the brain morphology of individuals with Turner and Klinefelter syndromes, magnetic resonance imaging and proton magnetic resonance spectroscopy studies have demonstrated significant differences in regional gray matter volumes and/or neuronal integrity, depending upon parental origin of X chromosome (Kesler *et al*, 2003; Cutter *et al*, 2006; Stemkens *et al*, 2006). Generally, in these studies, females whose X chromosome was paternally derived presented higher verbal and other behavioral skills, leading to the suspicion of the role of an "intelligence" imprinted gene which might be programmed to be inactive on a maternally X chromosome.

The prevalence of the X-linked mental retardation (XLMR) in the general population was estimated in 1,8/1000 during the 1980' decade (Herbst and Miller, 1980). In the same period, Fishburn and colleagues analyzed a cohort of mental handicapped males with affected brothers and found a frequency of 5/10000 for moderate to severe XLMR. Unfortunately, updated epidemiological data have not been reported since the publication of these surveys.

Traditionally, XLMR could be divided into two sub-groups: syndromic (MRXS or S-XLMR) or non-syndromic MR (MRX or NS-XLMR). In NS-XLMR, cognitive impairment is apparently the only event, not being associated to other recognizable clinical or biochemical features (somatic, neurological or metabolic findings) as in S-XLMR. However, at the molecular level this usual classification is questionable as mutations in a number of genes have been found to be present in both syndromic and non-syndromic XLMR.

The X chromosome is associated with over 300 Mendelian conditions, but genetic and epigenetic defects underlying XLMR are not evenly distributed along the X chromosome and seem to cluster in regions Xp11, Xp22 and Xq26-q28, with the Xp11 region carrying almost 30% of all gene mutations related to NS-XLMR (Ropers *et al*, 2003). About 209 entities of XLMR have been described so far, including malformations syndromes, neuromuscular disorders, metabolic conditions, dominant conditions and MRX traits, from which 65 had the underlying defect cloned (Table 1). Finding the molecular causative defect in NS-XLMR is intrinsically more difficult. To date, 85 families with NS-XLMR are recorded in the literature (XLMR Genes Update WebSite, 2006) as MRX numbered pedigrees, but only 35% of them have their causative mutations identified. This low diagnosis rate could be expected since NS-XLMR consists of numerous clinically indistinguishable mutations, in which the cognitive impairment is the only manifestation.

The diagnosis of XLMR is usually an exclusion procedure of other causes of developmental delay (Shevell *et al*, 2003). Chromosomal rearrangements have a prominent role in the etiology of MR and in almost all cases a >550 resolution banded karyotype is recommended to achieve detection of ~5-10 Mb large abnormalities. Thus, balanced rearrangements or small deletions involving X chromosome in mentally handicapped individuals led to the identification of many XLMR genes, mainly S-XLMR associated genes, because patients with S-XLMR are more likely to seek genetic services and undergo karyotyping than those with NS-XLMR. Of similar importance, submicroscope telomeric deletions have been detected in even 7% of patients with MR of idiopathic etiology (Flint and

Knight, 2003; Koolen *et al*, 2004), but its screening is not yet recommended in the routine diagnosis, at least in developing countries. After excluding chromosomal abnormalities, there are several XLMR genes, where mutations could result in S-XLMR or NS-XLMR. The choice for which gene will be initially tested depends on the identification of additional clinical features that could categorize the condition as syndromic (Table 2) and the relative prevalence of the specific gene mutation in the target population (Raymond, 2006). Generally, it is common to proceed to the Fragile X syndrome test in all males with syndromic and idiopathic MR, followed by *ARX* gene investigation. Therefore, searching for NS-XLMR causative defects could be more laborious and time-consuming due, mainly, to the absence of other clinical clues and the mutational heterogeneity.

Table 1. Total count of XLMR conditions

	Total	Mapped	Cloned
Malformations syndromes	82	30	17
Neuromuscular disorders	40	14	16
Metabolic conditions	13	1	12
Dominant conditions	8	3	4
Total MRXS	143	48	49
MRX	66	50	16
Total entries	209	98	65

Data from XLMR Genes Update WebSite (2006).

Table 2. Additional clinical features found in syndromic XLMR

Clinical features besides mental retardation	Potential gene involved
Microcephaly	*ATRX, MECP2, PQBP1, JARID1C*
Cleft lip and palate	*PQBP1*
Congenital heart disease	*PQBP1*
Spastic paraplegia	*SLC16A2, ATRX, JARID1C, MECP2*
Seizures	*AGTR2, ATRX, SLC6A8, ARX, JARID1C*
Absent speech	*ATRX, SLC16A2, SLC6A8*
Cerebellar hipoplasia	*OPHN1*
Short stature	*PQBP1, JARID1C*
Autistic behaviour	*NLGN3, NLGN4, AGTR2, SLC6A8*
Dystonia	*ARX*
Hypertelorism	*RPS6KA3*
Scoliosis	*RPS6KA3, ATRX*
Abnormal thyroid function	*SLC16A2*

Based on Raymond (2006).

Main Genes Involved Exclusively in S-XLMR

FMR1

FMR1, involved in the most common form of inherited MR (Fragile X syndrome), is the best-characterized gene associated to S-XLMR. Fragile X syndrome occurs in approximately 1 in 4000 males and 1 in 8000 females, accounting for 25% of the families with XLMR (Fishburn *et al*, 1983; Turner *et al*, 1996). The molecular basis for the disorder elapses from an expansion of 5'CGG 3' polymorphic repeats in the 5'UTR of the *FMR1* gene on Xq27.3. When the number of CGG exceeds 200 copies, cytosine methylation of the repeats and hypermethylation of the upstream CpG island in the promoter occurs associated to changes in the chromatin structure, which leads to transcriptional gene silencing. These aspects make Fragile X syndrome the best-characterized example of how DNA sequence alterations can modify the epigenetic code. The absence of FMRP protein, highly expressed at brain and testis, leads to MR in the moderate to severe range, macroorchidism (seen after pubertal age) and other behavioral and physical associated phenotypes (O'Donnell and Warren, 2002). Two main models for how the CGG repeats become de novo methylated are conceivable. In the first, the expanded number of repeats could be recognized as foreign and hence become methylated *de novo* like any other foreign DNA, e.g., integrated viral DNA (Genç *et al*, 2000). In another model, the expanded trinucleotide repeats are targeted through the formation of hairpin RNA from the transcribed repeat, which could recruit the post translation RNAi silencing machinery (Handa *et al*, 2003; Jin *et al*, 2004a). RNAi is a highly conserved silencing pathway triggered by double strand RNA (dsRNA), which regulates gene expression via targeted degradation of mRNAs and, subsequently, post transcriptional repression. The hallmark of this pathway involves the cleavage of dsRNAs into small interfering RNA molecules (siRNAs) by an Rnase-III-like enzyme called Dicer and the subsequent association of these siRNAs with a multiprotein RNAi effector complex called RISC (RNA induced silencing complex) to provide specificity for the degradation of complementary mRNAs (for review see Santos-Rebouças and Pimentel, 2007).

FMRP is an RNA binding protein involved in the control of local protein synthesis in the dendrites in response to synaptic activity (Bear *et al*, 2004). In Fragile X syndrome individuals, dendrites spines, in which synaptic transmission occurs, are abnormally long and immature (Irwin *et al*, 2000). Normally, FMRP shuttles from the nucleus to cytoplasm, where it forms messenger ribonucleoprotein complexes (mRNPs) (Feng *et al*, 1997) and binds to a specific group of mRNAs, suppressing their translation (Laggerbauer *et al*, 2001; Li *et al*, 2001). The identified target mRNAs, whose three dimensional structures generally presents an G-quartet (Darnell *et al*, 2001) and a FMRP-kissing complex (Darnell *et al*, 2005), include the *FMR1* mRNA itself, microtubule-associated protein 1B (MAP1B) and other important messages involved in neuronal development and plasticity (Brown *et al*, 2001; Darnell *et al*, 2001). Jin and colleagues (2004) demonstrated that FMRP can also interact with members of the Argonaute family of proteins and with the miRNA pathway, suggesting a novel mechanism of gene expression regulation by FMRP. Furthermore, there is several evidence that FMRP acts in the long term depression of transmission at hippocampal synapses triggered by metabolotropic glutamate receptors (mGluRs), suppressing mGluR-stimulated local protein translation (Weiler *et al*, 1997; Bear *et al*, 2004). Confirming these findings, loss of FMRP increases long term depression in mouse hippocampus (Huber *et al*, 2002) and many of the protein-synthesis-dependent functions of metabolotropic receptors are exaggerated in Fragile X syndrome patients (Bear *et al*, 2004).

Gathering from this and other recent evidence, Garber and colleagues (2006) proposed a more elucidative model, in which FMRP is transported to the nucleus, where it associates with specific transcripts and forms mRNPs, which migrate to cytoplasm and interact with RISC complex, inhibiting the translation of the target transcripts. Then, stimulation of neurons increases the transport of the silent complexes to the dendrites as granules and activates the proteosome to degrade the RISC complex, enabling rapid translation of the initially silent messages. When FMRP is absent, the cell lacks the opposing effect to mGluR stimulation, leading to an increase of the proteins normally stimulated by this system, which could result in the abnormal dendrite spine morphology seen in individuals and animal models with Fragile X syndrome.

As we could see, *FMR1* gene continues to be an exciting model about the role of chromatin changes, microRNA regulation, and synapse events. However, with the advent of high-throughput genomic technologies, the number of other cloned genes involved in syndromal forms of XLMR increased vertiginously (Figure 1).

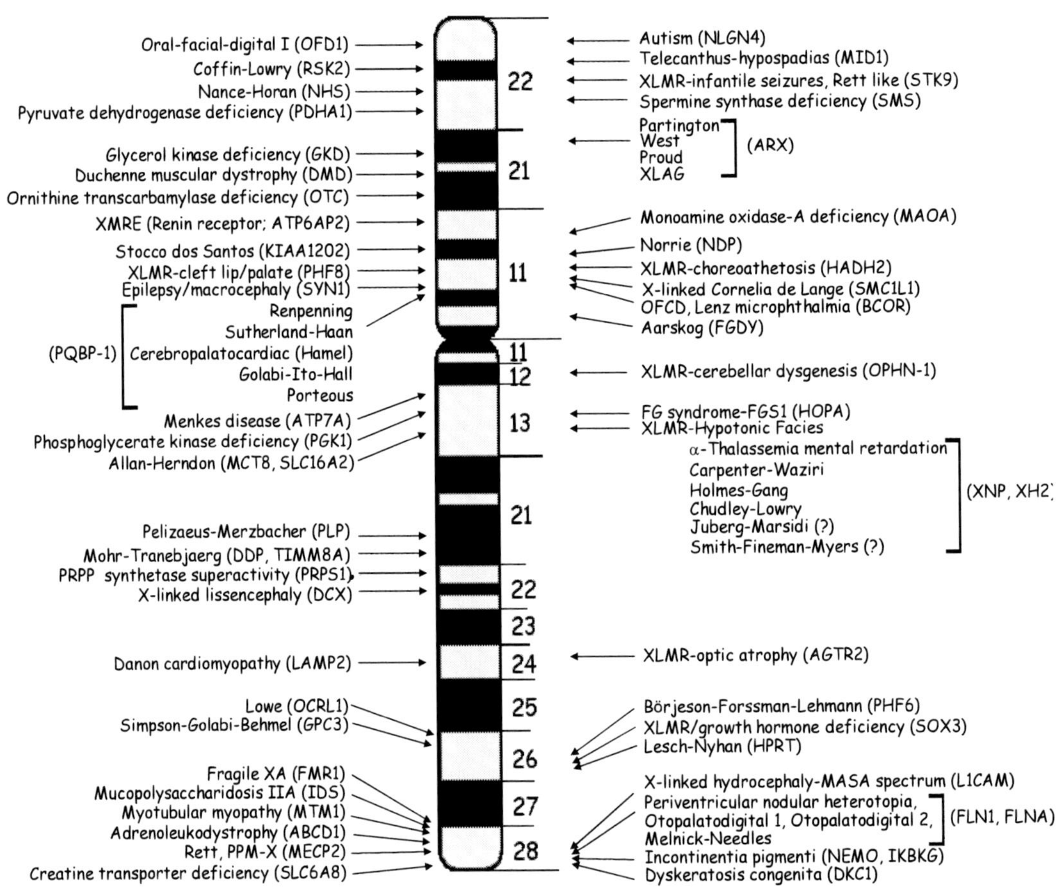

Figure 1. Genes involved in syndromic XLMR. Data from the Greenwood Genetic Center- XLMR update (2006).

L1CAM

L1 cell adhesion molecule gene (*L1CAM*) is another crucial factor in S-XLMR. The protein encoded by this gene is a neural recognition molecule belonging to a large class of immunoglobulin superfamily cell adhesion molecules that mediate cell-to-cell adhesion at the cell surface and is essential in the development of the nervous system (Kenwrick *et al*, 2000). It is mainly expressed on neurons and Schwann cells, and plays a key role in axon outgrowth and pathfinding through interactions with various extracellular ligands and intracellular second messenger systems (Fransen *et al*, 1997). Mutations in *L1CAM* gene are responsible for a wide spectrum of neurological abnormalities, including X-linked hydrocephalus, MASA syndrome (mental retardation, aphasia, shuffling gait, and adducted thumbs), X-linked complicated spastic paraplegia type 1 and X-linked agenesis of the corpus callosum. The main clinical features overlapping these disorders are MR, corpus callosum hypoplasia, adducted thumbs, spastic paraplegia and hydrocephalus, which could be recognized as a disorder named CRASH syndrome. Inter- and intrafamilial variability is a well-known feature of the *L1CAM* spectrum (Finckh *et al*, 2000). *L1CAM* mutations are distributed over the functional protein domains and there appears to be a relationship between the patients' clinical phenotype and the type of alteration. Most *L1CAM* mutations reported to date are point mutations (missense, nonsense, splice site) and only a few patients with larger rearrangements have been documented (Panayi *et al*, 2005). Missense mutations in extracellular domains or mutations in cytoplasmic regions cause milder phenotypes than those leading to truncation in extracellular domains or to non-detectable L1 protein (Weller and Gartner, 2001). Since there is no biochemically assayed disease marker, molecular analysis of the *L1CAM* gene is the only means of confirming a clinical diagnosis.

Although the wide mutational spectrum, many of the XLMR syndromes reported until this moment are caused by the loss of function of key genes essential to the early development processes or implicated in the transcriptional activation of other genes also involved in early developmental processes, cell proliferation and differentiation. This could explain the pleiotropic effects observed in syndromic cases of XLMR. Moreover, as exemplified by *L1CAM* mutations, in other S-XLMR disorders, even the same mutation in a single gene could produce a remarkable inter and intra-familial range of phenotypes between affected individuals, resulting apparently from differences in genetic background (Chelly, 1999).

Main Genes Involved Exclusively in NS-XLMR

NS-XLMR is twice more common than syndromic forms of XLMR (Fishburn *et al*, 1983) and this excessive frequency is particularly notable during early childhood, since at this stage a great proportion of apparently NS-XLMR patients does not exhibit yet some recognizable syndromic symptoms, as large testes in Fragile X syndrome. Therefore, as more elucidative molecular diagnosis analyses become available it is expected that the frequency of NS-XLMR decrease with a concomitant rise of the number of X-linked syndromic forms. Until this moment, at least 19 genes were exclusively associated to non-specific forms of XLMR (Table 3).

Table 3. Main genes exclusively involved in NS-XLMR

Gene	Name	Location	Potential Functions	Reference
ACS4 (FACL4)	Long-chain-fatty-acid--CoA ligase 4	Xq23	possible role in membrane synthesis and/or recycling	Meloni *et al*, 2002
AGTR2	angiotensin II receptor, type 2	Xq23	brain-expressed angiotensin receptor 2	Vervoort *et al*, 2002
ARHGEF6	Rho guanine nucleotide exchange factor 6	Xq26.3	integrin-mediated activation of Rac–cdc42; stimulation of neurite outgrowth	Yntema *et al*, 1998
ARHGEF9	Cdc42 guanine nucleotide exchange factor	Xq22.1	pivotal role in formation of postsynaptic glycine and GABA(A) receptor clusters	Marco *et al*, 2005
DLG3	Discs large homolog 3	Xq13.1	post-synaptic scaffolding protein linked to NMDA-type glutamatergic receptors	Tarpey *et al*, 2004
FMR2	Fragile mental retardation 2	Xq28	transcriptional regulator; possible role in long-term memory and enhanced long-term potentiation	Gecz *et al*, 1996
FTSJ1	FTSJ homolog 1	Xp11.23	RNA methyltransferase, possible role in tRNA modification and translation	Freude *et al*, 2004
GDI1	GDP dissociation inhibitor 1	Xq28	regulation of synaptosomal Rab4 and Rab5 pools; possible role in endocytosis	D'Adamo *et al*, 1998
GRIA3	AMPA receptor GLUR3	Xq25	mediates fast, synaptic transmission in central nervous system	Wu *et al*, 2005
IL1RAPL	IL-1 receptor accessory protein	Xp21.2	regulator of dense-core granule exocytosis; possible modulator of neurotransmitter release	Carrie *et al*, 1999
KLF8 / ZNF741	Kruppel-like Factor 8	Xp11.21	possible role in repress transcription mediated by a CACCC box-dependent promoter without using the CTBP2 contact motif	Lossi *et al*, 2002
NLGN3	neuroligin 3	Xq13	mediates cell-to-cell interactions between neurons	Jamain *et al*, 2003
PAK3	p21-activated kinase 3	Xq23	regulation of actin cytoskeleton; stimulation of neurite outgrowth	Allen *et al*, 1998
TM4SF2	tetraspanin	Xp11.4	modulation of integrin-mediated signalling; neurite outgrowth; possible role in synapse formation	Zemni *et al*, 2000
VCX-A	Variable Charge X A	Xp22.31	unknown	Fukami *et al*, 2000
ZDHHC15	Zinc finger, DHHC-type containing 15	Xq13.3	unknown	Mansouri *et al*, 2005

Table 3 (continued)

ZNF41	zinc-finger 41	Xp11.3	KRAB domain-containing zinc finger protein; putative transcriptional regulator; possible involvement in chromatin remodeling	Shoichet *et al*, 2003
ZNF81	zinc-finger 81	Xp11.23	KRAB domain-containing zinc finger protein; related to ZNF41 and ZNF674	Kleefstra *et al*, 2004b
ZNF674	zinc-finger 74	Xp11.3	KRAB domain-containing zinc finger protein; related to ZNF41 and ZNF81	Lugtenberg *et al*, 2006a

Data from Ropers (2006) and XLMR update website (2006).

FMR2

FRAXE fragile site associated MR affects 1 in 23423 males (Youings *et al*, 2000) and is a consequence of either a hypermethylation of the FRAXE CpG island, caused by an expansion of a CCG repeat near the 5'end of the *FMR2* gene, or internal *FMR2* gene deletions (Gecz, 2000). *FMR2* is a large gene (~650 kb), located in Xq28, 600 kb distal to FRAXA (*FMR1*), the Fragile X syndrome fragile site. It has a complex pattern of alternative splicing and encodes a conserved transcription co-activator protein. The major *FMR2* transcript is highly expressed in neurons of the neocortex, granular cell layer of the hippocampus and in Purkinje cells of the cerebellum. The cognitive impairment in FRAXE patients is due to *FMR2* loss of function and, although mild to-borderline non-syndromic MR is the most recognizable feature, the FRAXE phenotype could appears as learning difficulties, speech delay and behavioral problems (Gecz, 2000). Lilliputian (Lilli), a Drosophila *FMR2* orthologue, has been linked with several signal transduction pathways, including the transforming growth factor-beta (TGF-beta) pathway, the Raf/MEK/MAP kinase (MAPK) pathway, and the P13K/PKB pathway. Mutation of Lilli shows defects in germinal band extension, cytoskeletal structure, cell growth, and organ development (Gu and Nelson, 2003).

Unlike the individuals harboring full mutated alleles (>200 CCG repeats), it would be not expected that the bearers of FRAXE intermediate (31-60 CCG repeats) or premutated (61-200 CCG repeats) alleles exhibit FRAXE phenotype, since in these cases the *FMR2* gene is not turned off by the promoter hypermethylation. However, it is questioned whether FRAXE expanded unmethylated alleles (intermediate/premutated) are prone enough to cause an adverse effect in the intellectual and cognitive function. In 1996, Murray and colleagues verified an excess of FRAXE intermediate alleles in a population of English boys with learning disabilities attending special education classes, when compared to the maternal chromosome X used as control. Later, five other published studies accomplished in children with special education-needs or mentally retarded individuals did not corroborate the previous screenings, suggesting that the alleles in the intermediate zone did not play a role in intellectual disabilities (Mazzocco *et al*, 1997; Mornet *et al*, 1998; Patsalis *et al*, 1998; Crawford *et al*, 1999; Barros Santos and Gonçalves Pimentel, 2003). Therefore, more recently, Annesi and colleagues (2004) demonstrated a significant excess of FRAXE intermediate alleles among subjects with Parkinson disease (6,4%) than those found in healthy controls (0,27%), indicating that these relatively expanded alleles may be associated with this neurological disorder.

The identification of another FRAXE CpG island-associated gene, *FMR3*, transcribed in the opposite orientation to *FMR2*, and the lack of *FMR3* expression in FRAXE full mutation males suggests, that the *FMR3* gene might also contribute to the FRAXE mental retardation phenotype (Gecz, 2000a). Unlike *FMR2*, the *FMR3* gene is composed of only two exons and its putative transcription start site is located 23 bp proximal to the FRAXE CCG repeat, and only 3 bp from the putative *FMR2* transcription start site. Evidence showed that *FMR3* is likely a non-coding RNA gene, whose transcript was detected in adult brain (medulla and spinal cord), but its role is still unknown (Gecz, 2000a). Recently, we have identified a boy with a 58 pb deletion in the *FMR2* genc immediately distal to the FRAXE CCG repeat. RT-PCR studies on the *FMR2* and *FMR3* genes showed that only the *FMR3* expression was abolished, suggesting a possible causal relationship between the lack of *FMR3* expression and FRAXE mutation-likely phenotype in this patient (Santos-Rebouças *et al*, 2006). Unfortunately, due to the great length of the *FMR2* gene, almost all the screening studies focused only on FRAXE CCG repeats and flanking regions, making impossible the identification of other mutations along the gene, mainly short deletions affecting *FMR2/FMR3* expression. These deletions could be so or more frequent than expanded alleles and could be also associated to the FRAXE phenotype. Besides, it is tempting to speculate that individuals with *FMR2* mutations may well adapt to the environment and often escape ascertainment, especially as adults, contributing to a low prevalence of *FMR2* mutation.

The proximity of the FRAXE and FRAXA *loci* led some authors to speculate about possible effects on the *FMR1* or *FMR2* gene expression when one of them is expanded. Brown *et al* (1997) and Barros Santos and Gonçalves Pimentel (2003) have reported that large expansions at FRAXA are associated with expanded alleles at FRAXE, whereas Murray *et al* (1997) identified small alleles at FRAXE in subjects with expansions at the FRAXA *locus*. This effect between *FMR1/FMR2* genes could be explained by two mechanisms: a slipped strand mispairing in the FRAXE region during DNA replication due to the increased number of CGG repeats at the FRAXA *locus* or a potential disturbance of *cis*-acting factors.

Exception to *FMR2*, all the exclusively NS-XLMR genes identified represent rare causes of XLMR. Only few MRX families have been found to carry mutations in the same NS-XLMR gene and there remain a large number of families with XLMR in which the causative mutation has not been identified yet.

GDI1, DLG3 and IL1RAPL

GDP dissociation inhibitor 1 (*GDI1*) encodes alpha Gdi, one of the proteins controlling the activity of the small GTPases of the Rab family in vesicle fusion and intracellular trafficking (Novick *et al*, 1997). Only three MRX families and 1/164 males with non-familial MR were characterized as having *GDI1* mutations, suggesting that the prevalence of such alterations in NS-XLMR may be 0,5 to 1% (D'Adamo *et al*, 1998; Bienvenu *et al*, 1998). In the mouse, Gdi1 is expressed early in development and is upregulated at initial stages of brain differentiation, suggesting that it may also play a role in neuron migration and/or differentiation (D'Adamo *et al*, 1998). Although anatomically normal, Gdi1-deficient mice are impaired in tasks requiring formation of short-term temporal associations, suggesting a defect in short-term memory (D'Adamo *et al*, 2002).

Thus, changes in synaptic efficacy have been proposed as neural mechanisms underlying memory and learning. As *GDI1* gene, *DLG3* and *IL1RAPL* are also involved in the establishment and modulation of synapses. *DLG3 (*neuroendocrine dlg) gene encodes synapse-associated protein 102 (SAP102). Neuronal SAP102 is expressed during early brain development and is localized to the postsynaptic density of excitatory synapses (Muller *et al*, 1996; Makino *et al*, 1997). Tarpey *et al* (2004) identified four mutations in 329 families with a history of at least two males with significant non-syndromic intellectual impairment (1.2%). All of the mutations truncated SAP102 within or before its third PDZ domain, probably impairing the protein's ability to interact with NMDA receptors, which have been implicated in the induction of certain forms of synaptic plasticity, such as long-term potentiation and long-term depression in the hippocampus. IL1RAPL (IL1 receptor accessory protein like) interacts with neuronal calcium sensor-1, and is potentially implicated in the regulation of exocytosis and therefore in synaptic transmission (Bahi *et al*, 2003). Signal transduction through multifunctional proteins of the immune system, like IL1RAPL, appears to be critical for the development of physiological processes underlying cognitive function (Carrie *et al*, 1999). Mutations in *IL1RAPL* gene were already described in two unrelated families with NS-XLMR, both resulting in premature stop codons (Carrie *et al*, 1999; Tabolacci *et al*, 2006).

NLGN3

Neuroligins constitute a family of proteins thought to mediate cell-to-cell interactions between neurons. Mutations in *NLGN3* (neuroligin 3) and *NLGN4* (neuroligin 4- associated to both NS-XLMR and S-XLMR) were previously described as a cause of autism (Jamain *et al*, 2003; Laumonnier *et al*, 2004), but severe MR was also seen in the many of the affected individuals. Therefore, some recent studies suggest that neuroligin mutations most probably represent rare causes of autism (Gauthier *et al*, 2005; Ylisaukko-oja *et al*, 2005; Blasi *et al*, 2006).

Zinc Finger Protein-coding Genes

ZNF41 (zing finger protein 41), *ZNF81* (zing finger protein 81) and *ZNF674* (zing finger protein 674) contain a transcriptional repressor domain that is linked to mechanisms of chromatin remodeling, acting in transcription regulation. Mutations in these genes were found through the molecular investigation of non-syndromic MR individuals bearing balanced X translocations (Shoichet *et al*, 2003; Kleefstra *et al*, 2004b) or analysis of NS-XLMR families that show linkage to Xp11 (Lugtenberg *et al*, 2006a). The involvement of *ZNF41*, *ZNF81* and *ZNF674* in XLMR indicate a common role for these zinc-finger genes, crucial for DNA binding, in human cognitive functioning. Reinforcing this evidence, *ZNF41* and *ZNF81* do not have orthologues in the mouse, which signals that these genes are indispensable for normal human brain function (Ropers, 2006).

Table 4. Genes implicated in both S-XLMR and NS-XLMR

Gene	Name	Location	Potential Functions	Reference
ARX	Aristaless-related homeobox	Xp22.1	transcription factor with possible role in the maintenance of specific neuronal subtypes in the cerebral cortex and axonal guidance in the floorplate. Neuronal proliferation, differentiation of GABA-ergic neurons	Stromme *et al*, 2002; Poirier *et al*, 2006
ATRX	alpha-thalassemia/mental retardation syndrome gene	Xq13.3	DNA-binding helicase, involved in chromatin remodelling, DNA methylation and regulation of gene expression; intrinsic regulator of cortical size	Guerrini *et al*, 2000; Badens *et al*, 2006
FGD1	RhoGEF	Xp11.2	possible role in stimulation of neurite outgrowth	Lebel *et al*, 2002; Orrico *et al*, 2004
JARID1C (SMCX)	Jumonji, AT-rich interactive domain 1C	Xp11.22	role in chromatin remodelling	Jensen *et al*, 2005
MECP2	methyl-CpG binding protein	Xq28	serine–threonine protein kinase; CREB phosphorylation; role in long-term memory formation	Orrico *et al*, 2000; Christodoulou *et al*, 2003
NLGN4	neuroligin 4	Xp22.3	postsynaptic membrane protein; involved in induction of presynaptic structures; linked to NMDA-type glutamatergic receptors	Jamain *et al*, 2003; Laumonnier *et al*, 2004
OPHN1	oligophrenin-1	Xq12	oligophrenin-1 repress the Rho signaling pathway to maintain dendritic spine length	Billuart *et al*, 1998; Bergmann *et al*, 2003
PQBP1	polyglutamine-binding protein 1	Xp11.23	putative role in transcription and mRNA splicing	Deqaqi *et al*, 1998; Cason *et al*, 2003
RPS6KA3 (RSK2)	serine–threonine protein kinase	Xp22.1	CREB phosphorylation; role in long-term memory formation	Tivier *et al*, 1996; Merienne *et al*, 1999
SLC6A8	solute carrier family 6	Xq28	creatine transporter required for maintenance of (phospho) creatine pools in the brain	Rosenberg *et al*, 2004; Clark *et al*, 2006
SLC16A2 (MCT8)	solute carrier family 16, member 2	Xq13.2	thyroid hormone transport function	Friesema *et al*, 2003; Schwartz *et al*, 2005

Data from Ropers (2006) and XLMR update website (2006)

MAIN GENES INVOLVED IN BOTH S-XLMR AND NS-XLMR

To date, genetic linkage studies or characterization of chromosomal rearrangements have allowed the identification of at least 11 different genes responsible for syndromic forms of MR, in which the mildest mutations, with a certain remaining functional activity, cause non-specific MR (Table 4).

ARX

Aristaless Related Homeobox gene (*ARX*) mutations are considered to be the second most common cause of XLMR, accounting for ~10% of the MRX families published. The *ARX* gene is ortholog to the Drosophila melanogaster aristaless homeobox gene and encodes a bifunctional transcription factor (activator and repressor), expressed predominantly in the cerebral forebrain and floor plate, pancreas and testes (Stromme *et al*, 2002; Gecz *et al*, 2006). The ARX protein belongs to the class of homeoprotein, the paired (Prd) class, characterized by six invariant amino acids residues and a glutamine or serine residue at the critical position 50 (Q50/K50) of their homeodomain, and exerts primary developmental functions (Bienvenu *et al*, 2002; Stromme *et al*, 2002). This protein contains four polyalanine tracts (poly A), not seen in zebrafish and fly orthologues, and three highly conserved domains: a homeodomain, an aristaless domain (also called C peptide domain) and an octapeptide domain located near the N-terminus. The expression pattern suggests that ARX is involved in the differentiation and maintenance of specific neuronal cell types in the central nervous system (Ohira *et al*, 2002; Poirier *et al*, 2004; Suri, 2005). A wide spectrum of abnormal phenotypes were associated to *ARX* gene, including various forms of epilepsy, myoclonic seizures, dystonia, autism, lissencephaly, as well as syndromic and non-syndromic XLMR (Bienvenu *et al*, 2002; Kitamura *et al*, 2002; Stromme *et al*, 2002; Poirier *et al*, 2006; Gestinari-Duarte *et al*, 2006). This considerable pleiotropy is a result of the high rate of mutations (~59) that have been described in the *ARX* gene, which leads *ARX* to be called as a "gene for all seasons" (Gecz *et al*, 2006). Various approaches have been taken to identify the ARX target genes, but until now only Pax4 was found to be regulated by Arx (and vice-versa) at least in the pancreas, controlling cell fate specification (Collombat *et al*, 2003, 2005). The majority of the mutations identified in *ARX* gene represents deletions and duplications, mainly occurring in the exon 2, which indicates that these alterations might be a consequence of the same molecular event, including that seen in dynamic mutations (Kato *et al*, 2003; Pearson *et al*, 2005). The most frequent mutation already identified in the *ARX* gene (found in more than 40% of the unrelated individuals with *ARX* mutations) is a duplication of 24 bp (c.428–451dup) at the exon 2, that causes an expansion of the second poly A tract of the ARX protein (Stromme *et al*, 2002; Gecz *et al*, 2006). This duplication was detected in 6.5% of the XLMR families published (Poirier *et al*, 2006) and is likely to be present in 1/12,000 males, which is about one third of the established frequency for the Fragile X syndrome (Partington *et al*, 2004). Thus, it is acceptable that the c.428–451dup has a significant frequency among XLMR families, but its incidence in sporadic males with MR appears to be low (Stepp *et al*, 2005; Poirier *et al*, 2006; Gestinari-Duarte *et al*, 2006). However, one should keep in mind that in almost all the screening studies proceeded until this moment, only the DNA sequence of coding regions and flanking intronic regions of *ARX* were considered. Therefore, there are several ultraconserved elements near the exons, that were speculate to represent clusters of *ARX* enhancers (Bejerano *et al*, 2004) and when mutated could also contribute to *ARX* phenotypes. Recently, mutations in cyclin-dependent kinase-like 5 (*CDKL5*), also located within the Xp22, have been associated with a broad range of clinical manifestations, which overlaps the *ARX* mutations phenotype, including seizures/epilepsy, autism, and MR (Kalscheuer *et al*, 2003; Mari *et al*, 2005; Scala *et al*, 2005). By this way, *CDKL5* is, perhaps, another gene that should be screened in patients presenting MR associated with seizures/epilepsy and autism, particularly in XLMR families, who have negative results for *ARX* mutations.

SLC6A8

Of the genes involved in NS-XLMR and epilepsy, the most notable are *ARX* and solute carrier family 6 (*SLC6A8*), a creatine transporter gene. Mutations in the *SLC6A8* result in creatine deficiency in the brain and are also described to be associated to other phenotypes as developmental delay and hypotonia (Salomons *et al*, 2001), severe neurological disturbances including seizures, behavioral problems, speech delay, and inability to engage in structured play (Bizzi *et al*, 2002), MR with seizures (Hahn *et al*, 2002), truncal hypotonia, impaired eye-hand coordination, severe cognitive and language retardation (Schiaffino *et al*, 2005) and microcephaly, long and narrow face, and prominent chin (Clark *et al*, 2006). The data about the prevalence of *SLC6A8* mutations are still controversial. Rosenberg *et al* (2004) analyzed 290 patients with NS-XLMR archived by the European XLMR Consortium and found that the frequency of *SLC6A8* mutations (~2,1%) was close to that of CGG expansions in *FMR1* gene. However, Clark *et al* (2006) screened a large sample of males with idiopathic MR (n=478) and found pathogenic or potentially pathogenic *SLC6A8* mutations in only 1% of them. These frequency differences could be due to distinct discretions used to select the target populations. One should consider that analysis of urine creatine/creatinine ratio and cerebral creatine signal in proton magnetic resonance spectroscopy in males with MR of unknown cause could be great tools to assist the molecular diagnosis of *SLC6A8* mutations.

SLC16A2

Also known as *MCT8*, *SLC16A2* is another gene integrating solute carrier family that is related to both forms of XLMR. The protein encoded by *SLC16A2* demonstrates thyroid hormone transport function (Friesema *et al*, 2003), highly expressed in different brain areas (Heuer *et al*, 2005). Abnormal transporter function due to *SLC16A2* mutations is reflected in elevated free triiodothyronine and lowered free thyroxine levels in the blood. Besides high serum triiodothyronine (T3) concentrations, males with *SLC16A2* mutations generally exhibit severe MR and other neurological abnormalities, whereas heterozygous females appear to have a milder or any thyroid phenotype and no neurological defects (Friesema *et al*, 2003; Dumitrescu *et al*, 2004). The severe neurological phenotype in males and the lack of neurological improvement even after the normalization of serum TSH during treatment with thyroid hormone reinforce a possible preferential function of them in brain tissue (Dumitrescu *et al*, 2004). The phenotype of the *SLC16A2* mutations overlaps that seen in Allan-Herndon-Dudley syndrome (AHDS), characterized by severe MR associated with lack of speech, elevated serum T3 and rather low levels of the prohormone thyroxine (T4), hypotonia, reduced muscle mass, spastic paraplegia, involuntary movements, among others (Schwartz *et al*, 2005). In this way, families with AHDS have been also found to carry *SLC16A2* mutations (Schwartz *et al*, 2005; Maranduba *et al*, 2006). The disturbances of thyroid hormones levels in blood related to *SLC16A2* mutations could be used as a functional and cheap systematic detection method allied to molecular analysis.

MECP2

Methyl-CpG-binding protein 2 gene (*MECP2*), located in Xq28, encodes a multifunctional protein (MeCP2), which selectively binds to methylated cytosines and acts as an stable methylation-dependent transcriptional repressor via effects on chromatin structure (Nan *et al*, 1997) and also as a RNA splicing regulator (Young *et al*, 2005). This gene is expressed in almost all cells of the body, and has two separate isoforms: MeCP2_e2 (encoded by exons 2, 3, and 4) and MeCP2_e1 (encoded by exons 1, 3, and 4), which is the predominant isoform in human brain (Kriaucionis and Bird, 2004; Mnatzakanian *et al*, 2004) The principal isoform possesses three main functional domains: the MBD, responsible for binding to 5-methyl-CpG; the TRD, that mediates transcriptional repression through its interaction with a co-repressor protein complex and histone deacetylases; and the C-terminal domain, involved in protein stability (Nan *et al*, 1997, 1998; Jones *et al*, 1998). The initiation of *MECP2* expression is coincident with the synaptogenesis process, suggesting that MeCP2 plays an important role in neuronal maturation (Shahbazian *et al*, 2002). Some genes were found to be regulated by *MECP2*, like *BDNF* that codifies the brain-derived neurotrophic factor, crucial for learning and memory (Martinowich *et al*, 2003), and the genes *UBE3A* and *GABRB3* (Samaco *et al*, 2005), both genes involved in neurodevelopmental disorders, highlighting the importance of the *MECP2* gene in the development of the central nervous system.

Loss-of-function mutations in the *MECP2* gene were firstly described to cause Rett syndrome, the most common sporadically inherited form of MR in females, with an incidence of 1 in 10000-15000 (Percy, 2002). This postnatal neurodevelopmental disorder is characterized by degeneration of acquired motor and language skills around 6-18 months of age, severe mental impairment, seizures, autistic features, hand stereotypic movements, microcephaly, jerky truncal ataxia and other related neurological symptoms (Hagberg *et al*, 1983). Rett syndrome shows to be letal in hemizygous males, but boys that have a 47,XXY karyotype or are somatic mosaic could carry the same *MECP2* mutations seen in girls with the classic Rett phenotype. Nonsense, missense, frameshift mutations and intragenic deletions found in Rett patients are scattered all over the *MECP2* gene and there seems to be a strict correlation between the position of the mutation and the severity of the symptoms (Free *et al*, 2001; Lee *et al*, 2001). Nearly 70% of the mutations arise from C>T transitions at eight CpG nucleotides and seems to occurs preferentially either within the MBD or the TRD (Christodoulou *et al*, 2003; Ballestar *et al*, 2005), whereas carboxy-terminal deletions are estimated to occur in 10-15% of the Rett patients (Moretti and Zoghbi, 2006). In large panels of typical Rett, mutations affecting exon 1 of *MECP2* seems to be rare, representing only

0,47-1% of the deleterious alleles and exon 2 mutations are even less common (Philippe *et al*, 2006; Quenard *et al*, 2006). Recently, Philippe and colleagues (2006) screened a large cohort of French Rett syndrome patients and found that large and complex rearrangements not previously detected using only a PCR-based strategy represent 5.8% of the *MECP2* mutations found. These data suggest that quantitative analysis of this gene should be also considered as a routine proceeding. Generally, *MECP2* mutations were identified in approximately 80% of Rett patients suggesting that the remaining 20% may have mutations in other unexplored regions of this gene, like the carboxy-terminal sequence or in other genes. In this context, mutations in *CDKL5* gene have been found in female patients with a phenotype overlapping with that of Rett syndrome (Scala *et al*, 2005). Mari and colleagues (2005) showed that *CDKL5* product is a nuclear putative kinase whose expression in the nervous system overlaps that of MeCP2, during neural maturation and synaptogenesis. Besides, they demonstrated that MeCP2 and CDKL5 proteins interact both *in vivo* and *in vitro* and that CDKL5 is able to phosphorylate itself and to mediate MeCP2 phosphorylation, suggesting that these two proteins belong to the same molecular pathway. After the association of *MECP2* to Rett syndrome, mutations in this gene were reported to cause a wide range of human neurodevelopmental disorders in both females and males, including, autism, syndromic and non-syndromic XLMR, Angelman syndrome phenotype, PPM-X syndrome and other psychiatric disorders (Amir *et al*, 1999, 2000; Lam *et al*, 2000; Meloni *et al*, 2000; Orrico *et al*, 2000; Watson *et al*, 2001; Dotti *et al*, 2002; Klauck *et al*, 2002; Carney *et al*, 2003; Kleefstra *et al*, 2004a).

Interestingly, a mild over-expression of MeCP2 in neurons is also detrimental and leads to symptoms of severe motor dysfunction and seizures, suggesting that a proper dosage of MeCP2 is critical for neuronal function and that levels of MeCP2 in the nervous system are tightly regulated (Collins *et al*, 2004). *MECP2* duplications were identified in a girl with the phenotype of Rett syndrome with preserved language (Ariani *et al*, 2004), a boy with severe MR and some clinical features of Rett syndrome (Meins *et al*, 2005), in individuals with severe MR and progressive spasticity (Van Esch *et al*, 2005) and in patients with NS-XLMR (Lugtenberg *et al*, 2006).

JARID1C

Jumonji AT-rich interactive domain 1C (*JARID1C/SMCX*) is a relatively new gene among the known XLMR causes. It encodes for a member of a recently discovered protein family that harbors conserved DNA-biding motifs, suggesting a potential role in transcriptional regulation and in the modification of chromatin structure. A predominant transcript was identified in many human adult tissues, but the strongest expression was observed in brain and skeletal muscle (Jensen *et al*, 2005). To date, thirteen *JARID1C* mutations were identified to be causative of XLMR (Jensen *et al*, 2005; Tzschach *et al*, 2006; Santos *et al*, 2006). The degree of MR in the affected males ranges from mild to severe, and some patients exhibited additional features, such as, epilepsy, short stature or behavioral problems. Furthermore, in some of the families analyzed, expression studies revealed the almost complete absence of the mutated *JARID1C* transcript, suggesting that the phenotype in these families resulted from functional loss of the JARID1C protein (Jensen *et al*, 2005). The frequency of mutations in the *JARID1C* gene was estimated to account for 2.8% to 3.3% of families with XLMR.

PQBP1

Like *JARID1C*, another gene involved in XLMR associated to microcephaly and short stature is *PQBP1* (polyglutamine binding protein 1), which maps on Xp11.23 and codes a nuclear polyglutamine-binding protein that contains a WW domain. This domain has been shown to play an important role in the regulation of transcription by interacting with the PPxY motif commonly found in transcription factors (Lubs *et al*, 2006). Recently, evidence indicated that *PQBP1* is expressed predominantly in the central nervous system during development and might be involved in neuronal proliferation and/or maturation (Qi *et al*, 2005). Mutations in *PQBP1* have been reported in a moderately retarded family (MRX55) without any other clinical signs, except for a somewhat smaller body size in one individual (Deqaqi *et al*, 1998). Later, *PQBP1* was linked to five syndromic XLMR disorders (Golabi-Ito-Hall, Renpenning, Hamel cerebro-palatocardiac, Sutherland-Haan, and Porteous syndromes) and to several small families with similar clinical findings (Cason *et al*, 2003; Kalscheuer *et al*, 2003a; Lenski *et al*, 2004; Kleefstra *et al*, 2004; Lubs *et al*, 2006). Although, *PQBP1* has been linked to S-XLMR, additional studies of *PQBP1* mutations among sporadic males with NS-XLMR are needed to re-evaluate the role of this gene in non-specific MR.

OPHN1

OPHN1 encodes oligophrenin-1, which is a Rho-GTPase-activating protein (rhoGAP) expressed at low levels in all tissues, but highly expressed in fetal brain (Billuart *et al*, 1998). *OPHN1* mutations were primarily described as been a exclusively cause of NS-XLMR (Billuart *et al*, 1998), but the re-evaluation of the affected individuals brains using neuroimaging displayed fronto-temporal atrophy with rostral enlargement of the lateral ventricles, lower vermian agenesis and asymmetric cerebellar hypoplasia (Bergmann *et al*, 2003; Philip *et al*, 2003; Des Portes *et al*, 2004). Reduced oligophrenin-1 levels affect spine length by increasing RhoA and Rho-kinase activities (Govek *et al*, 2004). Interestingly, it appears that oligophrenin-1 shares the same Rho signaling pathways with other genes involved in XLMR. *OPHN1*, *OCRL*-1 (involved in S-XLMR), *ARHGEF6* (involved in NS-XLMR) and *FGD1* (involved in both S-XLMR and NS-XLMR) act as regulators of the Rho GTPases, whereas *PAK3* (involved in NS-XLMR) and *FMR1* (involved in Fragile X syndrome) act as effectors of this pathway (Billuart *et al*, 2005). Rho GTPases are key signaling proteins that integrate extracellular and intracellular signals to orchestrate coordinated changes in the actin cytoskeleton essential for directed neurite outgrowth and the regulation of synaptic connectivity (Ramakers, 2002). The association between mutations in Rho-linked genes and XLMR highlights the importance of Rho proteins in neuronal function.

ATRX

Likewise *FMR1*, associated to Fragile X syndrome, the *ATRX* gene is another example of how abnormal epigenetic patterns can lead to a XLMR phenotype. The *ATRX* gene is located on Xq13, undergoes X inactivation and codes for a nuclear protein supposed to be involved in chromatin remodeling and regulation of protein/protein or protein/DNA interactions. ATRX protein is widely expressed during development (Stayton *et al*, 1994) and presents a PHD-like domain (plant homeodomain), which is encountered in many chromatin-associated proteins. Moreover, ATRX protein contains a carboxi-terminal domain, which identifies it as a member of the SNF2-like subgroup of a superfamily of ATPases and helicase (Picketts *et al*, 1996). Both major functional domains appear to act as chromatin remodellers (Gibbons *et al*, 2000). In humans, ATRX is associated to highly repetitive DNA (McDowell *et al*, 1999) and *ATRX* mutations cause aberrant methylation of several repeated sequences including the rDNA arrays, a Y-specific satellite and subtelomeric repeats (Gibbons *et al*, 2000). This evidence suggests that *ATRX* is involved in the regulation of repressed chromatin and explains the high level of clinical heterogeneity among the phenotypes resulting from *ATRX* mutations.

To date, 66 *ATRX* mutations have been reported so far, mainly (~76%) located in the PHD-like domain (Badens *et al*, 2006). These alterations were reported in a wide and clinically heterogeneous spectrum of XLMR syndromes, including the X-linked alpha-thalassemia/mental retardation syndrome (ATRX syndrome), Juberg-Marsidi syndrome, Sutherland-Haan syndrome and Smith-Fineman-Myers syndrome (Gibbons *et al*, 1995; Vilard *et al*, 1996, 2000; Lossi *et al*, 1999). Besides MR, other common phenotypes include absent speech, hypotonia, microcephaly, spasticity, or seizures and growth retardation with midface hypoplasia and skeletal abnormalities (Raymond, 2006). Only one family with a nonsense *ATRX* mutation and NS-XLMR was reported (Guerrini *et al*, 2000), but although the proband did not manifest the *ATRX*-related syndromic features, other affected members of this family exhibited them, pointing also to the existence of intrafamilial heterogeneity.

RPS6KA3

Ribosomal protein S6 kinase family is implicated in the activation of the mitogen-activated kinase cascade and the stimulation of cell proliferation and differentiation. *RPS6KA3* (ribosomal protein S6 kinase), also known as *RSK2*, encodes a growth-factor regulated protein kinase, though to be involved in the regulation of excitatory synaptic transmission (Thomas *et al*, 2005). Loss-of-function mutations in *RPS6KA3* are responsible for a syndromic MR, Coffin-Lowry syndrome (CLS) (Trivier *et al*, 1996). Affected males exhibit characteristic facial and digital abnormalities, psychomotor retardation, progressive skeletal deformations and generally severe mental handicap. Mutations associated to CLS are extremely heterogeneous and lead to premature stop codons and/or to loss of phosphotransferase activity. However, no correlation between the type and location of mutation and the clinical phenotype is evident (Jacquot *et al*, 2002). A single family was reported (MRX19), in which a *RPS6KA3* missense mutation was associated solely with mild MR and no other clinical features (Merienne *et al*, 1999). So, further *RPS6KA3* testing is required to elucidate the genotype/phenotype correlation between the mutation and this unusual clinical presentation.

Future Directions and Therapeutic Tools

Recent advances in genomic sequence annotation and the availability of large cohorts of MR families have enabled an exponentially characterization of functional XLMR candidate genes. Large-scale mutational screening of mentally retarded individuals by high throughput molecular methods as high-resolution comparative genomic hybridization (Ishkanian *et al*, 2004) has provided a genome-wide detection of innumerous submicroscopic deletions and duplications. For NS-XLMR families that are too small for linkage analysis, Jensen LR, Chen W, Ropers HH and Kuss AW (*apud* Ropers, 2006) developed an oligonucleotide chip as a diagnostic tool. Moreover, after the observation that nerve cells in the central nervous system interact with a high plasticity, new therapeutic possibilities emerged for treat MR even after birth (Bonhoeffer and Yuste, 2002; Jin and Warren, 2003; McBride *et al*, 2005). In this context, once again Fragile X syndrome appears as a central role in XLMR. Since loss of FMRP protein leads to overexpression of group I metabotropic glutamate receptors (mGluRs), and subsequently, long-term depression, altered synaptic plasticity and dysgenesis of dendritic spines (Huber *et al*, 2002; Jin and Warren, 2003), antagonists of mGluRs has being successfully used in a Drosophila model for Fragile X syndrome, restoring short-term memory and central nervous defects. Thus, most human genes implicated in MR have orthologues in Drosophila, making it an ideal model organism for studying new therapeutic treatments for XLMR (Inlow and Restifo, 2004). Moreover, treatment of *FMR1*-methylated fragile X cell lines with 5-aza-2-deoxycytidine induced a decrease of H3-K9 methylation, an increase of H3 and H4 acetylation and an increase of H3-K4 methylation, resulting in *FMR1* transcriptional reactivation (Tabolacci *et al*, 2005). On the other hand, several studies have shown that DNA methylation is essential for normal function and development of neurons in the brain (Fan *et al*, 2001; Takizawa *et al*, 2001). In this way, since it should be considered that, in theory, it is probably easier to treat an epigenetic disease than a DNA sequence mutation disorder, epigenetic therapy might be also a good strategy for treating females bearing X-linked dominant disorders, like Rett syndrome and others chromatin remodeling disorders. As X-inactivation is random, 50% of the Rett females' cells harbour an unused but intact copy of the gene, which can be reactivated, ameliorating the clinical phenotype of the disorder (Egger *et al*, 2004).

Conclusion

Because of the haploid status of most genes on the X chromosome in males, they are ~1,4-fold more likely to have severe MR and, perhaps as much as 1,9-fold more likely to have mild MR than females (Leonard and Wen, 2002). By many years, this well-documented disproportional ratio was attributed solely to the presence of XLMR genes. However, although it is likely that the prevalence of mutations in XLMR genes could be higher, since several of them have been identified so recently and have still not been screened in large cohorts, some recent research demonstrated that the cumulative frequency of monogenic XLMR might not exceed 10% (Mandel and Chelly, 2004). Thus, X-linked recessive forms of MR could explain, in part the skewed male-female ratio. Besides, hormonal effects and distinct sex-specific gene-dosage might also be responsible for such excess. The dissimilarity in sex chromosome size is accompanied by substantial disparity in gene content (X chromosome codes for more than 800 proteins versus ~60 from Y), as a consequence of their different molecular evolution. As many as 20% of the genes on X chromosome, mainly located on the short arm (Xp), escape from inactivation and for most of these, there is no functionally equivalent homologue on the Y chromosome (Carrel *et al*, 1999; Brown and Greally, 2003). Evidence has demonstrated yet that some X-linked genes have different expression levels, depending if they are present in male or in female brains. In mice, six X-linked genes (Usp9x, Ube1x, Smcx, Eif2s3x, Utx and Dbs), orthologues of human X-chromosome, were significantly highly expressed in the brain of adulthood females than males, irrespective of their X-inactivation status (Xu and Burgoyne, 2002). Interestingly, three of them, that have homologues in both X and Y chromosomes (Usp9x/y, Ube1x/y and Eif2s3x/y), may have acquired different functions in the two genders. Therefore, there is not yet a plausible answer to explain why mild MR is apparently more associated to X-linked genes than severe MR. One hypothesis is the possible existence of X chromosome polymorphisms that lower IQ, but are not sufficient to cause MR, acting as X-linked genes modifiers of the intelligence (Mandel and Chelly, 2004).

One should keep in mind that although mutation screening research has so far been confined to chromosome X coding regions, it is becoming more and more clear that microRNAs, frequently located at intronic and intergenic regions (Ying and Lin, 2006), could be potentially related to MR. Among other biological and essential functions, miRNAs have been considered as regulators of neuronal gene expression and mediators of neuronal identity (Krichevsky *et al*, 2003). Many miRNAs have been isolated from mammalian embryonic neurons and mature brain, and some of them are neuronal-specific (Lagos-Quintana *et al*, 2002; Dostie *et al*, 2003; Krichevsky *et al*, 2003; Frederikse *et al*, 2006). Recently, Schratt and colleagues (2006) showed that a miRNA, named miR-134, has the capacity of inhibit the translation of Lim-domain-containing protein kinase 1 (limK1), which controls spine development. Using brain-derived neurotrophic factor (BDNF) for neuronal stimulation they relieved the inhibition and enabled the dendritic spine growth.

In XLMR, the role of miRNAs is more prominent. Besides the involvement of miRNAs with fragile mental retardation protein, to date, from the 462 Homo sapiens miRNAs sequences described in the MirBase, more than 10% are located in the X chromosome and are potential candidates to be involved in XLMR. Chen and colleagues (unpublished – *apud* Ropers, 2006) screened 13 brain-expressed X-linked miRNA genes in 400 families with a minimum of two mental handicapped males and found three variants not presented among the control healthy sample. Considering that multiple miRNAs can be generated from the same cluster and that each miRNA could regulates the expression of about 200 genes, certainly, prediction of other XLMR microRNAs using computer programming are needed to bring new insights on the mechanisms by which miRNAs are involved in cognitive functions.

Proper functioning of the nervous system requires high precision and the identification of further XLMR genes promises to be a significant contribution to the understanding of brain functions. Until all the XLMR genes already identified and still ignored have been screened in large sample cohorts, the importance and mutations prevalence of each XLMR gene will remain unknown. The future challenge is to provide cost-effective, accurate and rapid methods for detection of X-linked mutations in families with MR.

REFERENCES

Allen, KM; Gleeson, JG; Bagrodia, S; *et al.* PAK3 mutation in nonsyndromic X-linked mental retardation. *Nat Genet,* 1998, 20, 25-30.

Amir, RE; Van den Veyver, IB; Wan, M; *et al.* Rett syndrome is caused by mutations in X-linked MECP2, encoding methyl-CpG-binding protein 2. *Nat Genet,* 1999, 23, 185-188.

Amir RE, Zoghbi HY. Rett syndrome, methyl-CpG-binding protein 2 mutations and phenotype-genotype correlations. *Am J Med Genet,* 2000, 97, 147-152.

Annesi, G; Nicoletti, G; Tarantino, P; *et al.* FRAXE intermediate alleles are associated with Parkinson's disease. *Neurosci Lett,* 2004, 368, 21-24.

Ariani, F; Mari, F; Pescucci, C; *et al.* Real-time quantitative PCR as a routine method for screening large rearrangements in Rett syndrome, Report of one case of MECP2 deletion and one case of MECP2 duplication. *Hum Mutat,* 2004, 24, 172-177.

Badens, C; Lacoste, C; Philip, N; *et al.* Mutations in PHD-like domain of the ATRX gene correlate with severe psychomotor impairment and severe urogenital abnormalities in patients with ATRX syndrome. *Clin Genet,* 2006, 70, 57-62.

Bahi, N; Friocourt, G; Carrie, A; *et al.* IL1 receptor accessory protein like, a protein involved in X-linked mental retardation, interacts with neuronal calcium sensor-1 and regulates exocytosis. *Hum Molec Genet,* 2003, 12, 1415-1425.

Ballestar, E; Ropero, S; Alaminos, M; *et al.* The impact of MECP2 mutations in the expression patterns of Rett syndrome patients. *Hum Genet,* 2005,116, 91-104.

Barros Santos, C; Gonçalves Pimentel, MM. The influence of expanded unmethylated alleles for FRAXA/FRAXE loci in the intellectual performance among Brazilian mentally impaired males. *Int J Mol Medicine,* 2003, 12, 385-389.

Bear, MF, Huber, KM; Warren, ST. The mGluR theory of fragile X mental retardation. *Trends Neurosci,* 2004, 27, 370-377.

Bejerano, G; Pheasant, M; Makunin, I; *et al.* Ultraconserved elements in the human genome *Science*, 2004, 304, 1321-1325.

Bergmann, C; Zerres, K; Senderek, J; *et al.* Oligophrenin 1 (OPHN1) gene mutation causes syndromic X-linked mental retardation with epilepsy, rostral ventricular enlargement and cerebellar hypoplasia. *Brain*, 2003, 126, 1537-1544.

Bienvenu, T.; des Portes, V.; Saint Martin, A.; *et al.* Non-specific X-linked semidominant mental retardation by mutations in a Rab GDP-dissociation inhibitor. *Hum Molec Genet,* 1998, 7, 1311-1315.

Bienvenu, T; Poirier, K; Friocourt, G; *et al.* ARX, a novel Prd-class-homeobox gene highly expressed in the telencephalon, is mutated in X-linked mental retardation. *Hum Mol Genet*, 2002, 11, 981–991.

Billuart, P; Bienvenu, T; Ronce, N; *et al.* Oligophrenin 1 encodes a rho-GAP protein involved in X-linked mental retardation. *Pathol Biol (Paris),* 1998, 46, 678.

Billuart, P; Chelly, J; Gilgenkrantz, S. X-linked mental retardation. *Med Sci (Paris),* 2005, 21, 947-953.

Bizzi, A; Bugiani, M.; Salomons, GS; *et al.* X-linked creatine deficiency syndrome: a novel mutation in creatine transporter gene SLC6A8. *Ann Neurol,* 2002, 52, 227-231.

Blasi, F; Bacchelli, E; Pesaresi, G; *et al.* Absence of coding mutations in the X-linked genes neuroligin 3 and neuroligin 4 in individuals with autism from the IMGSAC collection. *Am J Med Genet B Neuropsychiatr Genet,* 2006,141, 220-221.

Bonhoeffer, T; Yuste R. Spine motility. Phenomenology, mechanisms, and function. *Neuron,* 2002, 35, 1019-1027.

Brown, CJ; Greally, JM. A stain upon the silence: genes escaping X inactivation. *Trends Genet,* 2003, 19, 432-438.

Brown, V; Jin, P; Ceman, S; *et al.* Microarray identification of FMRP-associated brain mRNAs and altered mRNA translational profiles in fragile X syndrome. *Cell,* 2001, 107, 477-487.

Brown, TC; Tarleton, JC; Go, RCP; *et al.* Instability of the FMR2 trinucleotide repeat region associated with expanded FMR1 alleles. *Am J Med Genet,* 1997, 73, 447-455.

Carney, RM; Wolpert, CM; Ravan, SA; *et al.* Identification of MeCP2 mutations in a series of females with autistic disorder. *Pediatr Neurol,* 2003, 28, 205-211.

Carrel, L; Cottle, AA; Goglin, KC; Willard, H. A first-generation X-inactivation profile of the human X chromosome. *Proc Natl Acad Sci USA*, 1999, 96, 14440-14444.

Carrie, A; Jun, L; Bienvenu, T; *et al.* A new member of the IL-1 receptor family highly expressed in hippocampus and involved in X-linked mental retardation. *Nat Genet,* 1999, 23, 25-31.

Cason, AL; Ikeguchi, Y; Skinner, C; *et al.* X-linked spermine synthase gene (SMS) defect: the first polyamine deficiency syndrome. *Eur J Hum Genet,* 2003, 11, 937–977.

Chelly, J. Breakthroughs in molecular and cellular mechanisms underlying X-linked mental retardation. *Hum Mol Genet,* 1999, 8, 1833-1838.

Christodoulou, J; Grimm, A; Maher, T; Bennetts, B. RettBASE: The IRSA MECP2 variation database-a new mutation database in evolution. *Hum Mutat,* 2003, 21, 466-472.

Clark, AJ; Rosenberg, EH; Almeida, LS; *et al.* X-linked creatine transporter (SLC6A8) mutations in about 1% of males with mental retardation of unknown etiology. *Hum Genet,* 2006, 119, 604-610.

Collins, AL; Levenson, JM; Vilaythong, AP; *et al.* Mild overexpression of MeCP2 causes a progressive neurological disorder in mice. *Hum Mol Genet,* 2004, 13, 2679-2689.

Collombat, P; Hecksher-Sorensen, J; Broccoli, V; *et al.* The simultaneous loss of Arx and Pax4 genes promotes a somatostatin-producing cell fate specification at the expense of the alpha- and beta-cell lineages in the mouse endocrine pancreas. *Development*, 2005, 132, 2969-2980.

Collombat, P; Mansouri, A; Hecksher-Sorensen, J; *et al.* Opposing actions of Arx and Pax4 in endocrine pancreas development. *Genes Dev,* 2003, 17, 2591-2603.

Crawford, DC; Meadows, KL; Newman, JL; *et al.* Prevalence and phenotype consequence of FRAXA and FRAXE alleles in a large, ethnically diverse, special education-needs population. *Am J Hum Genet,* 1999, 64, 495-507.

Cutter, WJ; Daly, EM; Robertson, DM; *et al.* Influence of X chromosome and hormones on human brain development: a magnetic resonance imaging and proton magnetic resonance spectroscopy study of Turner syndrome. *Biol Psychiatry,* 2006, 59, 273-83.

D'Adamo, P; Menegon, A; Lo Nigro, C; *et al.* Mutations in GDI1 are responsible for X-linked non-specific mental retardation. Mutations in GDI1 are responsible for X-linked non-specific mental retardation. *Nat Genet,* 1998, 19, 134–139.

D'Adamo, P; Welzl, H; Papadimitriou, S; *et al.* Deletion of the mental retardation gene Gdi1 impairs associative memory and alters social behavior in mice. *Hum Mol Genet,* 2002, 11, 2567-2580.

Darnell, JC; Fraser, CE; Mostovetsky, O; *et al.* Kissing complex RNAs mediate interaction between the Fragile-X mental retardation protein KH2 domain and brain polyribosomes. *Genes Dev,* 2005, 19, 903-918.

Darnell, JC; Jensen, KB; Jin, P; *et al.* Fragile X mental retardation protein targets G quartet mRNAs important for neuronal function. *Cell,* 2001, 107, 489-499.

Deqaqi, SC; N'Guessan, M; Forner, J; *et al.* A gene for non-specific X-linked mental retardation (MRX55) is located in Xp11. *Ann Genet,* 1998, 41, 11-16.

Des Portes, V; Boddaert, N; Sacco, S; *et al.* Specific clinical and brain MRI features in mentally retarded patients with mutations in the Oligophrenin-1 gene. *Am J Med Genet,* 2004, 124A, 364-371.

Dotti, MT; Orrico, A; De Stefano, N; *et al.* A Rett syndrome MECP2 mutation that causes mental retardation in men. *Neurology,* 2002, 58, 226-230.

Dostie, J; Mourelatos, Z; Yang, M; *et al.* Numerous microRNPs in neuronal cells containing novel microRNAs. *RNA*, 2003, 9, 180-186.

Dumitrescu, AM; Liao, XH; Best, TB; *et al.* A novel syndrome combining thyroid and neurological abnormalities is associated with mutations in a monocarboxylate transporter gene. *Am J Hum Genet,* 2004, 74, 168-175.

Egger, G; Liang, G; Aparicio, A; Jones PA. Epigenetics in human disease and prospects for epigenetic therapy. *Nature*, 2004, 429, 457-463.

Fan, G; Beard, C; Chen, RZ; *et al.* DNA hypomethylation perturbs the function and survival of CNS neurons in postnatal animals. *J Neurosci,* 2001, 21, 788-797.

Feng, Y; Absher, D, Eberhart, DE, *et al.* FMRP associates with polyribosomes as an mRNP, and the I304N mutation of severe fragile X syndrome abolishes this association. *Mol Cell,* 1997, 1, 109-118.

Finckh, U; Schroder, J; Ressler, B; *et al.* Spectrum and detection rate of L1CAM mutations in isolated and familial cases with clinically suspected L1-disease. *Am J Med Genet*, 2000, 92, 40–46.

Fishburn, J; Turner, G; Daniel, A; Brookwell, R. The diagnosis and frequency of X-linked conditions in a cohort of moderately retarded males with affected brothers. *Am J Med Genet,* 1983, 14, 713-724.

Flint, J; Knight, S. The use of telomere probes to investigate submicroscopic rearrangements associated with mental retardation. *Curr Opin Genet Dev,* 2003, 13, 310-316.

Fransen, E; Van Camp, G; Vits, L; Willems PJ. L1-associated diseases: clinical geneticists divide, molecular geneticists unite. *Hum Mol Genet,* 1997, 6, 1625-1632.

Frederikse, PH; Donnelly, R; Partyka, LM. miRNA and Dicer in the mammalian lens: expression of brain-specific miRNAs in the lens. *Histochem Cell Biol,* 2006, 126, 1-8.

Free, A; Wakefield, RI; Smith, BO; *et al.* DNA recognition by the methyl-CpG binding domain of MeCP2. *J Bio Chem,* 2001, 276, 3353-3360.

Freude, K; Hoffmann, K; Jensen, LR; *et al.* Mutations in the FTSJ1 gene coding for a novel S-adenosylmethionine-binding protein cause nonsyndromic X-linked mental retardation. *Am J Hum Genet,* 2004, 75, 305-309.

Friesema, ECH; Ganguly, S; Abdalla, A; *et al.* Identification of monocarboxylate transporter 8 as a specific thyroid hormone transporter. *J Biol Chem,* 2003, 278, 40128-40135.

Fukami, M; Kirsch, S; Schiller, S; *et al.* A member of a gene family on Xp22.3, VCX-A, is deleted in patients with X-linked nonspecific mental retardation. *Am J Hum Genet,* 2000, 67, 563-573.

Garber, K; Smith, KT; Reines, D; Warren, ST. Transcription, translation and fragile X syndrome. *Curr Opin Genet Dev,* 2006, 16, 270-275.

Gecz, J. The FMR2 gene, FRAXE and non-specific X-linked mental retardation: clinical and molecular aspects. *Ann. Hum Genet,* 2000, 64, 95–106.

Gecz, J. FMR3 is a novel gene associated with FRAXE CpG island and transcriptionally silent in FRAXE full mutations. *J. Med. Genet,* 2000a, 37, 782–784.

Gecz, J; Cloosterman, D; Partington, M. ARX: a gene for all seasons. *Curr Opin Genet Dev,* 2006, 16, 308-316.

Gecz, J; Gedeon, AK; Sutherland, GR; Mulley, JC. Identification of the gene FMR2, associated with FRAXE mental retardation. *Nat Genet,* 1996, 13, 105-118.

Genç, B; Muller-Hartmann, H; Zeschnigk, M; *et al.* Methylation mosaicism of 5'-(CGG)(n)-3' repeats in fragile X, premutation and normal individuals. *Nucleic Acids Res,* 2000, 28, 2141-2152.

Gestinari-Duarte, RS; Santos-Rebouças, CB; Pimentel, MMG. Mutational screening of ARX gene in Brazilian males with mental retardation of unknown etiology. *J Hum Genet,* 2006, 51, 737-740.

Gibbons, RJ; McDowell, TL; Raman, S; *et al.* Mutations in ATRX, encoding a SWI/SNF-like protein, cause diverse changes in the pattern of DNA methylation. *Nat Genet,* 2000, 24, 368-371.

Gibbons, RJ; Picketts, DJ; Villard, L; Higgs, DR. Mutations in a putative global transcriptional regulator cause X-linked mental retardation with alpha-thalassemia (ATR-X syndrome). *Cell,* 1995, 80, 837-845.

Govek, EE; Newey, SE; Akerman, CJ; *et al.* The X-linked mental retardation protein oligophrenin-1 is required for dendritic spine morphogenesis. *Nat Neurosci,* 2004, 7, 364-372.

Graves, JA; Koina, E; Sankovic N. How the gene content of human sex chromosomes evolved. *Curr Opin Genet Dev,* 2006, 16, 219-224.

Greenwood Genetic Center, 2006 (accessed on October, 2006). Available from http://www.ggc.org/xlmr.htm.

Gu, Y; Nelson, DL. FMR2 function: insight from a mouse knockout model. *Cytogenet Genome Res, 2003*, 100, 129-139.

Guerrini, R; Shanahan, JL; Carrozzo, R; *et al.* A nonsense mutation of the ATRX gene causing mild mental retardation and epilepsy. *Ann Neurol,* 2000, 47, 117-121.

Hagberg, B; Aicardi, J; Dias, K; Ramos, O. A progressive syndrome of autism, dementia, ataxia, and loss of purposeful hand use in girls: Rett's syndrome: report of 35 cases. *Ann. Neurol,* 1983, 14, 471-479.

Hahn, KA; Salomons, GS; Tackels-Horne, D; *et al.* X-linked mental retardation with seizures and carrier manifestations is caused by a mutation in the creatine-transporter gene (SLC6A8) located in Xq28. *Am J Hum Genet,* 2002, 70, 1349-1356.

Handa, V; Saha, T; Usdin, K. The fragile X syndrome repeats form RNA hairpins that do not activate the interferon-inducible protein kinase, PKR, but are cut by Dicer. *Nucleic Acids Res,* 2003, 31, 6243-6248.

Harsha, HC; Suresh S; Amanchy, R *et al.* A manually curated functional annotation of the human X chromosome. *Nat Genet,* 2005, 37, 331-332.

Herbst DS; Miller JR. Nonspecific X-linked mental retardation II: the frequency in British Columbia. *Am J Med Genet,* 1980, 7, 461–469.

Heuer, H; Maier, MK; Iden, S; *et al.* The monocarboxylate transporter 8 linked to human psychomotor retardation is highly expressed in thyroid hormone sensitive neuron populations. *Endocrinology,* 2005, 46, 1701–1706.

Huber, K; Gallagher, SM; Warren, ST; Bear, MF. Altered synaptic plasticity in a mouse model of fragile X mental retardation. *Proc Natl Acd Sci USA,* 2002, 99, 7746-7750.

Inlow, JK; Restifo, LL. Molecular and comparative genetics of mental retardation. *Genetics,* 2004, 16, 835-881.

Irwin, SA; Galvez, R; Greenough, WT. Dendritic spine structural anomalies in fragile-X mental retardation syndrome. *Cereb Cortex,* 2000, 10, 1038-1044.

Ishkanian, AS; Malloff, CA; Watson, SK; *et al.* A tiling resolution DNA microarray with complete coverage of the human genome. *Nature Genet,* 2004, 36, 299-303.

Jacquot, S; Zeniou, M; Touraine, R; Hanauer, A. X-linked Coffin-Lowry syndrome (CLS, MIM 303600, RPS6KA3 gene, protein product known under various names: pp90(rsk2), RSK2, ISPK, MAPKAP1). *Eur J Hum Genet,* 2002, 10, 2-5.

Jamain, S; Quach, H; Betancur, C; *et al.* Mutations of the X-linked genes encoding neuroligins NLGN3 and NLGN4 are associated with autism. *Nat Genet,* 2003, 34, 27-29.

Jensen, LR; Amende, M; Gurok, U; *et al.* Mutations in the JARID1C gene, which is involved in transcriptional regulation and chromatin remodeling, cause X-linked mental retardation. *Am J Hum Genet,* 2005, 76, 227-236.

Jin, P; Alisch, RS; Warren, ST. RNA and microRNAs in fragile X mental retardation. *Nat Cell Biol,* 2004, 6, 1048-1053.

Jin, P; Warren, ST. New insights into fragile X syndrome: from molecules to neurobehaviors. *Trends Biochem Sci,* 2003, 28, 152-158.

Jin, P; Zarnescu, DC; Ceman, S; *et al.* Biochemical and genetic interaction between the fragile X mental retardation protein and the microRNA pathway. *Nat Neurosci,* 2004a, 7, 113-117.

Jones, PL; Veenstra, GJ; Wade, PA. Methylated DNA and MeCP2 recruit histone deacetylase to repress transcription. *Nat Genet,* 1998, 19, 187–191.

Kalscheuer, VM; Freude, K; Musante, L; *et al.* Mutations in the polyglutamine-binding protein 1 gene cause X- linked mental retardation. *Nat Genet,* 2003a, 35, 313–315.

Kalscheuer, VM; Tao, J; Donnelly, A; *et al.* Disruption of the serine/threonine kinase 9 gene causes severe X-linked infantile spasms and mental retardation. *Am J Hum Genet,* 2003, 72, 1401–1411.

Kato, M; Das, S; Petras, K; *et al.* Polyalanine expansion of ARX associated with cryptogenic West syndrome. *Neurology,* 2003, 61, 267-276.

Kenwrick, S.; Watkins, A.; De Angelis, E. Neural cell recognition molecule L1: relating biological complexity to human disease mutations. *Hum Molec Genet,* 2000, 9, 879-886.

Kesler, SR; Blasey, CM; Brown,WE; *et al.* Effects of X-monosomy and X-linked imprinting on superior temporal gyrus morphology in Turner syndrome. *Biol Psychiatry,* 2003, 54, 636-646.

Kitamura, K; Yanazawa, M; Sugiyama, N; *et al.* Mutation of ARX causes abnormal development of forebrain and testes in mice and X-linked lissencephaly with abnormal genitalia in humans. *Nat Genet,* 2002, 32, 359–369.

Klauck, SM; Lindsay, S; Beyer, KS; *et al.* A mutation hot spot for nonspecific X-linked mental retardation in the MECP2 gene causes the PPM-X syndrome. *Am J Hum Genet,* 2002, 70, 1034-1037.

Kleefstra, T; Franken, CE; Arens, YH; *et al.* Genotype-phenotype studies in three families with mutations in the polyglutamine-binding protein 1 gene (PQBP1). *Clin Genet,* 2004, 66, 318–326.

Kleefstra, T; Yntema, HG; Nillesen, WM; *et al.* MECP2 analysis in mentally retarded patients: implications for routine DNA diagnostics. *Eur J Hum Genet,* 2004a,12, 24-28.

Kleefstra, T; Yntema, HG; Oudakker, AR; *et al.* Zinc finger 81 (ZNF81) mutations associated with X-linked mental retardation. *J Med Genet,* 2004b, 41, 394-399.

Koolen, DA; Nillesen, WM; Versteeg, MH; *et al.* Screening for subtelomeric rearrangements in 210 patients with unexplained mental retardation using multiplex ligation dependent probe amplification (MLPA). *J Med Genet,* 2004, 41, 892-899.

Kriaucionis, S; Bird, A. The major form of MeCP2 has a novel N-terminus generated by alternative splicing. *Nucleic Acids Res,* 2004, 32, 1818-1823.

Krichevsky, A; King, K; Donahue, C; *et al.* A microRNA array reveals extensive regulation of microRNAs during brain development. *RNA*, 2003, 9, 1274-1281.

Laggerbauer, B; Ostareck, D; Keidel, EM; *et al.* Evidence that fragile X mental retardation protein is a negative regulator of translation. *Hum Mol Genet,* 2001, 10, 329-338.

Lagos-Quintana, M; Rauhut, R; Yalcin, A; *et al.* Identification of tissue-specific microRNAs from mouse. *Curr Biol,* 2002, 12, 735-739.

Lam, CW; Yeung, WL; Ko, CH; *et al.* Spectrum of mutations in the MECP2 gene in patients with infantile autism and Rett syndrome. *J Med Genet,* 2000, 37, E41.

Laumonnier, F; Bonnet-Brilhault, F; Gomot, M; *et al.* X-linked mental retardation and autism are associated with a mutation in the NLGN4 gene, a member of the neuroligin family. *Am J Hum Genet,* 2004, 74, 552-557.

Lebel, RR; May, M; Pouls, S; *et al.* Non-syndromic X-linked mental retardation associated with a missense mutation (P312L) in the FGD1 gene. *Clin Genet,* 2002, 61, 139-145.

Lee, SS; Wan, M; Francke, U. Spectrum of MECP2 mutations in Rett syndrome. *Brain Dev,* 2001, 23 Suppl 1, S138-143.

Lenski, C; Abidi, F; Meindl, A; *et al.* Novel truncating mutations in the polyglutamine tract binding protein 1 gene (PQBP1) cause Renpenning syndrome and X-linked mental retardation in another family with microcephaly. *Am J Hum Genet,* 2004, 74, 777–780.

Leonard, H; Wen, X. The epidemiology of mental retardation: challenges and opportunities in the new millennium. *Ment Retard Dev Disabil Res Rev,* 2002, 8, 117-134.

Li, Z; Zhang, Y; Ku, L; *et al.* The fragile X mental retardation protein inhibits translation via interacting with mRNA. *Nucleic Acids Res,* 2001, 29, 2276-2283.

Lossi, AM; Laugier-Anfossi, F; Depetris, D; *et al.* Abnormal expression of the KLF8 (ZNF741) gene in a female patient with an X;autosome translocation t(X;21)(p11.2;q22.3) and non-syndromic mental retardation. *J Med Genet,* 2002, 39, 113-117.

Lossi, AM; Millan, JM; Villard, L; *et al.* Mutation of the XNP/ATR-X gene in a family with severe mental retardation, spastic paraplegia and skewed pattern of X inactivation:

demonstration that the mutation is involved in the inactivation bias. *Am J Hum Genet,* 1999, 65, 558-562.

Lubs HA. The other side of the coin: a hypothesis concerning the importance of genes for high intelligence and evolution of the X chromosome. *Am J Med Genet,* 1999, 85, 206–208.

Lubs, H; Abidi, FE; Echeverri, R; *et al.* Golabi-Ito-Hal syndrome results rom a missense mutation in the WW domain of the PQBP1 gene. *J Med Genet,* 2006, 43, e30.

Lugtenberg D; de Brouwer, AP; Kleefstra, T; *et al.* Chromosomal copy number changes in patients with non-syndromic X linked mental retardation detected by array CGH. *J Med Genet,* 2006, 43, 362-370.

Lugtenberg, D; Yntema, HG; Banning, MJ; *et al.* ZNF674: A New Kruppel-Associated Box-Containing Zinc-Finger Gene Involved in Nonsyndromic X-Linked Mental Retardation. *Am J Hum Genet,* 2006a, 78, 265-278.

McBride, SMJ; Choi, CH; Wang, Y; *et al.* Pharmacological rescue of synaptic plasticity, courtship behavior, and mushroom body defects in a Drosophila model of fragile X syndrome. *Neuron*, 2005, 45, 753-764.

McDowell, TL; Gibbons, RJ; Sutherland, H; *et al.* Localization of a putative transcriptional regulator (ATRX) at pericentromeric heterochromatin and the short arms of acrocentric chromosomes. *Proc Natl Acad Sci USA,* 1999, 96, 13983-13988.

Makino, K; Kuwahara, H; Masuko, N; *et al.* Cloning and characterization of NE-dlg: a novel human homolog of the Drosophila discs large (dlg) tumor suppressor protein interacts with the APC protein. *Oncogene*, 1997, 14, 2425–2433.

Mandel, JL; Chelly, J. Monogenic X-linked mental retardation: is it as frequent as currently estimated? The paradox of the ARX (Aristaless X) mutations. *Eur J Hum Genet,* 2004, 12, 689-693.

Mansouri, MR; Marklund, L; Gustavsson, P; *et al.* Loss of ZDHHC15 expression in a woman with a balanced translocation t(X;15)(q13.3;cen) and severe mental retardation. *Eur J Hum Genet,* 2005,13, 970-977.

Maranduba, CMC; Friesema, ECH; Kok, F; *et al.* Decreased cellular uptake and metabolism in Allan-Herndon-Dudley syndrome (AHDS) due to a novel mutation in the MCT8 thyroid hormone transporter. *J Med Genet,* 2006, 43, 457-460.

Marco, EJ; Bristow, J; Cotter, PD; *et al.* ARHGEF9: an "X" cellent mental retardation candidate gene (abstract). In 55th American Society of Human Genetics Meeting, 2241/T; Salt Lake City: 2005, 406.

Mari, F; Azimonti, S; Bertani, I; *et al.* CDKL5 belongs to the same molecular pathway of MeCP2 and it is responsible for the early-onset seizure variant of Rett syndrome. *Hum Mol Genet,* 2005, 14, 1935–1946.

Martinowich, K; Hattori, D; Wu, H; *et al.* DNA methylation-related chromatin remodeling in activity-dependent BDNF gene regulation. *Science*, 2003, 302, 890-893.

Mattson, MP. Methylation and acetylation in nervous system development and neurodegenerative disorders. *Ageing Res Rev,* 2003, 2, 329-342.

Mazzocco, MM; Sonna, NL; Teis, JT; *et al.* The FMR1 and FMR2 mutations are not common etiologies of academic difficulty among school-age children. *J Dev Behav Pediatr,* 1997, 18, 392-398.

Meins, M; Lehmann, J; Gerresheim, F; *et al.* Submicroscopic duplication in Xq28 causes increased expression of the MECP2 gene in a boy with severe mental retardation and features of Rett syndrome. *J Med Genet,* 2005, 42, e12.

Meloni, I; Bruttini, M; Longo, I; *et al.* A mutation in the rett syndrome gene, MECP2, causes X-linked mental retardation and progressive spasticity in males. *Am J Hum Genet,* 2000, 67, 982-985.

Meloni, I; Muscettola, M; Raynaud, M; *et al.* FACL4, encoding fatty acid-CoA ligase 4, is mutated in nonspecific X-linked mental retardation. *Nat Genet,* 2002, 30, 436-440.

Merienne, K; Jacquot, S; Pannetier, S; *et al.* A missense mutation in RPS6KA3 (RSK2) responsible for non-specific mental retardation. *Nat Genet,* 1999, 22, 13-14.

MiRBase: the home of microRNA data, 2006 (accessed on October, 2006). Available from http://microRNA.sanger.ac.uk.

Mnatzakanian, GN; Lohi, H; Munteanu, I; *et al.* A previously unidentified MECP2 open reading frame defines a new protein isoform relevant to Rett syndrome. *Nat Genet,* 2004, 36, 339-341.

Moretti, P; Zoghbi, HY. MeCP2 dysfunction in Rett syndrome and related disorders. *Curr Opin Genet Dev,* 2006, 16, 276-281.

Mornet, E; Chateau, C; Simon-Bouy, B; Serre, JL. The intermediate alleles of the fragile X CGG repeat in patients with mental retardation. *Clin Genet,* 1998, 53, 200-201.

Muller, BM; Kistner, U; Kindler, S; *et al.* SAP102, a novel postsynaptic protein that interacts with NMDA receptor complexes in vivo. *Neuron*, 1996, 17, 255–265.

Murray, A; Macpherson, JN; Pound, M; *et al.* The role of size, sequence and haplotype in the stability of FRAXA and FRAXE alleles during transmission. *Hum Mol Genet,* 1997, 6, 173-184.

Murray, A; Youings, S; Dennis, N; *et al.* Population screening at the FRAXA and FRAXE loci: molecular analyses of boys with learning difficulties and their mothers. *Hum Mol Genet*, 1996, 5, 727-735.

Nan, X; Campoy, FJ; Bird, A. MeCP2 is a transcriptional repressor with abundant binding sites in genomic chromatin. *Cell,* 1997, 88, 471-481.

Nan, X; Ng, HH; Johnson, CA; *et al.* Transcriptional repression by the methyl-CpG-binding protein MeCP2 involves a histone deacetylase complex. *Nature*, 1998, 393, 386–389.

Nguyen, DK; Disteche, CM. Dosage compensation of the active X chromosome in mammals. *Nat Genet,* 2006, 38, 47-53.

Novick, P; Zerial, M. The diversity of Rab proteins in vesicle transport. *Curr Opin Cell Biol,* 1997, 9, 496–504.

O'Donnell, WT; Warren, ST. A decade of molecular studies of fragile X syndrome. *Annu Rev Neurosci,* 2002, 25, 315-338.

Ohira, R; Zhang, YH; Guo, W; *et al.* Human ARX gene: genomic characterization and expression. *Mol Genet Metab,* 2002, 77, 179–188.

Orrico, A; Galli, L; Cavaliere, ML; *et al.* Phenotypic and molecular characterisation of the Aarskog-Scott syndrome: a survey of the clinical variability in light of FGD1 mutation analysis in 46 patients. *Eur J Hum Genet,* 2004, 12, 16-23.

Orrico, A; Lam, C; Galli, L; *et al.* MECP2 mutation in male patients with non-specific X-linked mental retardation. *FEBS Lett,* 2000, 481, 285-288.

Panayi, M; Gokhale, D; Mansour, S; Elles R. Prenatal diagnosis in a family with X-linked hydrocephalus.*Prenat Diagn,* 2005, 25, 930-933.

Partington, MW; Turner, G; Boyle, J; Gecz, J. Three new families with X-linked mental retardation caused by the 428-451dup(24bp) mutation in ARX. *Clin Genet,* 2004, 66, 39-45.

Patsalis, PC; Sismani, C; Hettinger, JA; *et al.* Molecular screening of fragile X (FRAXA) and FRAXE mental retardation syndromes in the Hellenic population of Greece and Cyprus: incidence, genetic variation, and stability. *Am J Med Genet,* 1999, 84, 184-190.

Pearson, CE; Nichol Edamura, K; Cleary, JD. Repeat instability: mechanisms of dynamic mutations. *Nat Rev Genet,* 2005, 6, 729-742.

Percy, AK. Rett syndrome. Current status and new vistas. *Neurol Clin,* 2002, 20, 1125-1141.

Philip, N; Chabrol, B; Lossi, AM; *et al.* Mutations in the oligophrenin-1 gene (OPHN1) cause X linked congenital cerebellar hypoplasia. *J Med Genet,* 2003, 40, 441-446.

Philippe, C; Villard, L; De Roux, N; *et al.* Spectrum and distribution of MECP2 mutations in 424 Rett syndrome patients: a molecular update. *Eur J Med Genet,* 2006, 49, 9-18.

Picketts, DJ; Higgs, DR; Bachoo, S; *et al.* ATRX encodes a novel member of the SNF2 family of proteins: mutations point to a common mechanism underlying the ATR-X syndrome. *Hum Mol Genet,* 1996, 5, 1899-1907.

Poirier, K; Lacombe, D; Gilbert-Dussardier, B; *et al.* Screening of ARX in mental retardation families: consequences for the strategy of molecular diagnosis. *Neurogenetics*, 2006, 7, 39–46.

Poirier, K; van Esch, H; Friocourt, G; *et al.* Neuroanatomical distribution of ARX in brain and its localisation in GABAergic neurons. *Brain Res Mol Brain Res,* 2004, 122, 35–46.

Qi, Y; Hoshino, M; Wada, Y; *et al.* PQBP-1 is expressed predominantly in the central nervous system during development. *Eur J Neurosci,* 2005, 22, 1277-1286.

Quenard, A; Yilmaz, S; Fontaine, H; *et al.* Deleterious mutations in exon 1 of MECP2 in Rett syndrome. *Eur J Med Genet,* 2006, 49, 313-322.

Ramakers, GJ. Rho proteins, mental retardation and the cellular basis of cognition. *Trends Neurosci,* 2002, 25, 191-199.

Raymond, FL. X linked mental retardation: a clinical guide. J Med Genet, 2006, 43, 193-200.

Ropers, HH. X-linked mental retardation: many genes for a complex disorder. *Curr Opin Genet Dev,* 2006, 1, 260-269.

Ropers, HH; Hoeltzenbein, M; Kalscheuer, V; *et al.* Nonsyndromic X-linked mental retardation: where are the missing mutations? *Trends Genet,* 2003, 19, 316-320.

Rosenberg, EH; Almeida, LS; Kleefstra, T; *et al.* High prevalence of SLC6A8 deficiency in X-linked mental retardation. *Am J Hum Genet,* 2004, 75, 97-105.

Ross, MT; Grafham, DV; Coffey AJ, *et al.* The DNA sequence of the human X chromosome. *Nature*, 2005, 434, 325-337.

Salomons, GS; van Dooren, SJM; Verhoeven, NM; *et al.* X-linked creatine-transporter gene (SLC6A8) defect: a new creatine-deficiency syndrome. *Am J Hum Genet,* 2001, 68, 1497-1500.

Samaco, RC; Hogart, A; LaSalle, JM. Epigenetic overlap in autism-spectrum neurodevelopmental disorders: MECP2 deficiency causes reduced expression of UBE3A and GABRB3. *Hum Mol Genet,* 2005, 14, 483-492.

Santos, C; Rodriguez-Revenga, L; Madrigal, I; *et al.* A novel mutation in JARID1C gene associated with mental retardation. *Eur J Hum Genet,* 2006, 14, 583-586.

Santos-Reboucas, CB; Abdalla, CB; Fullston, T; *et al.* Lack of FMR3 expression in a male with non-syndromic mental retardation and a microdeletion immediately distal to FRAXE CCG repeat. *Neurosci Lett,* 2006, 397, 245-248.

Santos-Rebouças, CB; Pimentel, MMG. Implication of abnormal epigenetic patterns for human diseases. *Eur J Hum Genet.* 2007, 15, 10-17.

Scala, E; Ariani, F; Mari, F; *et al.* CDKL5/STK9 is mutated in Rett syndrome variant with infantile spasms. *J Med Genet,* 2005, 42, 103–107.

Schratt, GM; Tuebing, F; Nigh, EA; *et al.* A brain-specific microRNA regulates dendritic spine development. *Nature*, 2006, 439, 283-289.

Schiaffino, MC; Bellini, C; Costabello, L; *et al.* X-linked creatine transporter deficiency: clinical description of a patient with a novel SLC6A8 gene mutation. *Neurogenetics*, 2005, 6, 165-168.

Shoichet, AS; Hoffmann, K; Menzel, C; *et al.* Mutations in the ZNF41 gene are associated with cognitive deficits: identification of a new candidate for X-linked mental retardation. *Am J Hum Genet,* 2003, 73, 1341-1354.

Schwartz, CE; May, MM; Carpenter, NJ; *et al.* Allan-Herndon-Dudley syndrome and the monocarboxylate transporter 8 (MCT8) gene. *Am J Hum Genet,* 2005, 77, 41-53.

Shahbazian, MD; Antalffy, B; Armstrong, DL; Zoghbi, HY. Insight into Rett syndrome: MeCP2 levels display tissue- and cell-specific differences and correlate with neuronal maturation. *Hum Mol Genet*, 2002, 11, 115-124.

Shevell, M; Ashwal, S; Donley, D; *et al.* Practice parameter: evaluation of the child with global developmental delay: report of the Quality Standards Subcommittee of the American Academy of Neurology and The Practice Committee of the Child Neurology Society. *Neurology*, 2003, 60, 367-380.

Skuse, DH; James, RS, Bishop, DV, *et al.* Evidence from Turner's syndrome of an imprinted X-linked locus affecting cognitive function. *Nature,* 1997, 387, 705-708.

Stayton, CL; Dabovic, B; Gulisano, M; *et al.* Cloning and characterization of a new human Xq13 gene, encoding a putative helicase. *Hum Mol Genet,* 1994, 3, 1957-1964.

Stemkens, D; Roza, T; Verrij, L. Is there an influence of X-chromosomal imprinting on the phenotype in Klinefelter syndrome? A clinical and molecular genetic study of 61 cases. *Clin Genet,* 2006, 70, 43-48.

Stevenson, RE. Splitting and lumping in the nosology of XLMR. *Am J Med Genet,* 2000, 97, 174-182.

Stepp, ML; Cason, AL; Finnis, M; *et al.* XLMR in MRX families 29, 32, 33 and 38 results from the dup24 mutation in the ARX (Aristaless related homeobox) gene. *BMC Med Genet*, 2005, 6, 16.

Stromme, P; Mangelsdorf, ME; Shaw, MA; *et al.* Mutations in the human ortholog of Aristaless cause X-linked mental retardation and epilepsy. Nat Genet, 2002, 30, 441-445.

Suri, M. The phenotypic spectrum of ARX mutations. *Dev Med Child Neurol,* 2005, 47, 133–137.

Tabolacci, E; Pietrobono, R; Moscato, U; *et al.* Differential epigenetic modifications in the FMR1 gene of the fragile X syndrome after reactivating pharmacological treatments. *Eur J Hum Genet,* 2005, 13, 641-648.

Tabolacci, E; Pomponi, MG; Pietrobono, R; *et al.* A truncating mutation in the IL1RAPL1 gene is responsible for X-linked mental retardation in the MRX21 family. *Am J Med Genet A,* 2006, 140, 482-487.

Takizawa, T; Nakashima, K; Namihira, M; *et al.* DNA methylation is a critical cell-intrinsic determinant of astrocyte differentiation in the fetal brain. *Dev Cell*, 2001, 1, 749-758.

Tarpey, P; Parnau, J; Blow, M. Mutations in the DLG3 Gene cause Nonsyndromic X-Linked Mental Retardation. *Am. J. Hum. Genet,* 2004, 75, 318–324.

Thapar, A; Gottesman, II; Owen, MJ; *et al.* The genetics of mental retardation. *Br J Psychiatry,* 1994, 164, 747-758.

Thomas, GM; Rumbaugh, GR; Harrar, DB; Huganir, RL; Ribosomal S6 kinase 2 interacts with and phosphorylates PDZ domain-containing proteins and regulates AMPA receptor transmission. *Proc Nat Acad Sci,* 2005, 102, 15006-15011.

Trivier, E; De Cesare, D; Jacquot, S; *et al.* Mutations in the kinase Rsk-2 associated with Coffin-Lowry syndrome. *Nature,* 1996, 384, 567–570.

Turner, G.; Webb, T.; Wake, S.; Robinson, H. Prevalence of fragile X syndrome. *Am. J. Med. Genet,* 1996, 64, 196-197.

Tzschach, A; Lenzner, S; Moser, B; *et al.* Novel JARID1C/SMCX mutations in patients with X-linked mental retardation. *Hum Mutat,* 2006, 27, 389.

Van Esch, H; Bauters, M; Ignatius, J; *et al.* Duplication of the MECP2 region is a frequent cause of severe mental retardation and progressive neurological symptoms in males. *Am J Hum Genet,* 2005, 77, 442-453.

Vervoort, VS; Beachem, MA; Edwards, OS; *et al.* AGTR2 mutations in X-linked mental retardation. *Science*, 2002, 296, 2401-2403.

Villard, L; Gecz, J; Mattei, JF; *et al.* XNP mutation in a large family with Juberg-Marsidi syndrome. *Nat Genet* 1996, 12, 359-360.

Villard, L; Fontes, M; Ades, LC; Gecz, J. Identification of a mutation in the XNP/ATR-X gene in a family reported as Smith-Fineman-Myers syndrome. *Am J Med Genet,* 2000, 91, 83-85.

XLMR update website. Pietro Chiurazzi, 2005 (accessed in October, 2006). Available from http://xlmr.interfree.it/home.htm

Watson, P; Black, G; Ramsden, S; *et al.* Angelman syndrome phenotype associated with mutations in MECP2, a gene encoding a methyl CpG binding protein. *J Med Genet,* 2001, 38, 224-228.

Weiler, IJ; Irwin, SA; Klintsova, AY; *et al.* Fragile X mental retardation protein is translated near synapses in response to neurotransmitter activation. *Proc Natl Acad Sci USA,* 1997, 94, 5395-5400.

Weller S, Gartner J. Genetic and clinical aspects of X-linked hydrocephalus (L1 disease): Mutations in the L1CAM gene. *Hum Mutat,* 2001, 18, 1-12.

World Health Organization.International classification of impairments, disabilities and handicaps. (World Health Organization, Geneva, 1980).

Wu, Y; Jiang, Y; Zhang, L; *et al.* Mutations in ionotropic ampa receptor 3 (GLUR3) in males with X-linked mental retardation (abstract). In 12th International Workshop on Fragile X and X-linked mental retardation; Williamburg: 2005, 84.

Xu, J; Burgoyne, PS. Sex differences in sex chromosome gene expression in mouse brain. *Hum Mol Genet,* 2002, 11, 1409-1419.

Ying, SY; Lin SL. Current perspectives in intronic micro RNAs (miRNAs). *J Biomed Sci,* 2006, 13, 5-15.

Ylisaukko-oja, T; Rehnstrom, K; Auranen, M; *et al.* Analysis of four neuroligin genes as candidates for autism. *Eur J Hum Genet,* 2005, 13, 1285-1292.

Youings, SA; Murray, A; Dennis, N; *et al*. FRAXA and FRAXE: the results of a five year survey. *J Med Genet,* 2000, 37, 415–421.

Young, JI; Hong, EP; Castle, JC; *et al*. Regulation of RNA splicing by the methylation-dependent transcriptional repressor methyl-CpG binding protein 2. *Proc Natl Acad Sci U S A,* 2005, 102, 17551-17558.

Yntema, HG; Hamel, BC; Smits, AP; *et al*. Localization of a gene for non-specific X linked mental retardation (MRX46) to Xq25-q26. *J Med Genet,* 1998, 35, 801-805.

Zechner, U; Wilda, M; Kehrer-Sawatzki, H; *et al*. A high density of X-linked genes for general cognitive ability: a run-away process shaping human evolution? *Trends Genet,* 2001, 17, 697–701.

Zemni, R; Bienvenu, T; Vinct, MC; *et al*. A new gene involved in X-linked mental retardation identified by analysis of an X;2 balanced translocation. *Nat Genet,* 2000, 24, 167-170.

In: Focus on Mental Retardation Research
Editor: Marina I. Carson, pp. 185-208
ISBN: 978-1-60021-647-3

Chapter 7

CARDIAC DYSAUTONOMIA AND MENTAL RETARDATION

***Maurizio Acampa**[*,1,2] **and Francesca Guideri**[1,3.]*
[1]Department of Clinical Medicine and Immunological Sciences University of Siena, Siena, Italy; [2]Section of Internal Medicine, [3]Section of Clinical Immunology, Siena, Italy

ABSTRACT

Mental retardation is characterized by significantly sub-average intellectual functioning, existing concurrently with related limitations in two or more of the applicable adaptive skill areas (communication, self care, home living, social skills, community use, self-direction, health and safety, functional academics, leisure and work). Causes of mental retardation can be broken into several categories (chromosomal abnormalities, genetic and inherited metabolic disorders, trauma, infections, toxic, nutritional, environmental and unexplained causes). The autonomic control of cardiac and respiratory activity in children with mental retardation is defective but pathogenesis of this alteration depend on different causes of mental retardation. Physiological control mechanisms of cardiac autonomic activity (sympathetic and parasympathetic divisions) involve complex interactions between the central autonomic neuronal network, the cerebellum and the cerebral cortex. This network may be altered at various levels in relations to different causes of mental retardation with various clinical expression. Rett syndrome is a classical example of cardiac dysautonomia in mental retardation but many other diseases with mental retardation show clinical signs of alterations in sympatho-vagal balance.

* Correspondence to be sent to: Maurizio Acampa, MD; Dipartimento di Medicina Clinica e Scienze Immunologiche, Sezione di Medicina Interna, Policlinico 'Le Scotte', viale Bracci, 53100 Siena, Italy. Telephone number: +39(0)577585741; Fax number:+39(0)57744114; E-mail address: M.Acampa@ao-siena.toscana.it

INTRODUCTION

Mental retardation is a lifelong disability that presents in infancy or the early childhood years but cannot be diagnosed until the child is older than 5 years, when standardized measures of intelligence become reliable and valid. The American Association on Mental Retardation defines mental retardation by measures of 3 domains: intelligence (IQ), adaptive behaviour and systems of supports [1]. Causes of mental retardation can be broken into several categories: genetic disorders, malformations, external prenatal disorders, paranatal disorders, postnatal disorders, unknown causes (see Figure 1) [2].

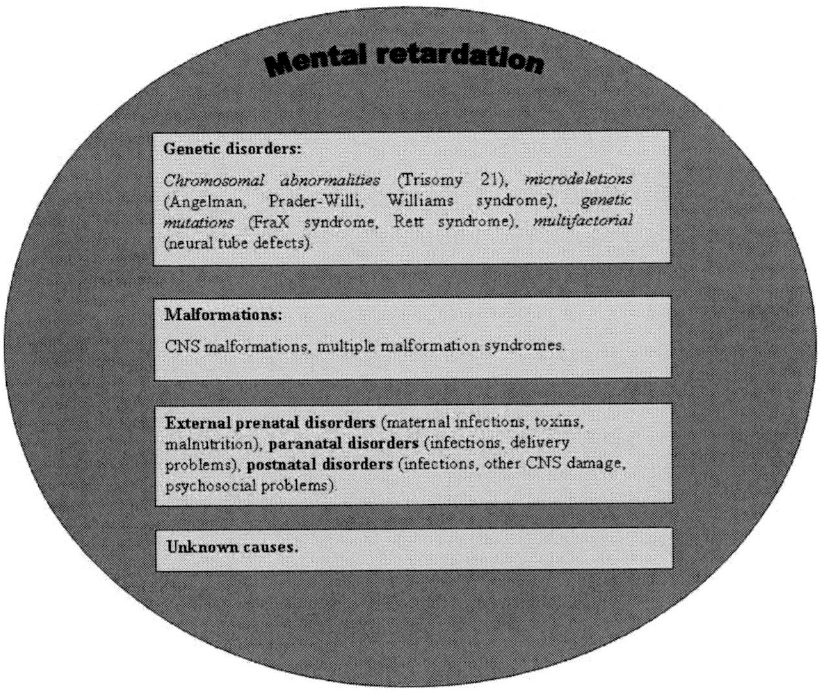

Figure 1. Aetiology of mental retardation.

An individual with mental retardation has a functionally abnormal brain, which may or may not have a developmental basis in morphogenesis or in histogenesis; structural brain abnormalities have been demonstrated in 34 to 98% of deceased severely retarded patients undergoing complete neuropathological study [3]. These defects include cortical malformations, neuronal circuitry disorders and perturbations of neuronal communication and synapse function [4].

In the last decade many studies showed that the autonomic nervous system is altered in various diseases with mental retardation [5, 6, 7]: in comparison with healthy subjects, in individuals with mental retardation there is a dysfunction of cardiac autonomic nervous system, a deficit of sympathetic influence and a prevalence of parasympathetic activity. Pathogenesis of this alteration vary according to different causes of mental retardation.

Understanding the anatomy and the physiology of the cardiac autonomic nervous system is relevant to the comprehension of the pathophysiology of heart rate control in these diseases because an alteration of the complex regulation of the cardiac autonomic nervous system may be the background for a higher risk of life-threatening cardiac arrhythmias and other cardiac disturbances [8].

Cardiac Autonomic Nervous System: Anatomy and Physiology

Anatomy

The autonomic nervous system (ANS) is a visceral and largely involuntary motor/effector system that is traditionally divided into sympathetic (thoracolumbar) and parasympathetic (craniosacral) divisions, each with a central and a peripheral component [9]. These divisions are closely integrated and regulated by a central autonomic neuronal network (CAN). The CAN maintains integral relationships with visceral sensory neurons via afferent input from the vagus nerve and relays transmission through the nucleus tractus solitarius to the hypothalamus, amygdala, and forebrain [10]. The ANS provides the main nerve supply to the heart, by means of its two anatomic branches: geographic proximity of nerve endings affects neural modulation; therefore, pathways of innervation are important [11].

The major sympathetic nerves arise from the stellate ganglion and lower cervical sympathetic trunk, with usually three right-sided and four left-sided nerves. Parasympathetic fibers leave the thoracic vagus nerves and recurrent laryngeal nerves. Parasympathetic and sympathetic nerves interconnect to form ventral and dorsal cardiopulmonary plexus, from which relatively large and discrete cardiac nerves emerge to supply the ventricles: the right and left coronary cardiac nerves and the left lateral cardiac nerves. A number of smaller nerves also supply the heart, and there are many anatomic variations among individuals with regard to the precise wiring diagram of the heart. In general, the right-sided sympathetic and vagal fibers are predominant at the sinus node, and fibers from the left sympathetic trunk and vagal nerves are predominant at the atrioventricular node. Parasympathetic pathways to the atria have been well characterized in dogs and, to some degree, in patients, with a concentration of ganglia in various fat pads directing innervation to specific sites. In the ventricles, major sympathetic trunks appear localized in the epicardium alongside coronary arteries, with transmural penetration to innervate the rest of the myocardium. In addition, the right-sided sympathetic nerves usually supply the anterior surface of the ventricle, while the left-sided sympathetic nerves supply the posterior surface. The major parasympathetic ventricular pathways are epicardial until crossing the AV groove, where vagal trunks appear to penetrate the myocardium to become located predominantly in the ventricular subendocardium.

Development of the ANS is intimately related to the development of the sensory nervous system; both have their embryonic origins in the multipotential neural crest cells [12]. These cells migrate and eventually evolve into sensory and autonomic ganglia as well as the adrenal chromaffin cells. Their differentiation and commitment to function in the mature nervous system is incumbent on exposure to growth factors released by structures along the migratory route and then within the target tissue. Eventually, specificity will be determined by their ability to produce specific neurotransmitters. Therefore, one could postulate that an early genetic error affecting initial migration would cause profound decreases in both sensory and autonomic populations, whereas a later genetic error might only affect cell survival to one or both populations, causing more erratic and varied clinical expression. Various factors promote normal progression from the embryonic to the mature autonomic and sensory nervous systems. Several key transcription factors have been identified that play critical roles in the development of the ANS (*MASH1* [mammalian achaete-scute homologue] and *PHOX* 2B [paired-like homeobox] genes) and in the differentiation of uncommitted neural crest cells to the developing ANS [13]. Another important regulator of development and survival is nerve growth factor (NGF), that promotes migration from the neural crest, enhances maturation through neurite outgrowth and neurotransmitter synthesis [14].

Physiology

For both the sympathetic and parasympathetic systems, the preganglionic innervation is largely cholinergic, with terminals releasing acetylcholine at the ganglion synapses. For the sympathetic system, norepinephrine is the major neurotransmitter, but other postganglionic neurotransmitters are also important, among which are substance P, dopamine, and vasoactive intestinal polypeptide [15, 16]. Regulation of cardiac neural activity is highly integrated and is achieved by circuitry at multiple levels; higher brain centers operate through elaborate pathways within the hypothalamus and medullary cardiovascular regulatory sites. Baroreceptor mechanisms have long been recognized as integral to autonomic control of the cardiovascular system, and significant clinical applications of this knowledge have been realized through heart rate variability and baroreceptor sensitivity testing. The intrinsic cardiac nerves and fat pads appear to provide local neural coordination independent of higher brain centers. At the level of the myocardial cell, considerable progress has been made to define the intimate role of the autonomic receptors as they influence G proteins to control ionic channels, pumps, and exchangers. Finally, studies of behavioral state provide evidence that markers of arrhythmia vulnerability can be monitored during emotional and physical stressors and sleep states to identify individuals at heightened risk of lethal cardiac arrhythmias [17].

As with the Chinese philosophy of yin and yang so the vagal and sympathetic drives to the heart can be characterized as polar opposites [18]. At the sinus node, parasympathetic stimulation is prepotent, whereas the reverse occurs in the ventricles, where sympathetic effects dominate. Parasympathetic stimulation reduces norepinephrine release from sympathetic nerve terminals while also opposing postganglionic sympathetic actions. Sympathetic stimulation counters vagal effects primarily by direct stimulation of α and β receptors. However, a more subtle interpretation of the yin–yang principle shows that it is the interrelation of the opposites that is crucial. So with the autonomic control of the heart, the interaction between sympathetic and parasympathetic, which is classically characterized as opposite and reciprocal, can under physiological and pathophysiological circumstances be both synchronous and synergistic.

In the normal ventricle, sympathetic stimulation shortens action potential duration and the QT interval in the scalar ECG and can reduce the dispersion of repolarization. However, in pathologic states associated with reduced repolarization reserve (e.g., heart failure and channelopathies such as the long QT syndrome [LQTS]), sympathetic stimulation is a potent stimulus for the generation of arrhythmias, perhaps by enhancing the dispersion of repolarization or by generation of afterdepolarizations. Parasympathetic stimulation modestly prolongs ventricular refractoriness and the QT interval in the normal heart, reflected by a longer QT interval during vagal stimulation in animal studies and during sleep in humans. The neurotransmitters epinephrine and norepinephrine activate cardiac adrenergic receptors, increasing systolic contractility and diastolic relaxation rate as well as accelerating heart rate and AV conduction. Beta-adrenergic receptor stimulation activates the G protein–adenylyl cyclase–cAMP–protein kinase A pathway to alter the activity of a number of ion channels and transporters. This in turn increases both peak amplitude and rate of decline of the $[Ca^{2+}]_i$ transient via stimulation of key Ca^{2+} handling proteins and shortens action potential duration via augmentation of K^+ outward currents. When action potential is prolonged (as in heart failure and LQTS, or in mutations of the ryanodine receptor in catecholaminergic ventricular tachycardia [VT]), intracellular calcium overload can augment ionic currents underlying afterdepolarizations. Sympathetic stimulation can enhance this response and, if calcium-regulated currents linked to repolarization, such as the Na/Ca exchanger, become dispersed heterogeneously, can contribute to arrhythmogenesis via increased dispersion of repolarization [19].

ASSESEMENT OF CARDIAC AUTONOMIC ACTIVITY

Autonomic assessment has played an important role in elucidating the role of the autonomic nervous system in diverse clinical and research settings [20].

Because the anatomic location of the cardiovascular autonomic nervous system renders it inaccessible to simple direct physiological testing, a group of clinical tests measuring cardiovascular autonomic function and dysfunction has been developed to circumvent this problem by measuring the end-organ responses to various physiological and pharmacological perturbations.

In recent years non-invasive techniques based on the electrocardiogram (ECG) have been used as markers of autonomic modulation of the heart [21], these include heart rate variability (HRV), baroreflex sensitivity (BRS), QT interval, and heart rate turbulence (HRT), a new method based on fluctuations of sinus rhythm cycle length after a single premature ventricular contraction. Among these techniques analysis of HRV has emerged as a simple, noninvasive method to evaluate the sympatho-vagal balance at the sinoatrial level.

Autonomic nervous system tone has been studied primarily in human subjects by employing the tool of HRV, which relies on the principle that the pattern of beat-to-beat control of the sinoatrial node provides a reflection of autonomic activity. Heart rate responds dynamically to physiologic perturbations mediated by the autonomic nervous system via efferent vagal and sympathetic nerve impulses. Even at rest heart rate fluctuates cyclically. High frequency (HF) cyclic fluctuations are modulated by ventilation, mediated entirely by changes in vagal outflow. Slower fluctuations occur due to baroreflexes or due to thermoregulation. The greatest variation of heart rate occurs with circadian changes, particularly the difference between night and day heart rate, mediated by complex and poorly understood neurohormonal rhythms. Exercise and emotion also have profound effects on heart rate. Fluctuations in heart rate reflect autonomic modulation and have prognostic significance in pathological states. On the basis of the different frequency response characteristics of sympathetic and parasympathetic modulation of heart rate, frequency analysis of heart rate variability is often used as a tool to determine "autonomic balance" or sympathetic and parasympathetic nervous system activity.

There are two common settings in which HRV is measured. First, HRV is assessed under controlled laboratory conditions with short-term measurements before and after tilt, drugs, controlled ventilation, or other maneuvers selected to challenge the autonomic system. Secondly, HRV can be determined from 24-hour electrocardiographic (ECG) recordings made while subjects perform their usual daily activities. Twenty-four-hour ECG recordings are particularly useful for risk stratification in a variety of pathological entities, but can also be useful for quantifying autonomic dysfunction. Methods for quantifying HRV are categorized as: time domain, spectral or frequency domain, geometric, and nonlinear. A short discussion of each will follow.

Time domain measures of HRV	
Statistical measures	
SDNN (ms)	Standard deviation of all NN intervals
SDANN (ms)	Standard deviation of the averages of NN intervals in all 5-minute segments of the entire recording
RMSSD (ms)	The square root of the mean of the sum of the squares of differences between adjacent NN intervals
SDNN index (ms)	Mean of the standard deviations of all NN intervals for all 5-minute segments of the entire recording
SDSD (ms)	Standard deviation of differences between adjacent NN intervals
NN50 count	Number of pairs of adjacent NN intervals differing by more than 50 ms in the entire recording;
pNN50%	NN50 count divided by the total number of all NN intervals
Geometric measures	
HRV triangular index	Total number of all NN intervals divided by the height of the histogram of all NN intervals measured on a discrete scale with bins of 7.8125 ms (1/128 seconds)
TINN (ms)	Baseline width of the minimum square difference triangular interpolation of the highest peak of the histogram of all NN intervals
Frequency domain measures of HRV	
Total power (ms2)	Variance of all NN intervals (≤0.4 Hz)
ULF (ms2)	Power in the ULF (range ≤0.003 Hz)
VLF (ms2)	Power in the VLF (range 0.003-0.04 Hz)
LF (ms2)	Power in the LF (range 0.04-0.15 Hz)
HF (ms2)	Power in the HF (range 0.15-0.4 Hz)
LF/HF Ratio	LF [ms2]/HF[ms2]

Figure 2. Time and Frequency Domain Measures of HRV.

Methods of Measurements of Cardiac Autonomic Activity

The variations in heart rate may be evaluated by a number of methods [22] (Figure 2). Perhaps the simplest to perform are the time domain measures. In *time domain analysis*, the intervals between adjacent normal R waves (NN intervals) are measured over the period of recording. A variety of statistical variables can be calculated from the intervals directly and others can be derived from the differences between intervals.

Either fast Fourier transformation or autoregression techniques can be used to quantify cyclic fluctuations of R-R intervals. Traditionally, *spectral analysis* has been done in short-term laboratory studies; often standard 5-minute ECG segments are analyzed. According to the Task Force of The European Society of Cardiology and The North American Society of Pacing and Electrophysiology these frequencies are classified into *1*) ultra-low frequencies (ULF; 5-h cycle length) that include the circadian rhythm; *2*) very low frequencies (VLF; 25-s cycle length) that are supposed to be affected by temperature regulation and humoral systems; *3*) low frequencies (LF; 6-s cycle length in humans) that are sensitive to changes in cardiac sympathetic (and presumably parasympathetic) nerve activity; and *4*) high frequencies (HF; 2.5- to 6.0-s cycle length in humans) that are synchronized to the respiratory rhythm and are primarily modulated by cardiac parasympathetic innervation.

The exact physiologic mechanism responsible for VLF is a matter of dispute [23], but, like most other forms of HRV, VLF power is abolished by atropine, suggesting that it uses a parasympathetic efferent limb. Very low frequency power is also reduced by about 20% by ACE inhibition, suggesting that, at least in part, it reflects the activity of the renin-aldosterone system. Others have suggested that VLF power reflects thermoregulation or vasomotor activity. Bernardi [24] showed that physical activity can exert a large effect on VLF power. In addition, sleep-disordered breathing can cause exaggerated values for VLF power, seen as clear peaks on plots of the HRV power spectrum during the night. The HF component corresponds to the frequency of respiration and is driven by the vagus as indicated by the strong respiratory pattern of cardiac vagal motoneurons in the nucleus ambiguus. The LF component has been ascribed to sympathetic modulation of cardiac pacemaker activity, because a variety of studies demonstrated that acute interventions that increase sympathetic nervous system activity, such as orthostatic perturbations, mental stress, or handgrip exercise increases LF spectral power of heart rate. In addition to acute perturbations of cardiac sympathetic nerve activity, feedback oscillations generated by the baroreceptor reflex also appear to contribute to LF spectral power of heart rate as it was demonstrated that sinoaortic denervation markedly reduces the LF component [23].

R-R interval power spectra also have been computed using data from 24-hour ECG recordings and categorized into total power and four mutually exclusive power bands, ultra low, very low, low, and HF power. Total and ultra-low frequency power are best calculated from a R-R interval tachogram of the entire 24-hour recording. Instead of computing the 24-hour power spectrum, spectral analysis often is performed on 5-minute segments from 24-hour recordings. The lowest frequency band in the 24-hour R-R interval power spectrum is ULF power, which quantifies fluctuations in R-R intervals with periods between every 5 minutes and once per 24 hours (ULF <0.003 Hz). Although the physiologic basis for ULF and VLF power are far less clear than HF and LF power, they have proven to be more powerful risk predictors in cardiovascular diseases.

Nonlinear phenomena are certainly involved in the genesis of HRV. They are determined by complex interactions of hemodynamic, electrophysiological, and humoral variables as well as by the autonomic and central nervous regulations. It has been speculated that analysis of HRV based on the *methods of nonlinear dynamics* might elicit valuable information for physiological interpretation of HRV and for the assessment of the risk of sudden death.

Nonlinear methods are based on the chaos theory and fractals. Chaos has been defined as the study of multivariable, nonlinear and nonperiodic systems. Chaos describes natural systems in a different way because it can account for nature's randomness and nonperiodicity [25]. Perhaps the theory of chaos may help in better understanding HR dynamics, taking into account that the healthy heartbeat is slightly irregular and to some extent chaotic. In the near future nonlinear fractal methods may give new insights into HR dynamics in the context of physiological changes and in high risk situations, particularly in patients after myocardial infarction or in the context of sudden death [25]. Recent data suggest that fractal analysis in comparison to standard HRV measurements seems to detect abnormal patterns of RR fluctuations more efficiently. The parameters that have been used to measure nonlinear properties of HRV include 1/f scaling of Fourier spectra, H scaling exponent, and Coarse Graining Spectral Analysis (CGSA) [26]. For data representation, Poincaré sections, low-dimension attractor plots, singular value decomposition, and attractor trajectories have been used. For other quantitative descriptions, the D_2 correlation dimension, Lyapunov exponents, and Kolmogorov entropy have been used.

Modern techniques for the estimation of *spontaneous baroreceptor reflex sensitivity (BRS)* are based on a variety of signal processing schemes and derive information on the baroreflex function from different perspectives [27]. Thus factors such as respiration and other non-stationary agents may have different influences on the estimates provided by each of these approaches. Notwithstanding such individual specificity, however, it has been observed that in several physiological and pathophysiological conditions these techniques often provide comparable information on BRS changes over time, particularly when the estimates are averaged over time windows of a few minutes. The tilting test is used to evaluate blood pressure variability and autonomic nervous responses, especially BRS during changes of body position. In this instance, BRS is expressed as the ratio between heart rate variation and systolic blood pressure variation (delta RR/delta SBP). The results were the same as those produced by all other tests including sequential method, squatting test, the neck chamber method, and tilting test.

PHYSIOPATHOLOGY

Many diseases with mental retardation are associated with autonomic disorders apparent at birth or within the first year of life [28]. Pathogenesis of these alteration vary according to causes of mental retardation: some of these disorders occur as a result of developmental abnormalities caused by specific genetic mutations required for neural crest cell migration and maturation; others occur as a result of prematurity or generalized central dysfunction. Those disorders that occur as a result of biochemical errors causing neurotransmitter deficiencies or inefficient mitochondrial metabolism can be more insidious and later in their presentation.

Chromosomal disorders usually have multisystem perturbations, and it is increasingly appreciated that autonomic dysfunction can be a feature of many of these disorders because of either expansions or deletions of particular genes. Infact, mental retardation caused by chromosomal alterations (for example Down syndrome, fragile X syndrome, Prader-Willi syndrome) produce an alteration of the varied functions of the CAN that integrated and regulated peripheral ANS function, involving the extensive circuitry of which ranges from the forebrain to the brainstem.

Disorders in the forebrain circuits, such as ischemia secondary to blood-flow disturbance, intracranial hemorrhage before or after birth, severe head injury, can cause autonomic dysfunction with cardiac arrhythmia; within this circuitry, the nucleus tractus solitarius in the medulla oblongata, which receives input from the vagus and glossopharyngeal nerves, functions as a major relay station, allowing continuous feedback and integration.

The peripheral ANS provides physiologic responses that are critical for homeostasis and acute adaptations to stressful circumstances via multiple transmitters and a chemical coding system of autonomic neurons. During the last 2 decades it has become clear that within a single neuron multiple transmitter systems coexist and that within a given ganglion the variety and pattern of neurotransmitters is extensive. Diseases with mental retardation may be associated with autonomic alterations caused by biochemical errors that include myopathies (mitochondrial myopathies: Leber hereditary optic neuropathy; X-linked kinky-hair disease; Leigh syndrome; Kerns-Sayre syndrome; myoneurogastrointestinal disorder with encephalopathy), neurotransmitters deficiencies (Dopamine-hydroxylase deficiency, Menkes), storage disorders (Fabry disease) and metabolic/endocrine disorders (diabetes, Addison disease, Cushing syndrome, thyroid disorders).

Because the ANS and its CAN component have pervasive effects that affect multiple other systems secondarily, clinical manifestations of cardiac dysautonomia may be associated with a multisystem involvement with a more global autonomic disorder and with symptoms extremely varied.

An involvement of cardiac autonomic nervous system may produce postural hypotension (with dizziness, lightheadedness, loss of consciousness/syncope), hypertension (with headache), cardiac arrhythmias with possible sudden death. A few representative disorders will be described.

Cardiac Dysautonomia in Specific Diseases with Mental Retardation

Genetic Disorders

Genetic disorders may be broken into 3 divisions: chromosomal abnormalities, genetic mutations and multifactorial causes [2, 29, 30] (Figure 1). *Chromosomal disorders* affect approximately 7 out of every 1,000 infants. The disorder results when a person has too many or too few chromosomes, or when there is a change in the structure of a chromosome. Half of all first-trimester miscarriages or spontaneous abortions occur as a result of a chromosome abnormality. If the child is born, he or she usually has multiple birth defects and mental retardation. Examples of chromosomal disorders include Down syndrome, Trisomy 13,

Trisomy 18 and Cri du chat. *Single-gene disorders* (sometimes called inborn errors of metabolism or Mendelian disorders) are caused by non-working genes. Disorders of metabolism occur when cells are unable to produce proteins or enzymes needed to change certain chemicals into others, or to carry substances from one place to another. The cell's inability to carry out these vital internal functions often results in mental retardation. Approximately 1 in 5,000 children are born with defective enzymes resulting in inborn errors of metabolism. Combinations of multiple gene and environmental factors leading to mental retardation are called *multifactorial disorders*. They are inherited but do not share the same inheritance patterns typically found in single-gene disorders. Their inheritance patterns are usually much more complex than those of single gene disorders because their existence depends on the simultaneous presence of heredity and environmental factors. Multifactorial disorders are very common and cause a majority of birth defects. Examples of multifactorial disorders include heart disease, diabetes, spina bifida, anencephaly, cleft lip and cleft palate, clubfoot and congenital heart defects.

Chromosomal Abnormalities

Down Syndrome

Down syndrome in humans, or trisomy of autosome 21, represents the hyperdiploidy that most frequently survives gestation, reaching an incidence of 1 in 700 live births. The condition is associated with multisystemic anomalies, including those affecting the central nervous system, determining a characteristic mental retardation [31]. At a neuronal level, Saud et al [32] have shown that the condition determines marked alterations of action potential and ionic current kinetics, which may underlie abnormal processing of information by the central nervous system.

Alterations in the autonomic nervous system have been reported in previous studies on individuals with Down syndrome evaluating the autonomic neurotransmitters: Yates CM [33] showed that norepinephrine levels measured in post-mortem brains from Down's syndrome were more markedly reduced; Schapiro MB [34] observed cerebrospinal fluid 5-hydroxyindoleacetic acid and norepinephrine levels significantly elevated with plasma levels unchanged; Eberhard et al. [35] showed reduced levels of circulating cathecolamine levels during exercise, suggesting a reduced sympathetic response to maximal exercise; Udeschini G [36] observed that plasma adrenaline tended to be higher in patients with Down syndrome, both in the standing and the cold pressor tests.

Recent studies showed that patients with Down syndrome, but without congenital heart disease, exhibit reduced heart rate and blood pressure responses to exercise, or chronotropic incompetence [37, 38]: the inability to adequately increase heart rate during aerobic exercise has been identified as the primary contributor to the low physical work capacity and cardiorespiratory fitness in these subjects [39] suggesting an autonomic dysfunction. Furthermore, there are reports of low blood pressure in Down syndrome, lower than in other forms of mental handicap and lower than in a normal population [40]; it is likely that blood pressure is lowered in DS by the widespread neuropathy [41]. This is apparent in fetal life and then later as a failure of growth and maturation in the brain, with loss of neurones [42] and dendrites [43]. Cholinergic nerves are particularly vulnerable [44]. Reports of postural hypotension [45] and the failure of heart rate and blood pressure to rise normally with maximum exercise [46] suggest autonomic failure in DS (Figure 3).

Chromosomal disorder	Pathogenesis	Clinical manifestations
Down syndrome	multisystemic anomalies in CNS and ANS with widespread neuropathy, blunted sympathetic activation and vagal withdrawal, plasma NE reduced during excercise.	hypotension, orthostatic hypotension, chronotropic incompetence.
Praeder-Willi syndrome	uncertain	equivocal findings (reduced vagal activity?).
Angelman disease	increased vagal activity	syncope, malaise, asystole.
Williams syndrome	elastin mutation with abnormal elastic fiber assembly at the arterial level, altered BRS.	hypotension, cardiac arrhythmias.

Figure 3. Clinical manifestations and pathogenesis of cardiac dysautonomia in chromosomal abnormalities with mental retardation.

The function of autonomic nervous system in Down syndrome is noninvasively assessed by heart rate variability analysis; preliminary studies conducted during sleep with subjects who have Down syndrome revealed equivocal findings: Sei [47] found reduced sympathetic nervous system activity during rapid eye movement sleep, whereas Ferri et al. [48] found increased sympathetic modulation and reduced vagal tone during sleep. However these studies included a small number of participants and used different methodological approaches for the heart rate variability analysis.

Recently Baynard et al. [49] demonstrated a greater vagal modulation at rest in patients with Down syndrome. Iellamo et al [50] studied cardiac autonomic activity in Down syndrome with autoregressive power spectral analysis to investigate heart rate variability, whereas he studied baroreflex modulation of sinus node by means of the spontaneous baroreflex sequences method: low-frequency and high-frequency (both expressed in normalized units) components of heart rate variability did not differ between individuals with Down syndrome and control subjects at rest, however, during standing, significant increase in LF and decrease in HF were observed in control subjects but not in Down syndrome subjects. Baroreflex sensitivity (BRS) did not differ between Down syndrome and control subjects at rest and underwent significant decrease on going from supine to upright in both groups. However, BRS was greater in subjects with Down syndrome during standing. These data indicate that in Down syndrome there is a reduced heart rate response to orthostatic stress associated with blunted sympathetic activation and vagal withdrawal and a lesser reduction in BRS in response to active orthostatism. These findings suggest overall impairment in autonomic cardiac regulation in Down syndrome and may help to explain the chronotropic incompetence typically reported during exercise in these subjects without congenital heart disease.

Prader-Willi Syndrome

The Prader-Willi syndrome is characterized by diminished fetal activity, obesity, muscular hypotonia, mental retardation, short stature, hypogonadotropic hypogonadism, and small hands and feet [51]. It can be considered to be an autosomal dominant disorder and is caused by deletion or disruption of a gene or several genes on the proximal long arm of the paternal chromosome 15 or maternal uniparental disomy 15, because the gene(s) on the maternal chromosome(s) 15 are virtually inactive through imprinting; Prader-Willi syndrome is a contiguous gene syndrome resulting from deletion of the paternal copies of the imprinted SNRPN_(small nuclear ribonucleoprotein polypeptide N) gene, the necdin gene and possibly other genes.

Studies of cardiac autonomic nervous system activity in this syndrome revealed equivocal findings: Di Mario FJ et al [52] evaluate simultaneous electrocardiography and serial recordings of pulse rate and systolic/diastolic mean arterial blood pressures during orthostatic maneuvers and measurements of plasma norepinephrine at rest and after standing in subjects with Prader-Willi syndrome, suggesting that these patients have a detectable underlying autonomic dysfunction characterized principally by diminished parasympathetic nervous system activity. However, Wade CK et al. [53] recorded electrocardiograms, beat-to-beat finger blood pressures, and respiration for several minutes in supine, standing, sitting position during Valsalva maneuver, during moderate exercise and recovery showing that cardiac autonomic modulation in patients with Prader-Willi syndrome does not differ from age and body mass index-matched subjects (Figure 3).

Angelman Syndrome

Angelman's syndrome [54] is an association of severe mental retardation with absence of language, ataxia, convulsions and hyperactive, joyful behaviour with frequent bouts of laughing. Genetic diagnosis is possible in about 80% of cases. Four known genetic mechanisms can cause Angelman syndrome: approximately 70% of the cases result from de novo maternal deletions involving chromosome 15q11.2-q13; approximately 2% result from paternal uniparental disomy of 15q11.2-q13; and 2 to 3% result from imprinting defects; a subset of the remaining 25% are caused by mutations in the gene encoding the ubiquitin-protein ligase E3A gene.

Analysis of Holter 24 hour ECG recording and oculo-cardiac reflex in these subjects [55] suggest the presence of an increased vagal tone, confirmed by clinical signs (malaise, syncope and asystole)[56] (Figure 3).

Williams Syndrome

Williams syndrome (WS) is a neurodevelopmental disorder caused by a hemizygous deletion on chromosome 7q11.23, encompassing the elastin locus. The incidence is usually given as 1 in 20,000 live births, but new prevalence estimates are as high as 1 in 7,500, which means that WS could account for 6% of all cases of mental retardation of genetic origin [57]. The study of baroreceptors and consequently the baroreflex sensitivity (BRS) in these individuals [58] showed that the amplitudes of the low frequency (LF) and high frequency

(HF) component were reduced in WS. The BRS obtained with the sequence technique was also reduced in WS. In conclusion a BRS reduction associated with a pulse rate elevation was observed in normotensive WS subjects. It is likely that abnormal elastic fiber assembly at the arterial level alters baroreceptor reflex (Figure 3).

Genetic Mutations

Rett Syndrome

Rett syndrome (RS) is one of the most common forms of childhood neurodevelopmental disorder affecting females; it affects approximately 1 in 10,000-15,000 females [59] and it is considered to be the second most common cause, after Down's syndrome, of severe mental retardation in females [60]. Mutations in the methyl-CpG-binding protein 2 gene (MECP2) are present in the majority of cases of RS, but a proportion of atypical cases may result from mutations in CDKL5, particularly the early onset seizure variant [61, 62]. RS consisted of profound and progressive loss of intellectual functioning occurring after a period (at least 6 months) of normal development with classic stereotype hand movements, gait ataxia, jerky truncal ataxia, deceleration of brain and body organ growth with many autistic features [62]. Clinical severity of the disease may vary with increasing age; these variations may be described by the four-stage model of Hagberg and Witt-Engerström [63]. The mortality rate in RS is 1.2% for year; of these deaths 48% occurs in debilitated people, 13% from natural causes, 13% with prior sever seizures, 26% were sudden unexpected death [64]. In comparison, the incidence of sudden death in the general population, between 1 and 22 years of age, was 1.3 in 100,000 patients for year [65].

There are clinical and experimental evidences that in Rett syndrome (RS) autonomic nervous system is abnormal at various levels from central to peripheral nervous system [66]. Julu [67] in 1997 measured the autonomic reactions to hyperventilation in RS to understand the interactions between medullary autonomic and cardiorespiratory neurons, suggesting that medullary cardioinhibition is immature in RS. In particular, measuring the cardiac response to baroreflex using the Neuroscope™ (MediFit Diagnostics, London, UK) which outputs a measure of cardiac vagal tone, Julu observed that cardiac vagal tone was invariably withdrawn at the height of sympathetic activity during both hyperventilation and breath holding in RS, leading to sympathovagal imbalance with the risk of cardiac arrhythmias and possibly sudden death.

In fact, it is well known a role for cardiac dysautonomia in the pathogenesis of lethal ventricular arrhythmias: sympathetic stimulation lowers the ventricular fibrillation threshold, whereas vagal stimulation antagonizes sympathetic activity and increases ventricular fibrillation threshold [68].

Johnsrude [69] studied HRV parameters from 24 h ECG ambulatory monitoring in 25 females with RS (3-27 years). Diminished HRV was demonstrated in RS females for the mean of standard deviation of normal RR for all 5 min. segments, for the root mean square successive differences, for the difference percentage between normal RR>50 msec and for the high frequency spectral component power.

Guideri [70, 71] studied the cardiac autonomic nervous system by means of HRV observing that: 1) the total power spectrum of HRV was significantly lower in children with Rett syndrome and this alteration progresses with age and with clinical stages of the syndrome; 2) the sympathovagal balance expressed by the ratio LF/HF (low frequency/high frequency) was significantly higher in RS, reflecting the prevalence of sympathetic activity; 3) girls with preserved speech variant showed a slight increase of sympathetic tone but a normal values of total power of HRV.

These results suggested that a loss of physiological HRV associated with an increase of adrenergic tone may represent the electrophysiological basis of cardiac instability and sudden death.

Pathogenesis of cardiac dysautonomia in RS is not well known [72] (figure 4); Julu observed that baseline brain stem functions (breathing rhythm, cardiac sensitivity to baroreflex and cardiac vagal tone which are maintained by complex integrative inhibition) are affected in RS, suggesting an insufficient rcciprocal innervation and leak of integrative inhibition within the cardiorespiratory neurons of the brain stem [73]; Weese-Mayer DE et al suggested that cardiorespiratory dysregulation may offer insight into the mechanisms that render girls with RS more vulnerable to sudden death [74].

Neurotransmitters may also have a role in the pathogenesis of cardiac dysautonomia (figure 4): substance P is deficient in the central nervous system of RS females and a deficiency of this substance may contribute to impairment of autonomic nervous system resulting in cardiac dysautonomia [75].

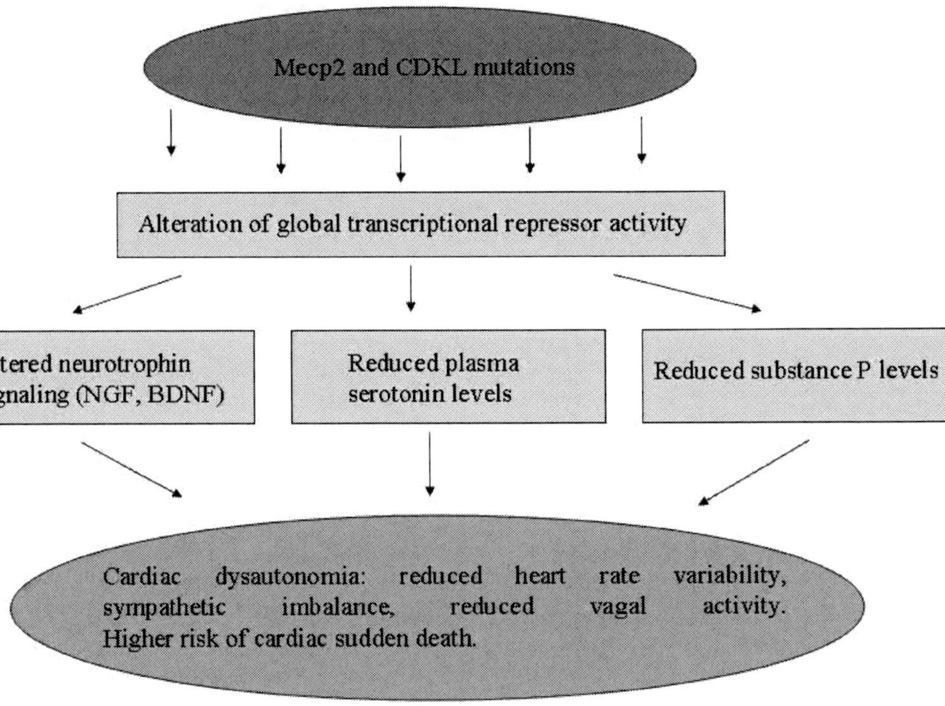

Figure 4. *hypothesis of pathogenetic mechanisms explaining cardiac dysautonomia in Rett syndrome.* The altered neurotrophin signalling, the serotoninergic dysfunction and the deficiency of substance P may contribute to impairment of autonomic nervous system resulting in cardiac dysautonomia with sympathetic imbalance. That may favour the onset of life-threatening ventricular arrhythmias with higher risk of sudden death.

Furthermore, recently Guideri [76] observed that serotonin plasma levels are low in RS and correlated positively with sympatho-vagal balance (LF/HF ratio), suggesting that cardiac dysautonomia could be linked to serotoninergic dysfunction. In fact, central serotoninergic pathways are known to innervate areas involved in cardiovascular regulation and various authors have provided different aspects of central serotonin's effects on the control of autonomic areas of the cardiovascular system [77]; previous studies suggested that an increase in central nervous system serotoninergic neurotransmission reduces the susceptibility to ventricular fibrillation [78], showing that this occurs because the increase in central serotonin produces a decrease in sympathetic nerve traffic to the heart [79]. Therefore, it seems likely that the brain's control of sympathetic output is closely linked with central serotoninergic mechanisms (high serotonin/low sympathetic output; low serotonin/high sympathetic output) [80].

An alteration of nerve growth factor levels may also contribute to an altered sympatho-vagal balance, because NGF also functions as a modulator of synaptic transmission between sympathetic neurons and cardiac myocytes [81] (figure 4).

Fragile X Syndrome

X-linked mental retardation associated with marXq28, or fragile X syndrome, is characterized by moderate to severe mental retardation, macroorchidism, large ears, prominent jaw, and high-pitched jocular speech. Expression is variable, with mental retardation being the most common feature. This phenotype is associated with mutations in the FMR1 gene [82].

Boccia ML and Roberts JE [83] observed a case of a boy with fragile X syndrome evaluating heart period with spectral analysis and suggesting a lower parasympathetic activity; further studies showed that young boys with Fragile X Syndrome display poorly modulated and low levels of vagal tone [84, 85].

However, Ferri R et al. [86] studied spontaneous heart rate variability on the recording night observing that all heart rate variability related parameters in the time and frequency domains showed no significant changes in these patients, suggesting that autonomic function has little relationship to the FMR-1 protein deficit that occurs in this syndrome.

Tay-Sachs Disease

Classic Tay-Sachs disease (GM2 gangliosidosis) caused by mutation in the alpha subunit of the hexosaminidase A gene is characterized by the onset in infancy of developmental retardation, followed by paralysis, dementia and blindness, with death in the second or third year of life [87].

A gray-white area around the retinal fovea centralis, due to lipid-laden ganglion cells, leaving a central 'cherry-red' spot is a typical funduscopic finding. Pathologic verification is provided by the finding of the typically ballooned neurons in the central nervous system. Tay-Sachs disease is characterized by a severe central nervous system involvement: a process of neurodegeneration that include inflammation as a factor leading to the precipitous loss of neurons in individuals with these disorders. Involvement of the peripheral and autonomic nervous system has been suspected and documented in published case reports in the chronic form of the disease. Salman MS [88] examined four patients, aged 24-29 years, with chronic GM2-gangliosidosis for evidence of peripheral and autonomic nervous system dysfunction by means of nerve conduction studies, sympathetic skin responses and cardiac monitoring during the head tilt-table test. Salman MS suggested that the peripheral and autonomic nervous system may be involved in patients with chronic GM2-gangliosidosis, but cardiovascular autonomic instability is apparently not a significant problem in young adult patients with the disease.

Mitochondrial Encephalomyopathies

Mitochondrial encephalomyopathies are heterogeneous group of diseases with multisystem presentations that affect mitochondrial ATP production. The defect in energy production may be caused by abnormalities in substrate transport or use (such as pyruvate dehydrogenase complex deficiency), Krebs cycle, oxidative phosphorylation, and defects of intergenomic signalling; most of these enzymes are encoded by nuclear genes, and are therefore transmitted by Mendelian inheritance, usually autosomal recessive. Common symptoms include hypotonia, ophthalmoplegia, seizures, pyramidal and extrapyramidal signs, psychomotor regression, ataxia, stroke-like episodes, lactic acidosis, and sometimes endocrinopathies. In general, involvement of the ANS has not been stressed; however, on occasion, the autonomic abnormalities can be so severe that they can overshadow the myopathic features and may delay definitive diagnosis [89]. Autonomic features including vomiting, impaired respiratory control, cardiovascular dysregulation with cardiac arrhythmia have been observed with Leigh syndrome and Kerns-Sayre syndrome and in myoneurogastrointestinal disorder with encephalopathy. In addition, autonomic or visceral features such as cardiac conduction defects or hypothermia and feeding problems may occasionally occur in other mitochondrial diseases including Leber hereditary optic neuropathy and X-linked recessive kinky-hair disease. In addition, decreased lacrimation, vasomotor disturbances characterized by blotchy erythema and skin mottling, altered sweating, and postural hypotension have also been noted in individuals in whom muscle biopsy has verified abnormal respiratory-chain enzymes. Because mitochondrial disorders are multisystem diseases, dysfunction of the ANS may be a result of structural abnormalities of mitochondria within the central or peripheral nervous system [90]. Diagnosis is verified by biochemical assays for mitochondrial enzyme activities.

Multifactorial Disorders

Neural Tube Defects

Neural tube defects have a birth incidence of approximately 1 in 1,000 in American Caucasians and are the second most common type of birth defect after congenital heart defects. The two most common neural tube defects are open spina bifida, also known as spina bifida cystica (SBC) or myelomeningocele, and anencephaly [91].

Previous study [92] showed diurnal variation in baseline fetal heart rate suggesting that these variations might be caused by maternal factors because present in the anencephalic fetuses that had no central nervous system having the oscillators of the circadian rhythm.

Recently Sohno [93] observed the relationship between fractal structure of fetal HRV and the developing central nervous system. In particular, the 1/f fluctuation of HR variability in an anencephalic fetus from the 1.25 to 13.8 s time scale might have a strong relation to the defect of the central nervous system.

Chiari malformation type II, also known as the Arnold-Chiari malformation, is often associated with open spina bifida. The study of the autonomic control of heart rate in patients with Arnold-Chiari deformity types I and II showed an abnormal decrease in low-frequency HRV or an abnormal increase in high-frequency HRV power. These observations suggest that patients with cervicomedullary anatomic abnormalities caused by Arnold-Chiari deformities may exhibit abnormal autonomic control of heart rate [94].

Infections

Mental retardation may be caused by infections involving central nervous system during pregnancy or in the period neonatal and postnatal. The neurologic sequelae form SNC infections (meningitis, encephalitis and meningoencephalitis) include varied symptoms such as involuntary movement, paresthesia and focal neurological deficits. Some of these patients have occasionally autonomic nervous system dysfunction [95, 96], with severe parasympathetic and sympathetic failure [97]: the characteristics features included severe orthostatic hypotension, impaired gastrointestinal and bladder motility, impaired light reflex, ptosis and accommodation difficulties.

Paranatal Disorders

Cerebral Palsy

CP is a common problem, the worldwide incidence being 2 to 2.5 per 1000 live births [98]. Cerebral palsy is primarily a disorder of movement and posture. It may be stated as a static encephalopathy in which, even though the primary lesion, anomaly or injury is static, the clinical pattern of presentation may change with time due to growth and developmental plasticity and maturation of the central nervous system. Mental retardation is common in CP in up to 60% of the cases [99].

The etiology of CP is very diverse and multifactorial. The causes are congenital, genetic, inflammatory, infectious, anoxic, traumatic and metabolic. The injury to the developing brain may be prenatal, natal or postnatal. The symptoms of autonomic dysfunction can be suspected in cases of bowel and bladder dysfunction, excessive sweating and tachycardia during walking; Yang reported that there were no significant differences of sympathetic skin response and mean RR interval between children with cerebral palsy and normal controls [100], but, by means of power spectrum analysis of HRV, performed under standardized conditions, he observed [101] a disturbed balance of activity between the sympathetic and parasympathetic nervous system suggesting a loss of hemispheric influence in patients with cerebral palsy. Park ES [102] investigated the function of the autonomic nervous system in children with spastic cerebral palsy through an analysis of HRV occurring with orthostatic stress: in the head-up tilt position, absolute and normalized LF were significantly increased and absolute HF was significantly decreased in the normal children, but not in the children with spastic cerebral palsy. These results suggested that cardiac autonomic functions, such as vagal withdrawal and sympathetic activation which occur during head-up tilt position, are not sufficient to overcome the orthostatic stress arising in spastic cerebral palsy children.

Intracranial Hemorrhage

Preterm newborns represent a high-risk population for brain damage which may result in neurodevelopmental disabilities of variable severity. Brain damage in preterm infants primarily affects the white matter; however, grey matter, basal ganglia, cerebellum, and brainstem can also be affected though to a lesser extent [103]. The most common type of damage, even though at variable rates in different studies, is represented by periventricular leukomalacia (PVL) and intraventricular hemorrhage (IVH). Determinants of brain damage have been extensively investigated, and several factors (including bleeding, abnormal weight gain during pregnancy, *abruptio placentae*, premature rupture of membranes, respiratory distress syndrome, and chorioamnionitis) have been frequently reported to be associated with brain damage in preterm newborns. Etiological pathways for brain damage in preterm newborns are complex and difficult to be explored. It is likely that different patterns of risk factors may act in different "susceptibility windows of pregnancy". Ischemic and inflammatory pathways can, to some extent, coexist: the ischemic theory focuses on the role of hypoxia-ischemia resulting from perinatal complication, often present in preterm newborns, as a determinant of a breakdown of neuronal metabolism and the subsequent cerebral damage; according to the inflammatory theory both brain damage and preterm birth may be caused by the microbial infection of the fetal membranes and by the secondary inflammatory response of mother/fetus [103]. White-Traut et al. [104] compared the developmental patterns of heart rate, respiratory rate, and hemoglobin oxygen saturation of premature infants with and without central nervous system injury observing that premature infants with periventricular leukomalacia and/or intraventricular hemorrhage present an altered maturation of the autonomic nervous system and an increase risk of decelerative heart rate changes with associated clinical compromise.

Robles P [105] recently observed the degree of central and autonomic dysfunction by means of electroencephalographic and cardio-pneumographic recording in infants with post-hemorrhagic hydrocephalus: he showed an absence of heart rate variability in these subjects (63%), suggesting a cortical-subcortical, and a brainstem dysfunction with severe encephalopathy and autonomic nervous dysfunction related to ventricular dilatation in these infants.

REFERENCES

[1] Moeschler JB, Shevell M. Clinical genetic evaluation of the child with mental retardation or development delays. Am Acad of Pediatrics 2006; 117: 2304-2316.

[2] Wilska ML, Kaski MK. Why and how to assess the aetiological diagnosis of children with intellectual disability/mental retardation and other neurodevelopmental disorders: description of the Finnish approach. *Eur J Paediatr Neurol* 2001; 5(1): 7-13.

[3] Curry CJ, Stevenson RE, Aughton D, Byrne J, Carey JC, Cassidy S, Cunniff C, Graham JM Jr, Jones MC, Kaback MM, Moeschler J, Schaefer GB, Schwartz S, Tarleton J, Opitz J. Evaluation of mental retardation: recommendation of a consensus conference. *Am J Med Gen* 1997; 72: 468-477.

[4] Francis F, Meyer G, Fallet-Bianco C, Moreno S, Kappeler C, Socorro AC, Tuy FP, Beldjord C, Chelly J. Human disorders of cortical development from past to present. *Eur J Neurosci* 2006; 23: 877-893.

[5] Napalkov DA, Shestova IA, Fonsova NA, Moskvitin AA, Shul'govskii VV. The characteristics of the autonomic reactions of healthy adolescents and of those with lowered intellectual productivity. *Zh Vyssh Nerv Deiat Im I P Pavolva* 1994; 44 (4-5):674-681.

[6] Porges SW, Humphrey MM. Cardiac and respiratory responses during visual search in nonretarded children and retarded adolescents. Am J Ment Defic 1977; 82(2):162-169.

[7] Shibagaki M. Heart-rate variability during nocturnal sleep in mentally retarded children. *Percept Mot Skills* 2001; 93(3):785-796.

[8] Armour JA. Cardiac neuronal hierarchy in health and disease. *Am J Physiol Regul Integr Comp Physiol* 2004; 287(2):R262-271.

[9] Barron KD, Chokrovrty S. Anatomy of the autonomic nervous system: brain and brainstem. In: Low PA eds. Clinical Autonomic Disorders. *Little, Brown and Company.* Boston Toronto London; 1993: 3-15.

[10] Loewy AS. *Central autonomic pathways*. In: Loewy AS, Spyer KM. eds. Central regulation of autonomic functions. New York, NY: Oxford University Press; 1990:88-103.

[11] Kawashima T. The autonomic nervous system of the human heart with special reference to its origin, course, and peripheral distribution. *Anat Embryol (Berl)* 2005; 209(6):425-438.

[12] Axelrod FB, Chelimsky GG, Weese-Mayer DE. Pediatric autonomic disorders. *Pediatrics* 2006; 118(1):309-321.

[13] Howard MJ. Mechanisms and perspectives on differentiation of autonomic neurons. *Dev Biol* 2005; 277(2):271-286.

[14] Lockhart ST, Turrigiano GG, Birren SJ. Nerve growth factor modulates synaptic transmission between sympathetic neurons and cardiac myocytes. *J Neurosci* 1997; 17:9573-9582.

[15] Ardell JL. Neurohumoral control of cardiac function. In: *Heart Physiology and Pathophysiology*, edited by Sperelakis N, Kurachi Y, Terzic A, and Cohen MV. New York: Academic, 2001, p. 45–59.

[16] Levy MN. Neural control of cardiac function. *Baillieres Clin Neurol* 1997; 6(2):227-244.

[17] Oppenheimer S. Cerebrogenic cardiac arrhythmias: cortical lateralization and clinical significance. *Clin Auton Res* 2006; 16(1):6-11.

[18] Paton JF, Boscan P, Pickering AE, Nalivaiko E. The yin and yang of cardiac autonomic control: vago-sympathetic interactions revisited. *Brain Res Brain Res Rev* 2005; 49(3):555-565.

[19] Zipes DB, Rubart M. Neural modulation of cardiac arrhythmias and sudden cardiac death. *Heart Rhythm* 2006; 3(1):108-113.

[20] Freeman R. Assessment of cardiovascular autonomic function. *Clin Neurophysiol* 2006; 117(4):716-730.

[21] Sztajzel J. Heart rate variability: a non-invasive electrocardiographic method to measure the autonomic nervous system. *Swiss Med Wkly* 2004; 134: 514-522.

[22] Task Force of the European Society of Cardiology and the North American Society of Pacing Electrophysiology. Heart rate variability: standards of measurement, physiological interpretation, and clinical use. *Circulation* 1996;93:1043–65.

[23] Eckberg DL. Physiological basis for human autonomic rhythms. *Ann Med* 2000; 32(5): 341-349.

[24] Bernardi L, Valle F, Coco M, Calciati A, Sleight P. Physical activity influences heart rate variability and very-low-frequency components in Holter electrocardiograms. *Cardiovasc Res* 1996; 32(2): 234-237.

[25] Lombardi F. Chaos theory, heart rate variability, and arrhythmic mortality. *Circulation* 2000; 101: 8-10.

[26] Huikuri HV, Makikallio TH, Perkiomaki J. Measurement of heart rate variability by methods based on nonlinear dynamics. *J Electrocardiol* 2003; 36 (Suppl): 95-99.

[27] Parati G, Di Rienzo M, Mancia G. How to measure baroreflex sensitivity: from the cardiovascular laboratory to daily life. *J Hypertension* 2000; 18: 7-19.

[28] Axelrod FB, Chelimsky GG, Weese-Mayer DE. Pediatric autonomic disorders. *Pediatrics* 2006; 118: 309-321.

[29] Greydanus DE, Pratt HD. Syndromes and disorders associated with mental retardation. *Indian J Pediatr* 2005; 72(10): 859-64.

[30] Kabra M, Gulati S. Mental retardation. *Indian J Pediatr* 2003; 70(2): 153-158.

[31] Roubertoux PL, Kerdelhue B. Trisomy 21: from chromosomes to mental retardation. *Behav Genet* 2006; 36(3): 346-354.

[32] Saud K, Arriagada C, Cardenas AM, Shimahara T, Allen DD, Caviedes R, Caviedes P. Neuronal dysfunction in Down syndrome: contribution of neuronal models in cell culture. *J Physiol Paris* 2006; 99 (2-3):201-210.

[33] Yates CM, Simpson J, Gordon A, Maloney AF, Allison Y, Ritchie IM, Urquhart A. Catecholamines and cholinergic enzymes in pre-senile and senile Alzheimer-type dementia and Down's syndrome. *Brain Res* 1983; 280 (1):119-126.

[34] Schapiro MB, Kay AD, May C, Ryker AK, Haxby JV, Kaufman S, Milstien S, Rapoport SI. Cerebrospinal fluid monoamines in Down's syndrome adults at different ages. *J Ment Defic Res* 1987; 31(Pt 3):259-269.

[35] Eberhard Y, Eterradossi J, Therminarias A. Biochemical changes and catecholamine responses in Down's syndrome adolescents in relation to incremental maximal exercise. *J Ment Defic Res* 1991; 35 (Pt 2):140-6.

[36] Udeschini G, Casati G, Bassani F, Picotti GB, Culotta P. Plasma catecholamines in Down's syndrome, at rest and during sympathetic stimulation. *J Neurol Neurosurg Psychiatry* 1985; 48(10):1060-1.

[37] Fernhall B, Otterstetter M. Attenuated responses to sympathoexcitation in individuals with Down syndrome. *J Appl Physiol.* 2003; 94(6):2158-2165.

[38] Guerra M, Llorens N, Fernhall B. Chronotropic incompetence in persons with down syndrome. *Arch Phys Med Rehabil.* 2003; 84(11):1604-1608.

[39] Fernhall B, Pitetti KH, Rimmer JH, McCubbin JA, Rintala P, Millar AL, Kittredge J, Burkett LN. Cardiorespiratory capacity of individuals with mental retardation including Down syndrome. *Med Sci Sports Exerc* 1996; 28(3):366-371.

[40] Richards BW, Enver F. Blood pressure in Down's syndrome. *J Ment Defic Res* 1979;23:123-135.

[41] Morrison RA, McGrath A, Davidson G, Brown JJ, Murray GD, Lever AF. Low blood pressure in Down's syndrome, A link with Alzheimer's disease? *Hypertension* 1996; 28(4): 569-75.

[42] Wisniewski KE. Down's syndrome children often have brain with maturation delay, retardation of growth and cortical dysgenesis. *Am J Genet Suppl* 1990;7: 274-281.

[43] Takashima S, Iida K, Mito T, Arima M. Dendritic and histochemical development and ageing in patients with Down's syndrome. *J Intellect Disabil Res* 1994;38: 265-273.

[44] Yates CM, Simpson J, Maloney AFJ, Gordon A, Reid AH. Alzheimer-like cholinergic deficiency in Down's syndrome. *Lancet.* 1980;2:979.

[45] Pavey RJ. Pretreatment systolic orthostatic blood pressure depression in Down's syndrome. *J Clin Psychopharmacol.* 1989;9:146-147. Letter.

[46] Pitetti KH, Climstein M, Campbell KD, Barrett PJ, Jackson JA. The cardiovascular capacities of adults with Down's syndrome: a comparative study. *Med Sci Sports Exerc.* 1992;24:13-19.

[47] Sei H, Enai T, Chang HY, Morita Y. Heart rate variability during sleep in Down's syndrome. *Physiol Behav* 1995; 58(6):1273-1276.

[48] Ferri R, Curzi-Dascalova L, Del Gracco S, Elia M, Musumeci SA, Pettinato S. Heart rate variability and apnea during sleep in Down's syndrome. *J Sleep Res* 1998; 7(4):282-287.

[49] Baynard T, Pitetti KH, Guerra M, Fernhall B. Heart rate variability at rest and during exercise in persons with Down syndrome. *Arch Phys Med Rehabil* 2004; 85(8):1285-1290.

[50] Iellamo F, Galante A, Legramante JM, Lippi ME, Condoluci C, Albertini G, Volterrani M. Altered autonomic cardiac regulation in individuals with Down syndrome. *Am J Physiol Heart Circ Physiol* 2005; 289(6): H2387-2391.

[51] Wattendorf DJ, Muenke M. Prader-Willi syndrome. *Am Fam Physician* 2005; 72(5): 827-30.

[52] Di Mario FJ Jr, Dunham B, Burleson JA, Moskovitz J, Cassidy SB. An evaluation of autonomic nervous system function in patients with Prader-Willi syndrome. *Pediatrics* 1994; 93(1):76-81.

[53] Wade CK, De Meersman RE, Angulo M, Lieberman JS, Downey JA. Prader-Willi syndrome fails to alter cardiac autonomic modulation. *Clin Auton Res* 2000; 10(4):203-206.

[54] Horsthemke B, Buiting K. Imprinting defects on human chromosome 15. *Cytogenet Genome Res* 2006; 113(1-4): 292-299.

[55] Douchin S, Do-Ngoc D, Rossignol AM, Lucet V, Joannard A, Jouk PS. [Angelman syndrome and severe vagal hypertonia. *Three pediatric case reports] Arch Mal Coeur Vaiss* 2000; 93(5):559-563.

[56] Vanagt WY, Pulles-Heintzberger CF, Vernooy K, Cornelussen RN, Delhaas T. Asystole during outbursts of laughing in a child with Angelman syndrome. *Pediatr Cardiol* 2005; 26(6):866-868.

[57] Meyer-Lindenberg A, Mervis CB, Berman KF. Neural mechanisms in Williams syndrome: a unique window to genetic influences on cognition and behaviour. *Nat Rev Neurosci* 2006; 7(5): 380-393.

[58] Girard A, Sidi D, Aggoun Y, Laude D, Bonnet D, Elghozi JL. Elastin mutation is associated with a reduced gain of the baroreceptor-heart rate reflex in patients with Williams syndrome. *Clin Auton Res* 2002; 12(2): 72-77.

[59] Witt-Engerström I, Gillberg C. Rett syndrome in Sweden. *J Autism Dev Disord* 1987; 17:149-150.

[60] Hagberg B. Rett syndrome: clinical peculiarities and biological mysteries. *Acta Pediatr* 1995; 84: 971-976.

[61] Weaving LS, Christodoulou J, Williamson SL, Friend KL, McKenzie OL, Archer H, Evans J, Clarke A, Pelka GJ, Tam PP, Watson C, Lahooti H, Ellaway CJ, Bennetts B, Leonard H, Gecz J. Mutations of CDKL5 cause a severe neurodevelopmental disorder with infantile spasms and mental retardation. *Am J Hum Genet* 2004; 75: 1079-1093.

[62] Weaving LS, Ellaway CJ, Christodoulou J. Rett syndrome: clinical review and genetic update. *J Med Genet* 2005; 42: 1-7.

[63] Hagberg B, Witt-Engerström I. Rett syndrome: a suggested staging system for describing impairment profile with increasing age towards adolescence. *Am J Med Genet* 1986; 24 (Suppl 1): 47-59.

[64] Kerr AM, Armstrong DD, Prescott RJ, Doyle D, Kearney D.L. Rett syndrome: analysis of deaths in the British survey. *Eur Chil Adolesc Psychiatry* 1997; 6 (Suppl 1):71-74.

[65] Driscoll DJ, Edwards WD. Sudden unexpected death in children and adolescents. *J Am Coll Cardiol* 1985; 5:118B-21B.

[66] Dahlström A. *The central and peripheral autonomic nervous system and possible implications in Rett syndrome patients.* In Kerr A and Witt-Engerström I (eds). Rett disorder and the developing brain. Oxford: Oxford University Press, 2001, 227-250.

[67] Julu POO, Kerr AM, Hansen S, Apartopoulos F, Jamal GA. Immaturity of medullary cardiorespiratory neurones leading to inappropiate autonomic reactions as a likely cause of sudden death in Rett's syndrome. *Arch Dis Child* 1997; 77: 464-465.

[68] Vanoli E, Schwartz PJ. Sympathetic-parasympathetic interaction and sudden death. *Basic Res Cardiol* 1990; 85: 305-321.

[69] Johnsrude C, Glaze D, Schultz R, Frideman R. Prolonged QT intervals and diminished heart rate variability in patients with Rett syndrome. *Pacing Clin Electophysiol* 1995; 18: 889 (Abstract).

[70] Guideri F, Acampa M, Hayek G, Zappella M, Di Perri T. Reduced heart rate variability in patients affected with Rett syndrome. A possible explanation for sudden death. *Neuropediatrics* 1999; 30:146-148.

[71] Guideri F, Acampa M, Di Perri T, Zappella M, Hayek G. Progressive cardiac dysautonomia observed in patients affected by classic Rett syndrome and not in the preserved speech variant. *J Child Neurol* 2001; 16:370-373.

[72] Acampa M, Guideri F. Cardiac disease and Rett syndrome. *Arch Dis Child* 2006;91: 440-443.

[73] Julu POO, Kerr AM, Apartopoulos F, Al-Rawas S, Witt-Engerström I, Witt-Engerström L, Jamal GA, Hansen S. Characterisation of breathing and associated central autonomic dysfunction in the Rett disorder. *Arch Dis Child* 2001; 85: 29-37.

[74] Weese-Mayer DE, Lieske SP, Boothby CM, Kenny AS, Bennett HL, Silvestri JM, Ramirez JM. Autonomic Nervous System Dysregulation: Breathing and Heart Rate Perturbation during Wakefulness in Young Girls with Rett Syndrome. *Pediatr Res* 2006; 60 (4):443-449.

[75] Deguichi K, Antalffy B, Twohill L, Chakrohorty S, Glaze D, Armstrong D. Substance P in Rett syndrome. Relation to autonomic dysfunction. *Pediatr Neurol* 2000; 22:259-266.

[76] Guideri F, Acampa M, Blardi P, De Lalla A, Zappella M, Hayek Y. Cardiac dysautonomia and serotonin plasma levels in Rett syndrome. *Neuropediatrics* 2004; 35:36-38.

[77] Ramage AG Central cardiovascular regulation and 5-hydroxytryptamine receptors. *Brain Res Bull* 2001; 56, 425-439.

[78] Lehnert H, Lobbardi F, Raeder EA, Lorenzo AV, Verrier RL, Lown B et al. Increased release of brain serotonin reduces vulnerability of ventricular fibrillation in the cat. *J Cardiovasc Pharmacol* 1987; 10:389-397.

[79] Verrier R. Neurochemical approaches to the prevention of ventricular fibrillation. *Fed Proc* 1986; 45:2191-2196.

[80] Blatt CM, Rabinowitz SH, Lown B. Central serotoninergic agents raise the repetitive extrasystole threshold of the vulnerable period of the canine ventricular myocardium. Circ Res 1979; 44:723-730.

[81] Guideri F, Acampa M, Calamendrei G, Aloe L, Zappella M, Hayeck Y. Nerve growth factor plasma levels and ventricular repolarization in Rett syndrome. Pediatr Cardiol 2004; 25:394-396.

[82] Ropers HH. X-linked mental retardation: many genes for a complex disorder. Curr *Opin Genet Dev* 2006; 16(3): 260-269.

[83] Boccia ML and Roberts JE. Behavior and autonomic nervous system function assessed via heart period measures: the case of hyperarousal in boys with fragile X syndrome. *Behav Res Methods Instrum Comput* 2000; 32(1):5-10.

[84] Roberts JE, Boccia ML, Bailey DB Jr, Hatton DD, Skinner M. Cardiovascular indices of physiological arousal in boys with fragile X syndrome. *Dev Psychobiol* 2001;39:107-123.

[85] Roberts JE, Boccia ML, Hatton DD, Skinner ML, Sideris J. Temperament and vagal tone in boys with fragile X syndrome. *J Dev Behav Pediatr* 2006; 27(3):193-201.

[86] Ferri R, Del Gracco S, Elia M, Musumeci SA, Pettinato S. Heart rate variability and autonomic function during sleep in fragile X syndrome. *Am J Med Genet* 1999 2; 83(4):296-297.

[87] Fernandes Filho JA, Shapiro BE. Tay-Sachs disease. *Arch Neurol* 2004; 61(9): 1466-1468.

[88] Salman MS, Clarke JT, Midroni G, Waxman MB. Peripheral and autonomic nervous system involvement in chronic GM2-gangliosidosis. *J Inherit Metab Dis* 2001; 24(1): 65-71.

[89] Zelnik N, Axelrod FB, Leshinsky E, Griebel ML, Kolodny E. Mitochondrial encephalopathies presenting with features of autonomic and visceral dysfunction. *Pediatr Neurol.* 1996;14: 251–254.

[90] Nissenkorn A, Zeharia A, Lev D, Fatal-Valevski A, Barash V, Gutman A, Harel S, Lerman-Sagie T. Multiple presentation of mitochondrial disorders. *Arch Dis Child* 1999; 81: 209-214.

[91] Detrait, E. R.; George, T. M.; Etchevers, H. C.; Gilbert, J. R.; Vekemans, M.; Speer, M. C. Human neural tube defects: developmental biology, epidemiology, and genetics. *Neurotox Teratol* 27: 515-524, 2005.

[92] Terao T, Kawashima Y, Noto H, Inamoto Y, Lin TY, Sumimoto K, Maeda M. Neurological control of fetal heart rate in 20 cases of anencephalic fetuses. *Am J Obstet Gynecol* 1984; 149(2):201-208.

[93] Shono H, Shono M, Iwasaka T, Sugimori H. Analysis of heart rate variability of an anencephalic fetus using a new method to determine a fractal dimension of non-stationary time-serial data. *Front Med Biol Eng* 2001; 10(4):337-44.

[94] Ireland PD, Mickelsen D, Rodenhouse TG, Bakos RS, Goldstein B. Evaluation of the autonomic cardiovascular response in Arnold-Chiari deformities and cough syncope syndrome. *Arch Neurol* 1996; 53(6):526-531.

[95] Tamura N, Shimazu K, Yamamoto T, Itokawa K, Hamaguchi K. [A case of sympathotonic orthostatic hypotension following herpes simplex encephalitis] *Rinsho Shinkeigaku*. 1996; 36(10):1161-1165.

[96] Dune X, Lee WT, Shen YZ. Postmeningoencephalitic dysautonomia: report of one case. *Pediatr Neurol* 2002; 26(2):161-163.

[97] Shimoda S, Ishibashi H, Niho Y. Acute autonomic neuropathy and the other related disease. *J Clin Med* 1992; 50:852-857.

[98] Rosen MG, Dickinson JC. The incidence of cerebral palsy. *Am J Obstet Gynecol* 1992; 167: 417-423.

[99] Sankar C, Mundkur N. Cerebral palsy-definition, classification, etiology and early diagnosis. *Indian J Pediatr* 2005; 72(10):865-868.

[100] Yang TF, Chan RC, Liao SF, Chuang TY, Liu TJ. Electrophysiologic evaluation of autonomic function in cerebral palsy. *Am J Phys Med Rehabil* 1997; 76(6): 458-461.

[101] Yang TF, Chan RC, Kao CL, Chiu JW, Liu TJ, Kao NT, Kuo TB. Power spectrum analysis of heart rate variability for cerebral palsy patients. *Am J Phys Med Rehabil* 2002; 81(5): 350-354.

[102] Park ES, Park CI, Cho SR, Lee JW, Kim EJ. Assessment of autonomic nervous system with analysis of heart rate variability in children with spastic cerebral palsy. *Yonsei Med J* 2002; 43(1): 65-72.

[103] Arpino C, D'Argenzio L, Ticconi C, Di Paolo A, Stellin V, Lopez L, Curatolo P. Brain damage in preterm infants: etiological pathways. *Ann Ist Super Sanita* 2005; 41(2): 229-237.

[104] White-Traut RC, Nelson MN, Silvestri JM, Patel M, Berbaum M, Gu GG, Rey PM. Developmental patterns of physiological response to a multisensory intervention in extremely premature and high-risk infants. *J Obstet Gynecol Neonatal Nurs* 2004; 33(2):266-275.

[105] Robles P, Poblano A, Hernandez G, Ibarra J, Guzman I, Sosa J. Cortical, brainstem and autonomic nervous system dysfunction in infants with post-hemorrhagic hydrocephalus. *Rev Invest Clin* 2002; 54(2):133-138.

INDEX

A

B

C

D

E

F

G

J

K

L

M

N

O

Q

R

T

U

V

W

X

Y

Z